OXFORD MEDICAL PUBLICATIONS

The facial nerve

The facial nerve

CHARLES DIAMOND
CONSULTANT E.N.T. SURGEON AND
CLINICAL TUTOR IN POSTGRADUATE MEDICINE,
NEWCASTLE GENERAL HOSPITAL;
CLINICAL LECTURER IN E.N.T. STUDIES
UNIVERSITY OF NEWCASTLE UPON TYNE

IVOR FREW
CONSULTANT E.N.T. SURGEON,
NEWCASTLE GENERAL HOSPITAL;
LECTURER AND EXAMINER IN E.N.T. STUDIES
UNIVERSITY OF NEWCASTLE UPON TYNE

OXFORD
OXFORD UNIVERSITY PRESS
NEW YORK TORONTO
1979

Oxford University Press, Walton Street, Oxford OP2 6DP
OXFORD LONDON GLASGOW NEW YORK
TORONTO MELBOURNE WELLINGTON CAPE TOWN
IBADAN NAIROBI DAR ES SALAAM LUSAKA ADDIS ABABA
KUALA LUMPUR SINGAPORE JAKARTA HONG KONG TOKYO
DELHI BOMBAY CALCUTTA MADRAS KARACHI

ISBN 0 19 261128 3

British Library Cataloguing in Publication Data
Diamond, Charles
The facial nerve. – (Oxford medical publications).
1. Facial nerve – Diseases
I. Title II. Frew, Ivor III. Series
616.8′7 RC418 78-40315
ISBN 0-19-261128-3

TYPESET BY ENSET LTD., MIDSOMER NORTON, BATH, AVON.
PRINTED IN GREAT BRITAIN BY
J. W. ARROWSMITH LTD., BRISTOL

TO OUR WIVES

Preface

DISEASES involving the facial nerve present problems to doctors in all branches of medicine. Information on the facial nerve is scattered throughout the textbooks and journals of many different specialities. No comprehensive book dealing with all aspects of the nerve exists, and this volume has been written in an attempt to fill that gap. The book has given us the opportunity of taking a fresh and critical look at the anatomy of the nerve, at the aetiology of Bell's palsy, and also at the vexed question of surgical treatment.

The book is not designed for the exclusive benefit of a single speciality. We hope that the chapter on trauma will satisfy physicians, and that the surgical treatment will be sufficient for the needs of neurologists. If our surgical colleagues find the sections on electrophysiology and medical diseases of the seventh nerve adequate for their purposes, we shall be more than satisfied.

The allocation of the chapters has been governed by the interest and experience of each author, and the opinions expressed in each chapter are those of the writer of that chapter.

Gathering the information for this book has been a very enjoyable and instructive experience. We hope that clinicians, for whom this volume is intended, will find as much pleasure in reading it as we had in writing it.

E.N.T. Department C.D.
Newcastle upon Tyne General Hospital I.F.

Acknowledgements

WE are indebted to the Department of Neuro-radiology at Newcastle General Hospital for the radiographs. Dr Singh and Mr East, F.R.C.S., also provided a photograph, and temporal bone dissections.

Dr D. Barwick, Consultant Neurologist at Newcastle General Hospital, very kindly read the section on electrical testing of the facial nerve, and we are grateful for the advice he gave us. We are also indebted to him for providing Figs 4.2, 4.6, 6.5, and 6.6. We would also like to express our thanks to Dr W. Sandford who read part of the manuscript.

Our work has been greatly facilitated by Miss Emmerson and her staff at the Newcastle University Library, and by Mrs Jeffries and her team in the Medical Library of Newcastle General Hospital. The Department of Photography at the Medical School produced our clinical photographs. To all those who have helped us, we express our sincere thanks.

Contents

1 Anatomy and physiology

1 Anatomy and physiology

General introduction

THE ANATOMY of the facial nerve is particularly interesting because this nerve has the longest and most tortuous course in bone of any cranial nerve, and also because it subserves a variety of functions. These functions have been the subject of debate over the years and some areas of uncertainty still persist. The distinction between the sensory nerve of the face (fifth cranial nerve) and the motor nerve of the face (seventh cranial nerve) was established by Sir Charles Bell (1821, 1829). He held the view that facial nerve function was principally respiratory and called it 'the respiratory nerve of the face'. This fitted in with his concept of the phrenic nerve as the 'great internal respiratory nerve' and the nerve to serratus anterior as the 'great external respiratory nerve'. Indeed this latter nerve is still called the long thoracic nerve of Bell. By establishing that the principal function of the nerve was motor, he helped to end the practice, prevalent at that time, of cutting the facial nerve for relief of tic douloureux.

The facial nerve has two motor or efferent components. The greater part of the nerve is composed of motor fibres to the muscles of facial expression, and in addition the nerve carries secretomotor fibres for the submandibular and sublingual salivary glands and the lacrimal gland. The facial nerve also has two sensory or afferent components. One carries taste sensation from the tongue and palate, and the other carries ordinary sensation from the skin in the region of the external ear.

Embryological considerations

Course of the motor root in the pons

The complex meandering of the motor fibres in the pons can be understood only in the light of the embryological development of the facial nucleus. The nucleus initially lies in the floor of the fourth ventricle, rostral or cephalic to the sixth nerve nucleus. After the fibres from the facial nucleus have been established, the nucleus undergoes a migration. Nerve cells can migrate only by lengthening their axons and the axons therefore trace the path taken by the nucleus from its original to its definitive position. The facial nucleus at first moves caudally and dorsally to the abducens nucleus, and then ventrally to reach its final position.

Some authors attempt to explain this migration by the theory of neurobiotaxis. According to this theory, the nucleus tends to remain as close as possible to its predominant source of stimulation and will migrate in the direction from which the greatest density of stimuli originate. On this basis, the facial nucleus is deemed to be attracted towards the spinal tract of the trigeminal and its nucleus. The abducens nucleus is drawn forward towards the position occupied by the other eye muscle nuclei and it carries the facial root fibres in front of it as it advances. In the opinion of Crosby and de Jonge (1963), the genu is formed in this way.

The theory of neurobiotaxis is not universally accepted, however, and many authors hold the view that this migration may be more apparent than

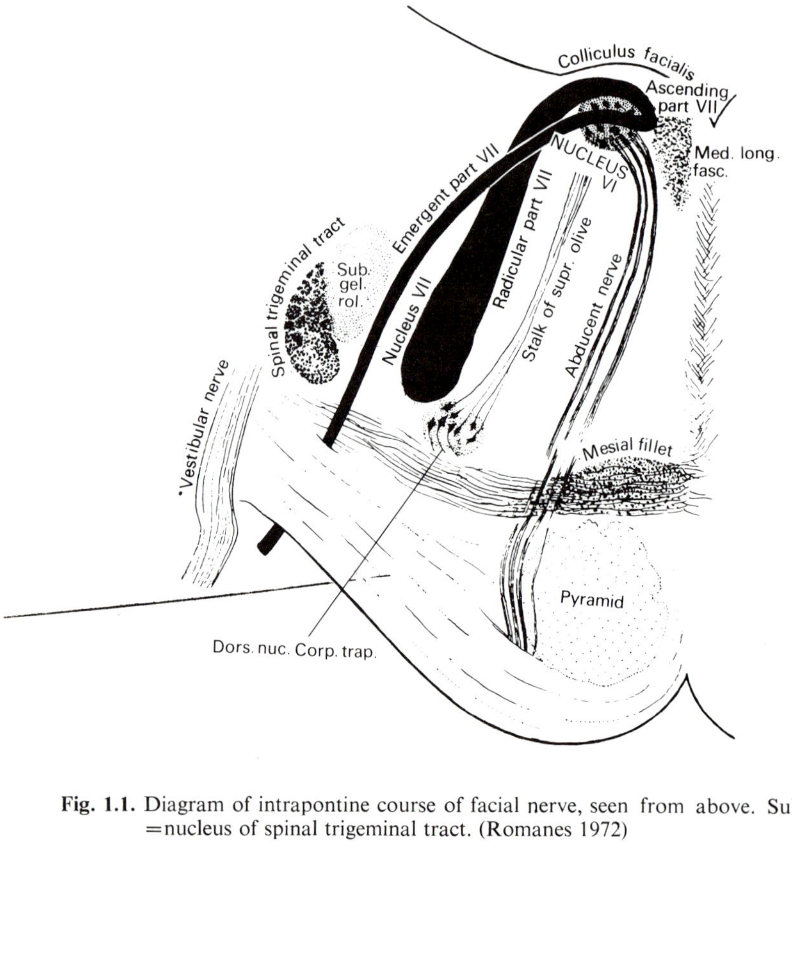

Fig. 1.1. Diagram of intrapontine course of facial nerve, seen from above. Sub.Gel.Rol. =nucleus of spinal trigeminal tract. (Romanes 1972)

real, and may merely be the result of differential growth patterns and displacement rather than active migration (Fig. 1.1). Be that as it may, this migration of the nucleus, whether active or passive, accounts for the highly unusual course of the facial motor root fibres in the pons.

Branchial arch system

By the fifth week of intra-uterine life the human embryo has a well-developed system of external branchial arches and grooves which will eventually intervene between the mouth and the thorax. These external branchial grooves are matched by a similar series of internal pharyngeal pouches (Fig. 1.2(a)). In fish, slits appear in the grooves and pouches to form the gill slits. In amphibia these openings disappear at metamorphosis. In humans the arches are present only in the embryo. Communication between groove and pouch does not take place, and the two remain separated by a layer of ectoderm externally, a layer of endoderm internally, and some mesenchymal tissue sandwiched between these two layers. The muscles of mastication are derived from the first (mandibular) arch, and its principal nerve is the mandibular division of the trigeminal. The muscles of facial expression originate from the second (hyoid) arch, and the nerve of the second arch is the facial nerve. Each arch also receives a branch from the nerve of the arch caudal to it. Thus the first arch receives a branch from the second arch nerve, the second arch receives a branch from the third arch nerve, and so on. These branches must cross over the branchial groove (*trema*: a cleft) separating the two arches and ultimately come to lie in front of that groove (pretrematic branch). The chorda tympani nerve is the pretrematic nerve of the first arch, and Jacobsen's nerve (tympanic branch of the glossopharyngeal nerve) is the pretrematic branch of the second arch (Fig. 1.2(b)). This explains why in the adult the chorda tympani nerve leaves the facial nerve to loop over the tympanic cavity (which incorporates the first pouch) to join the lingual division of the mandibular nerve.

There tends to be a distinct relationship between the nerve of an arch and the arch cartilage. The nerve descends into the arch posterior to the cartilage and then turns forward round its lateral aspect to reach the front of the arch. This relationship persists in the course of the facial nerve in the adult human where the nerve descends posterior both to the stapes and the styloid process and then reaches the facial muscles, by turning forward over the lateral aspect of the styloid. The stapes and styloid process are both derivatives of the second arch cartilage.

Relationship to the parotid gland

An interesting argument exists over the relationship of the facial nerve to the parotid gland. Bailey (1941, 1947) strongly advocated the view that the

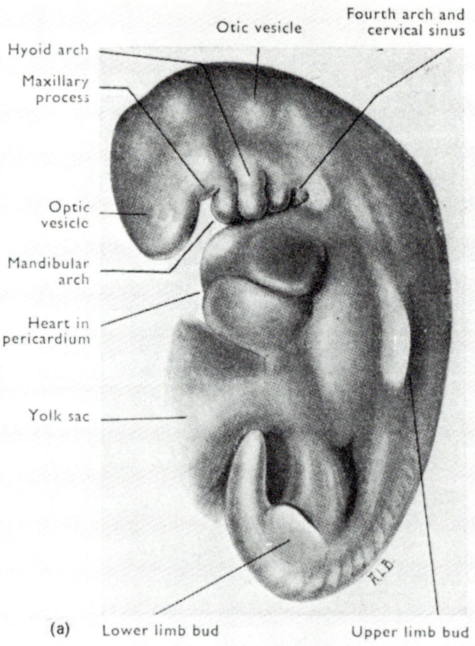

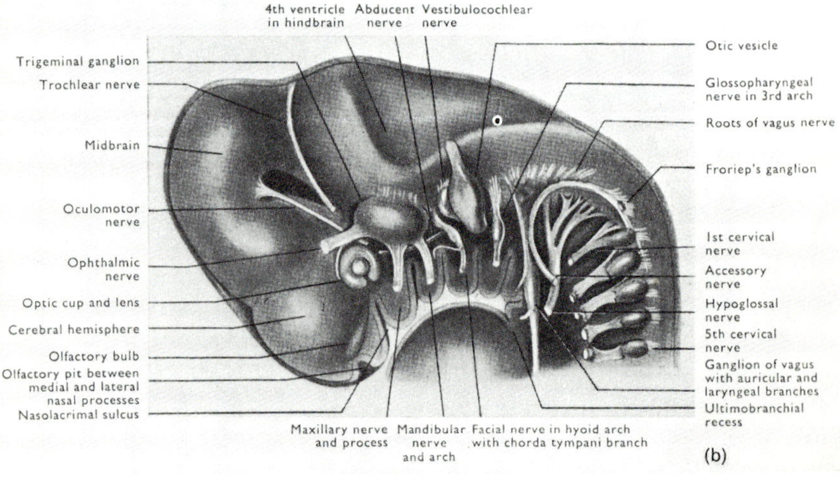

Fig. 1.2. (a) Head end of 5·3 mm long human embryo to show the development of the branchial arches. (Romanes 1972)
(b) Developmental arrangement of the cranial nerves. (Romanes 1972)

gland is a simple bilobed structure united by a single isthmus, which contains all the ducts that pass between the two lobes. According to him, the temporofacial and cervicofacial trunks embrace the isthmus and no part of the facial nerve runs actually in the gland substance. Instead all the branches lie in a plane between the two lobes. He vividly described this arrangement of the nerve in the gland as 'the meat in a parotid sandwich'. He stated that 'the anatomical classics are inaccurate in their descriptions of the facial nerve' and that the nerve does not plunge into the main body of the gland and then divide within the parenchyma as it is traditionally reputed to do. He claimed that surgical enterprise in the parotid region had been stultified by anatomical teaching, and he begged contemporary anatomists, 'to revise their teaching and alter their textbooks'. He was supported by McCormack *et al.* (1945), who carried out over a hundred parotid dissections in cadavers, and by the anatomists Hamilton and Harrison who wrote in Scott-Brown's *Diseases of the ear, nose and throat* (1971), 'The parotid gland is divided into two lobes, a superficial lobe and a deep lobe, by the main branches of the facial nerve which pass through it in a fascial plane'. If this is true, then surgical removal of the parotid gland with preservation of the facial nerve ought to be a very simple matter.

However, Patey and Ranger (1957), in their cadaver dissections, found no evidence to support the bilobar concept of the parotid gland. In an elegant experiment, McKenzie (1948) injected the parotid duct system of anatomical specimens and demonstrated that ducts passed between the superficial and

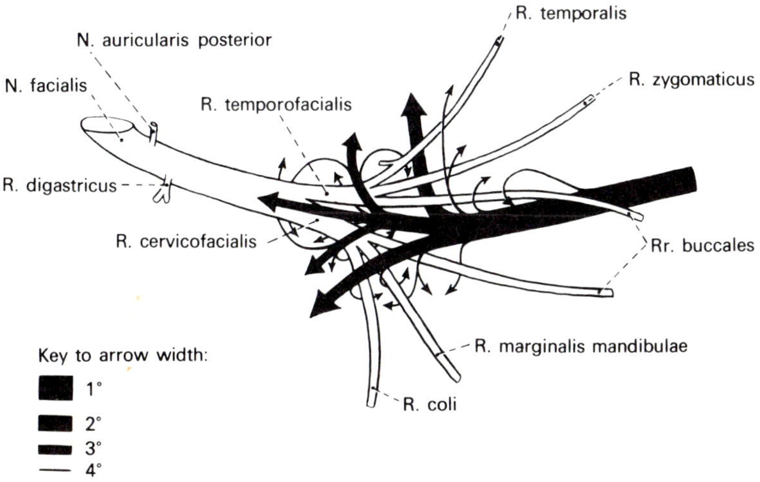

Fig. 1.3. General pattern of development of parotid gland. The black arrows indicate the direction of growth of the primordium of the parotid gland around the facial nerve and its branches. The width of the black arrows indicates the sequence of development. (Gasser 1970)

deep parts of the gland through several gaps in the facial nerve plexus. He concluded that the gland interdigitates with the nerve in an inconstant manner. Not to be outdone in the field of similes, he described the relationship of the gland to the nerve as that of 'a creeper weaving itself into the meshes of a trellis-work fence'. Having demonstrated that the gland was not

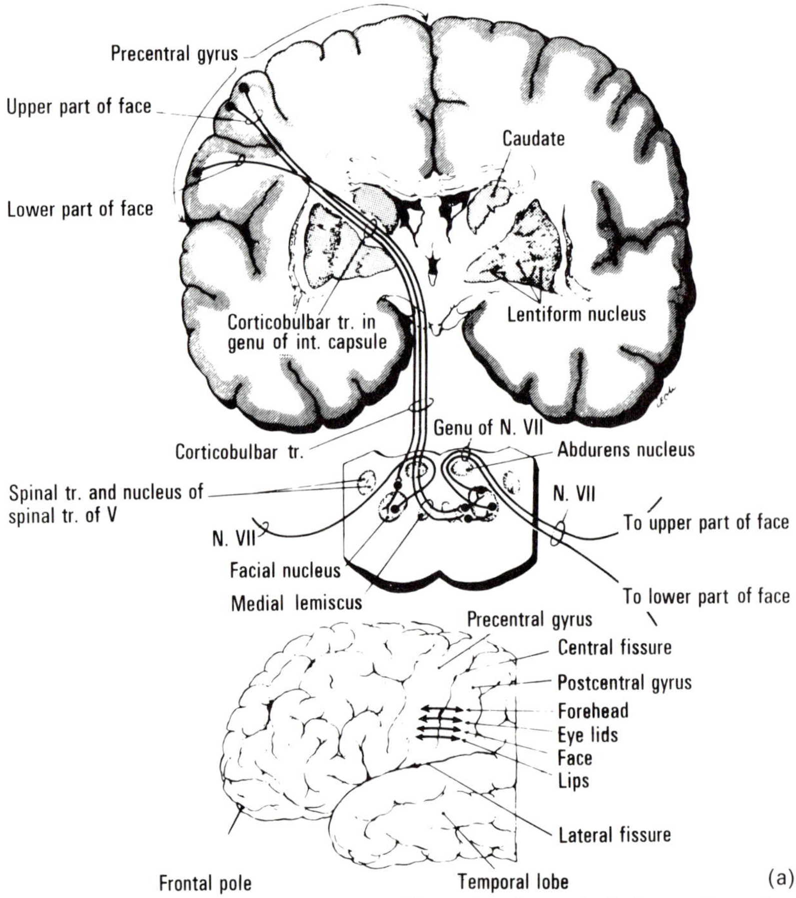

Fig. 1.4. Supranuclear pathways: (a) Diagram illustrating the corticobulbar pathway from the motor 'face' area of the cerebral cortex to the facial nucleus. The projection (largely by way of intercalate neurones) is bilateral to the lower part of the facial nucleus, which innervates the muscle of the upper part of the face. The projection is unilateral (contralateral) to the upper part of the facial nucleus, which innervates the muscles of the lower part of the face.

The diagram of the lateral wall of the hemisphere (which is in the lower part of the figure) shows the motor areas in the precentral gyrus and sensory areas in the postcentral gyrus associated with the different parts of the face. (Crosby and De Jonge 1963)

composed of two lobes, McKenzie suggested that the terms 'superficial and deep portions' of the parotid were more appropriate. These terms have now been accepted by *Nomina Anatomica* (1966). If McKenzie is correct, parotidectomy with preservation of the facial nerve becomes a more difficult surgical problem.

If knowledge of the embryological development of the parotid gland were complete, it would be of great help in understanding the relationship between gland and nerve in the adult. It has long been known that the gland develops as an outgrowth from the buccal cavity near the future angle of the mouth and travels backwards towards the ear as an elongated solid cord of cells. As it approaches the facial nerve, the cord of cells divides and branches repeatedly. The cells at the extremities of the branches differentiate and proliferate to form the acinar cells and the solid cords become hollowed out to form the duct system. More recently, Gasser (1970) has studied in great detail the early development of the parotid gland around the facial nerve in human embryos. He reported that a complete cleavage plane through the gland primordium with a single mass of ductules (single isthmus) was never observed. The main branches, or ducts, generally passed superficial to the

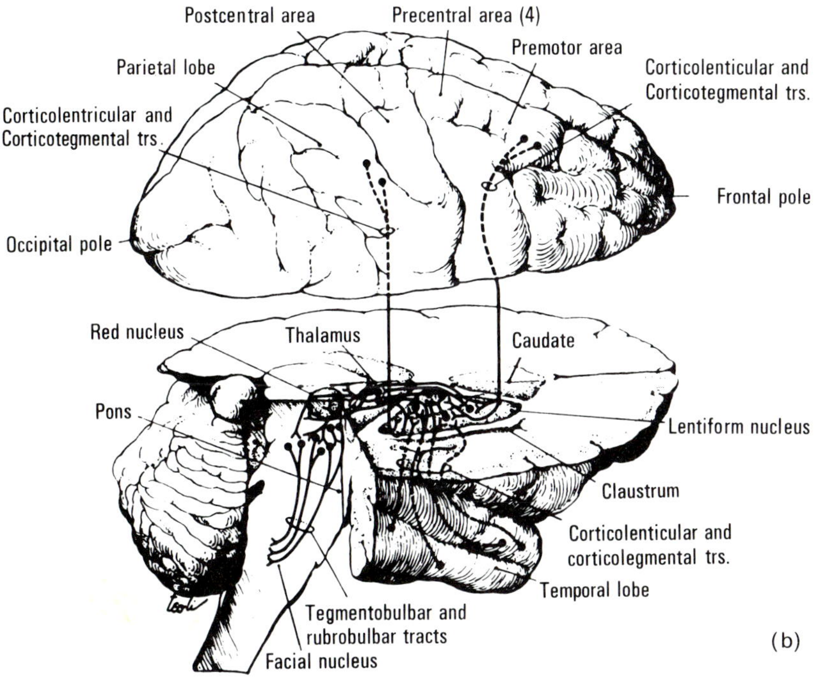

Fig. 1.4. (b) Diagram to illustrate some multisynaptic pathways from certain additional motor areas (premotor parietal and temporal) of the cerebral cortex to the facial nucleus. (Crosby and De Jonge 1963)

facial nerve and its cervicofacial division, but deep to the temporofacial division. Further subdivision of the gland ducts took place between the terminal branches of the facial nerve with which they intertwined (Fig. 1.3). Gasser's embryological studies reinforce the work of McKenzie and provide strong support for the traditional anatomical teaching, and they seriously undermine the position of Bailey and his supporters.

Upper motor neurones

The primary motor cortex for the face is in front of the central fissure in the precentral gyrus (Fig. 1.4). The size of the area of motor cortex representing the different members of the body is in direct proportion to the skills of movement employed by them, rather than to their muscle bulk. The face area of the motor cortex is therefore relatively large. Fibres from these cortical cells pass without synapse in the corticobulbar tracts to the motor nucleus in the pons. The majority of these fibres descend and cross the midline to synapse in the contralateral motor nucleus. Some descend without crossing to innervate the subnuclei responsible for the periorbital and frontalis muscles. These subnuclei thus have an ipsilateral and a contralateral cortical innervation, while the subnuclei for the lower half of the face receive contralateral corticobulbar fibres only.

In addition to the motor cortex for voluntary movement in the precentral gyrus, there are several other cortical areas concerned with the regulation of emotional and associated movements of the face. A number of these additional motor areas have been positively identified in man, e.g. in the preoccipital cortex, in the premotor cortex, and in the cingulate area, but documentation is not complete in man (Crosby and De Jonge 1963).

Unlike the direct corticonuclear tracts from the precentral gyrus, the pathways from these additional cortical motor areas to the facial nucleus contain numerous synapses. Some of these synaptic junctions are located in the hypothalamus, basal ganglia, and midbrain tegmentum. Emotional movements such as smiling at an amusing story, and automatic associated movements, e.g. unconsciously pursing the lips while concentrating on a problem, may thus persist in patients with a supranuclear facial palsy involving the direct corticobulbar pathway.

Hausman (1971) believes that irritation of the pyramidal (direct corticofacial) fibres produces convulsive twitching movements of the lower face on the opposite side, while involvement of the extrapyramidal (multisynaptic indirect) fibres to the facial nucleus results in a fixed facies, as in Parkinson's disease. However, the functional distinction between the pyramidal and the extrapyramidal systems is becoming blurred, and concepts based on them are gradually being abandoned, together with the terms pyramidal and extrapyramidal.

Facial nerve roots and associated nuclei

The nerve is usually described as consisting of two roots, a larger more medially placed motor root, and a smaller more laterally placed sensory root, which is called the nervus intermedius of Wrisberg. The two roots enter the lower lateral aspect of the pons between the inferior cerebellar peduncle and the olive, in the cerebellopontine angle (Fig. 1.5).

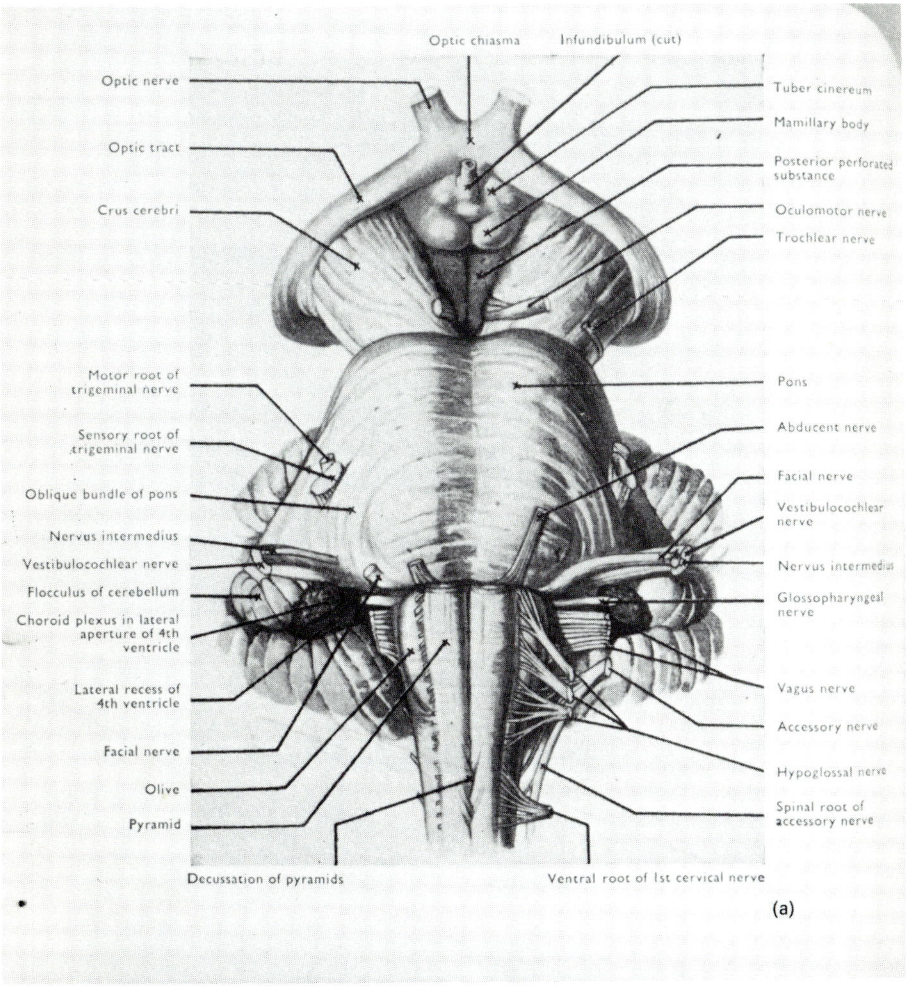

Fig. 1.5. (a) Anterior view of medulla oblongata and pons. (Romanes 1972)

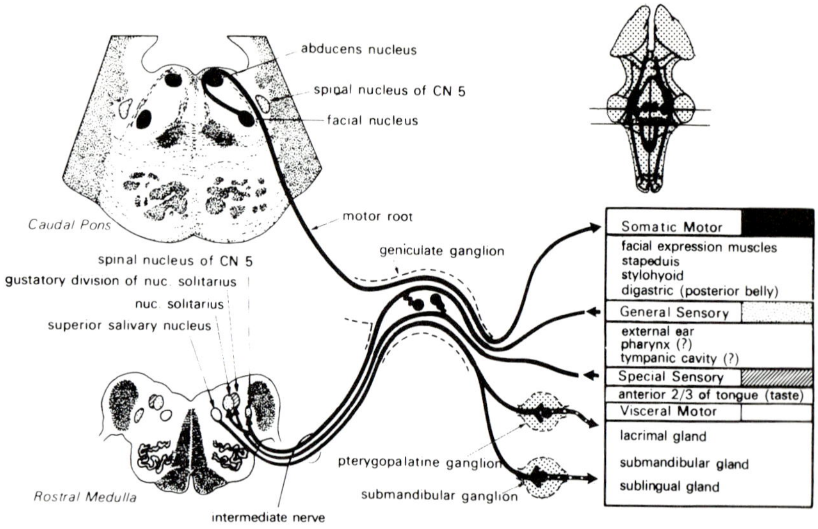

Fig. 1.5. (b) Scheme of central connections and peripheral distribution of facial nerve. (Dunkerley 1975)

The sensory root

The sensory root contains:

(1) efferent preganglionic parasympathetic fibres for the submandibular and sublingual salivary glands, the lacrimal gland, and the glands of the nasal, palatal, and pharyngeal mucosa, and

(2) central processes of the unipolar cells of the geniculate ganglion. The peripheral processes of these cells consist of some afferent taste fibres from the chorda tympani and greater petrosal nerves, and some afferent somatic fibres from the skin around the concha.

The sensory nucleus of the facial nerve

This nucleus lies in the upper part of the nucleus of the tractus solitarius in the medulla oblongata. It receives afferents from the sensory facial root and sends efferent fibres which run close to the midline to reach the thalamus of the opposite side. From the thalamus they are relayed to the inferior part of the postcentral gyrus.

The salivatory nuclei

The superior salivatory nucleus lies in close relation to the caudal end of the facial nucleus. Its nerve fibres loop around the abducens nucleus in the facial colliculus and travel via the sensory facial root and the chorda tympani nerve. The inferior salivatory nucleus lies more caudally and its fibres run with the glossopharyngeal nerve.

The motor nucleus and root

The cells of the motor nucleus lie in the lower third of the pons deep in the reticular formation. They are separated from the spinal tract of the trigeminal and its nucleus by the emerging facial root. The cells are arranged in small groups to form subnuclei each of which seems to be responsible for innervating the muscles supplied by an individual nerve branch. The subnuclei concerned with innervation of the frontalis and the muscles around the eye are thought to occupy the ventral part of the nucleus, while those innervating the lower half of the face are placed dorsally (Crosby and De Jonge 1963). Each nucleus receives fibres from both hemispheres. It has already been mentioned that the subnuclei serving the muscles of the lower half of the face receive contralateral corticonuclear fibres whilst the subnuclei for the muscles of the upper face receive both contralateral and ipsilateral cortical fibres. As a consequence of this bilateral innervation, the voluntary control of the muscles of the upper face is retained in upper motor neurone facial paralysis.

For reasons that were mentioned earlier the emerging fibres from the facial nucleus pursue an unusual path. At first, they run dorsally and medially to reach the posterior aspect of the abducens nucleus. Then they run forward between the dorsal aspect of this nucleus and the floor of the fourth ventricle, forming the facial colliculus. At the anterior end of the abducens nucleus they make a second bend and run ventrally and laterally to emerge from the pons between the olive and the inferior cerebellar peduncle. The loop around the abducens nucleus is often referred to as the internal genu in contrast to the external genu in the temporal bone, at the site of the geniculate ganglion (see Fig. 1.1).

Peripheral course of the facial nerve

It is customary to describe the peripheral course of the facial nerve in the following sections.

1. Course in the posterior fossa and internal auditory canal

This intrameningeal portion is approximately 30 mm long. From their attachment to the brain the two roots pass laterally and forward for a distance of 23 mm or so to the internal auditory meatus, accompanied by the eighth cranial (auditory) nerve. In the internal auditory canal, which is roughly 7 mm long, the motor root lies in a groove on the anterior and superior surface of the auditory nerve and the sensory root is placed between

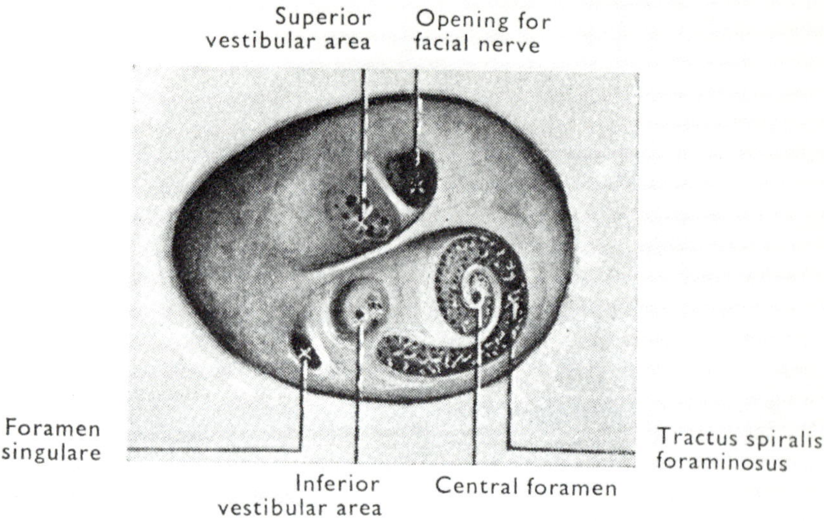

Fig. 1.6. Fundus of left internal auditory canal divided into upper and lower areas by the transverse crest. (Romanes 1972)

them. Both the facial and the auditory nerves are together surrounded by a sheath of meninges as they enter the meatus. This sheath extends to the lateral end of the canal. At the fundus of the canal the nerve pierces the dura and enters the facial nerve (Fallopian) canal. Occasionally the dural coverings extend beyond the internal auditory canal and may clothe the facial nerve as far as the geniculate ganglion (Perlman and Lindsay 1939). Of the four principal openings in the lateral end of the internal auditory canal, the antero-superior one transmits the facial nerve (Fig. 1.6).

2. Course in the Fallopian canal

That part of the facial nerve which runs in the Fallopian canal is approximately 30 mm long. It can be described in three sections: the labyrinthine section, the tympanic or horizontal section, and the mastoid or vertical section.

(a) The labyrinthine section is very short, only 3–4 mm in length. It starts at the opening of the Fallopian canal in the lateral end of the internal auditory canal, and runs laterally above the vestibule. It passes between the vestibule and the cochlea until it reaches the medial wall of the middle ear cleft. At this point the nerve is expanded by the geniculate ganglion which contains the unipolar cells of the sensory root (Fig. 1.7).

(b) The tympanic or horizontal portion begins at the ganglion. This is the place where the nerve makes an abrupt posterior bend of almost 90° to form

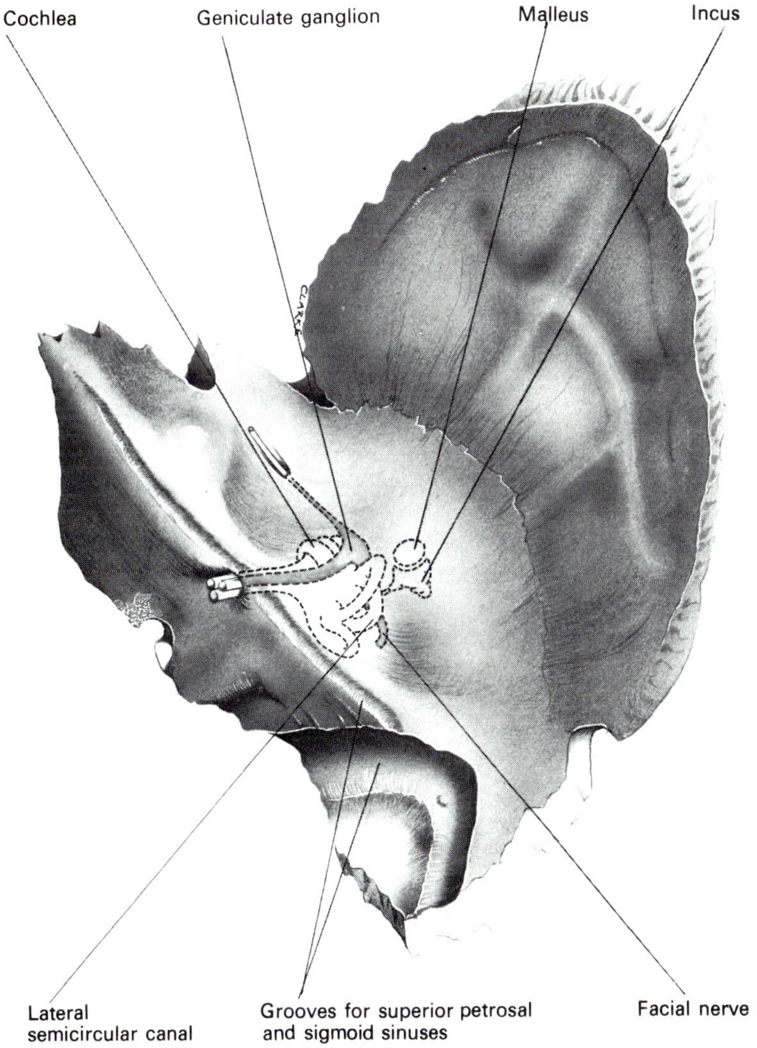

Fig. 1.7. Internal aspect of right temporal bone to show (i) facial nerve passing between cochlea and vestible; (ii) geniculate ganglion and position of greater petrosal nerve; (iii) pyramidal turn of facial nerve below lateral semi-circular canal. (Romanes 1972)

the external genu. The nerve then continues to run posteriorly and slightly downwards in the medial wall of the middle ear, above the oval window and below the prominence caused by the horizontal semicircular canal. This section extends for a length of approximately 12 mm.

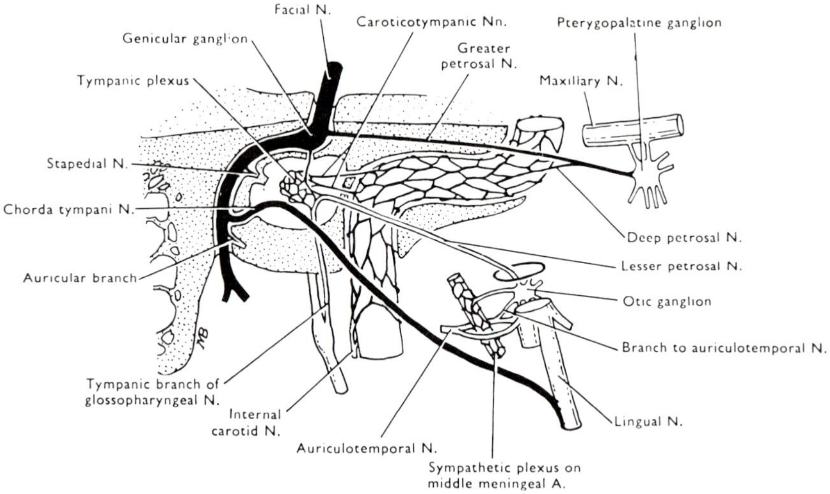

Fig. 1.8. Diagram of intratemporal part of facial nerve and its connections. (Romanes 1978)

(c) The mastoid or vertical portion then begins with a less abrupt, more obtuse-angled bend, called the pyramidal turn, in which the nerve passes below the semicircular canal to descend behind the pyramid. It then passes vertically downwards to reach the stylomastoid foramen. This section is roughly 15 mm long (Fig. 1.8).

3. Course in the neck and parotid gland

After the nerve has coursed through the Fallopian canal, it emerges from the stylomastoid foramen and passes downwards and forwards towards the parotid gland. After crossing the lateral surface of the styloid process and the external carotid artery the nerve reaches the parotid gland and divides behind the neck of the mandible into its two main branches, namely the temporofacial and cervicofacial trunks. These subdivide to form the five terminal branches called the temporal, zygomatic, buccal, marginal mandibular, and cervical branches. These five terminal branches are united to each other by vertical anastomotic branches to form a nerve plexus which has been named the pes anserinus because of its resemblance to the foot of a goose. The segment in the neck and parotid gland is 15–20 mm long.

Branches of the facial nerve

The facial nerve has numerous branches throughout its course and clarity might be served by tabulating the branches of communication, and the branches of distribution.

Branches of communication

1. In the internal auditory canal: with the auditory nerve
2. At the geniculate ganglion:
   (a) with pterygopalatine ganglion by the greater petrosal nerve
   (b) with the otic ganglion by a branch to the lesser petrosal nerve
   (c) with the sympathetic plexus on the middle meningeal artery
3. In the facial canal: with the auricular branch of the vagus by a branch sometimes called the external petrosal nerve
4. At the stylomastoid foramen: with glossopharyngeal, vagus, great auricular, and auriculotemporal nerves
5. Behind the ear: with the lesser occipital nerve
6. On the face: with the trigeminal nerve
7. In the neck: with the transverse cutaneous nerve of the neck.

Of these branches, only the petrosal nerves require further description (Fig. 1.8).

(a) The external petrosal nerve is simply a branch from the sympathetic plexus on the middle meningeal artery to the geniculate ganglion.
(b) The lesser petrosal nerve is essentially the continuation of the tympanic branch of the glossopharyngeal nerve through the tympanic plexus. It receives a branch from the geniculate ganglion, and runs to join the otic ganglion.
(c) The deep petrosal nerve is a branch from the sympathetic plexus on the internal carotid artery. It enters the foramen lacerum to join the greater petrosal nerve.
(d) The greater petrosal nerve arises from the geniculate ganglion, receives a twig from the tympanic plexus, and passes forward in a groove on the floor of the middle fossa. It passes beneath the trigeminal ganglion, and enters the foramen lacerum. There it joins the deep petrosal nerve to form the nerve of the pterygoid canal. It runs through the pterygoid canal, and ends in the pterygopalatine ganglion. The greater petrosal nerve is made up of taste fibres mainly, together with some preganglionic parasympathetic fibres destined for the pterygopalatine ganglion. The parasympathic fibres synapse in the pterygopalatine ganglion, and then pass to the lacrimal gland and the mucosal glands of the nose and palate. The taste fibres arise from the palate and pass through the pterygopalatine ganglion without synapse to reach their cell bodies in the geniculate ganglion.

Branches of distribution

1. Branches within temporal bone (a) *Nerve to stapedius muscle* The facial nerve lies immediately posterior to the pyramidal eminence through which the stapedius tendon emerges. The branch to the muslce leaves the facial nerve at this level and passes forward into the small canal which houses the stapedius muscle.

(b) *Chorda tympani nerve* This arises from the facial nerve about 6 mm above the stylomastoid foramen and runs upwards and forwards in its own canal, named the posterior canaliculus for the chorda tympani nerve. It emerges close to the posterior border of the tympanic membrane, at the level of the upper end of the malleus handle. Faithful to its embryonic position between first visceral groove and first pharyngeal pouch, it arches forward in

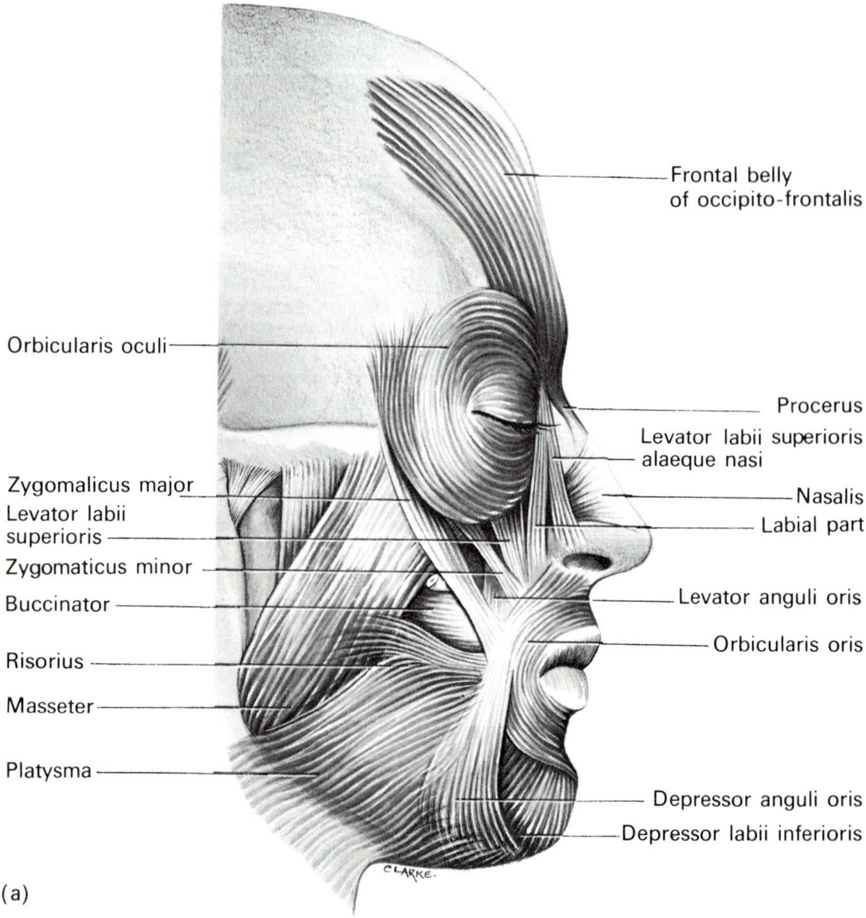

Fig. 1.9. (a) **The** facial muscles. (Romanes 1978)

a fold of the mucosal layer of the tympanic membrane to reach the anterior wall of the middle ear cleft. There it enters the anterior canaliculus for the chorda tympani nerve (sometimes called the canal of Huguier), which is separated from the Eustachian tube by the canal for the tensor tympani muscle. The nerve runs downwards and forwards from its canal and crosses the medial surface of the sphenoid spine, which it sometimes grooves, to join the lingual nerve on its posterior surface. This is at the level of the lower border of the lateral pterygoid muscle.

Most of the fibres of the chorda tympani nerve are taste fibres from the anterior two-thirds of the tongue. The nerve also contains efferent secretomotor parasympathetic fibres destined to synapse in the submandibular

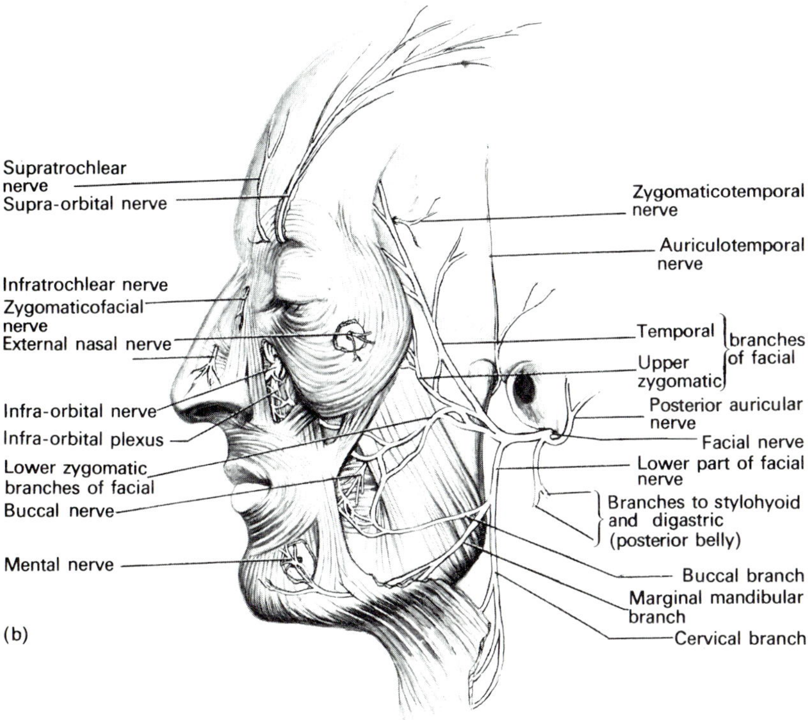

Fig. 1.9. (b) Distribution of the facial nerve branches (dark lines) and tregeminal nerve branches (light lines) on the face. (Romanes 1972)

ganglion, before passing on to the submandibular and sublingual salivary glands.

2. Branches in the neck

Nerve	*Muscles supplied*
Posterior auricular branch	(a) Auricular division to posterior auricular muscle. (b) Occipital division to occipital belly of occipitofrontalis muscle
Digastric branch	Posterior belly of digastric muscle
Stylohyoid branch	Stylohyoid muscle

3. Branches in the face

Nerve	*Muscles supplied*
(a) Temporal	Anterior and superior auricular muscles, frontal belly of occipitofrontalis, orbicularis oculi, and corrugator
(b) Zygomatic	Orbicularis oculi principally
(c) Buccal	Procerus, zygomaticus major and minor, levator labii superioris, levator anguli oris, levator labii superioris alaeque nasi, orbicularis oris, and buccinator
(d) Marginal mandibular	Risorius, depressor anguli oris, depressor labii inferioris, and mentalis
(e) Cervical	Platysma principally

(This represents a general pattern of innervation. Because the terminal branches of the facial nerve anastomose in a plexus, different patterns of innervation are possible.)

(f) Cutaneous fibres

It is recognized that cutaneous fibres of the facial nerve accompany the auricular branch of the vagus and probably innervate the skin over the conchal cartilage. Details of the innervation are uncertain, however.

Blood-supply of the facial nerve

The blood-supply of the nerve is of particular interest because some current theories state that ischaemia of the nerve is the cause of many cases of facial paralysis. In its course through the temporal bone, the nerve is supplied by three arteries, and the territories supplied by these arteries overlap, so that at least two vessels are involved in supplying any one portion of the nerve.

(a) The anterior inferior cerebellar artery supplies the nerve in the posterior fossa. Normally a branch of this vessel, the internal auditory artery, supplies the facial nerve in the internal auditory canal. Fine arterial branches extend to supply the nerve as far as the geniculate ganglion.

(b) The petrosal branch of the middle meningeal artery enters the Fallopian canal at the geniculate ganglion and divides into descending and ascending branches. The descending branch runs distally with the nerve to the stylomastoid foramen, while the ascending branch supplies the region proximal to the geniculate ganglion.

(c) The stylomastoid branch of the posterior auricular artery enters the facial canal through the stylomastoid foramen and soon also divides into an ascending and descending branch. The ascending branch runs with the nerve up to the geniculate ganglion level. The descending branch supplies the nerve down to the stylomastoid foramen and accompanies the posterior auricular nerve.

These arteries and their accompanying veins lie in the loose connective tissue (epineurium) between the periosteum of the canal wall and the nerve sheath proper. Blunt (1954) has shown that these vessels anastomose with each other and Anson *et al.* (1970) also noted numerous anastomoses with the marrow spaces of surrounding bone, and with the rich vascular plexus of the middle ear mucosa.

In its extracranial course, the facial nerve again derives its blood-supply from several sources. It is nourished by branches of the stylomastoid, posterior auricular, superficial temporal, and transverse facial arteries which send anastomosing branches to the nerve.

The blood-supply of the facial nerve would thus appear to be very secure. Blunt concluded that there is no anatomical evidence of precarious blood-supply to any part of the nerve below the geniculate ganglion which would especially predispose it to ischaemia from primary vascular spasm. Facial nerve paralysis due to primary ischaemia is no longer considered to be a likely hypothesis.

In a later article, however, Blunt (1965) supports the theory of 'combined primary and secondary ischaemia' as a cause of Bell's palsy. According to this view, vascular spasm of unknown aetiology, although incapable of producing sufficient primary ischaemia to cause nerve paralysis, can, however, cause tumescence or swelling of the nerve. This swelling of the nerve in the Fallopian canal can in turn be followed by 'compression ischaemia resulting in facial paralysis'.

At first sight, this may appear to be an exercise in splitting hairs. However, it really represents a radical alteration in the theory of a vascular cause of Bell's palsy. Blunt infers that the paralysis is not due to an anatomically inadequate blood-supply as such, but to the fact that the nerve, with its sheath and vessels, is incarcerated in a rigid bony tube. Since the cause of any primary ischaemia is unknown, supporters of the combined theory rely heavily on the assumption that passage through an intact bony canal in some way makes the nerve vulnerable. Clinical experience, however, shows that an intact bony canal often affords protection to the nerve. In otitis media, facial palsy does not occur if the Fallopian canal is intact. Indeed, the occurrence of facial palsy in otitis media indicates the presence of a congenital or acquired defect in the facial nerve canal (see Chapter 3). The Fallopian canal would seem to be sufficiently wide for the normal facial nerve does not occupy more than 50 per cent of the cross-sectional area available to it in the bony canal.

Facial nerve sheath

Most textbooks of otology state that the facial nerve sheath is composed of three layers, but there is some confusion about what these layers should be called. The outermost layer is the endosteum of the canal wall and is quite thin. The middle layer or epineurium is composed of loose connective tissue in which the blood-vessels course. The epineurium condenses around the perineurium to contribute to the nerve sheath proper. The perineurium invests the bundles of nerve fibres and forms the inner layer of the 'nerve sheath proper'. In the sheath, the perineurium merges with the epineurium without any abrupt line of demarcation. This is what produces the difficulty in nomenclature, with some authors labelling the sheath as epineurium (Sunderland 1968, Anson and Donaldson 1973) and others as perineurium (Karnes 1975). The essential point is that the sheath which invests the nerve bundles is composed of epineurium and perineurium blended together without any discernible plane of cleavage between them. This sheath is thickest around the vertical segment of the facial nerve and thins progressively as it travels proximally. Sunderland (1946) has shown that incising the perineurium of normal nerves caused a bulging and herniation of the underlying nerve fibres. This herniation will not occur if epineurium only is incised. Many surgeons have described a ballooning or herniation after incising 'the nerve sheath' in patients with Bell's palsy and have cited this as evidence of pathological oedema of the nerve. Sunderland's observations, therefore, cast doubt on the validity of such evidence.

Facial nerve reflexes

Often certain reflexes are tested to determine the integrity of the motor root of the facial nerve or facial nucleus. The reflexes depend equally on an intact afferent sensory loop.

1. Naso-lacrimal reflex Irritation of the nasal mucous membrane, e.g. by ammonia or benzene vapour, or by mechanical stimuli, induces a strong flow of tears. The afferent pathway is the trigeminal nerve, and the greater petrosal nerve forms the efferent path. Decreased lacrimation in lesions involving the facial nerve is the basis of Schirmer's test (see Chapter 6, p. 212).

2. Corneal reflex Gentle stimulation of the cornea by a wisp of cotton wool produces reflex blinking of the eyelids.

Again the afferent pathway is the trigeminal nerve. The efferent path is the facial nerve. In acoustic neuromas, if the facial nerve is obviously intact, the absence of a corneal reflex indicates involvement of the trigeminal sensory root. Although textbooks of neurology describe the loss of this reflex as an early sign in acoustic neuromas, it is in fact a late sign. It indicates that the tumour has reached a large size and has involved an additional cranial nerve, some distance from the auditory nerve.

3. Stapedius reflex Loud sounds elicit the protective reflex contraction of the stapedius muscle which reduces the transmission of sound waves by the stapes to the inner ear fluids. In this reflex the afferent route is the auditory nerve, and the efferent pathway is the facial nerve. The presence or absence of this reflex in patients with facial paralysis helps to determine the level of the nerve lesion (see Chapter 6).

4. Palpebral or blinking reflex This is the reflex contraction of the palpebral portion of the orbicularis oculi muscle in response to tactile, optic, or acoustic stimuli. Afferent stimuli can travel through the trigeminal, optic, or auditory nerves. The facial nerve forms the motor pathway. The blink test is performed by tapping with a finger on the supraorbital region, and thereby inducing a reflex blinking action.

5. Naso-mental reflex Tapping the side of the nose produces elevation of the upper lip and angle of the mouth. If the stimulus is increased, the lower lip may be raised and the skin of the chin will wrinkle (Crosby and De Jonge 1963).

Anatomical variations

The tortuous course of the facial nerve from the pons to the parotid is fairly constant from individual to individual, and, although several variations having clinical significance have been described, variation is the exception rather than the rule.

At birth, before the mastoid process has developed, the stylomastoid foramen is superficially placed and the facial nerve lies virtually in the subcutaneous plane. There it is susceptible to damage by obstetrical forceps and by post auricular incisions. As the mastoid process develops, it overlies the stylomastoid foramen and shields the nerve. This variation from the adult position is of course normal.

Variations within an intact Fallopian canal

An abnormal position of the facial nerve is more likely to be encountered in patients who have developmental anomalies of the first and second branchial arches. The presence of microtia, atresia of the pinna or external auditory canal, the Treacher Collins syndrome, a branchial fistula, or the history of thalidomide damage should alert the surgeon to the increased risk of facial nerve aberrations. Fortunately, the course of the Fallopian canal can now be demonstrated by the use of radiological tomography (Wright and Taylor 1972) and this examination can be carried out pre-operatively in suspected cases.

The vertical segment of the nerve was closely studied by Kettel (1946), who pointed out that it was not always truly vertical, although it is commonly reputed to lie perpendicularly between the most overhanging part of the lateral semicircular canal and the stylomastoid foramen. This perpendicular line is indicated by the tympanomastoid suture line which is easily located at operation. He quotes Batson's (1938) statement that 'the nerve is never posterior to this line', and goes on to show the different posterior positions it may take. Shambaugh (1967) states categorically that 'the never may lie posterior to the suture line but never anterior' and this is more generally accepted. It is also widely agreed that the nerve always lies deep or medial to the suture line and never superficial or lateral to it.

Fowler (1961) collected all the anomalies he had seen or could find in the literature, apart from dehiscence of the Fallopian canal, and made them into comparable diagrams which are reproduced here (Fig. 1.10).

Dehiscence of the Fallopian canal

Reichert's cartilage (second branchial arch cartilage) contributes to the structure of the Fallopian canal, and anomalies in the development of this cartilage can result in congenital dehiscence of the canal wall. Perhaps, strictly speaking, these deshiscences should not be regarded as true anomalies of the facial nerve, but they do allow the nerve to escape from the canal wall and to take an alarmingly aberrant course. Baxter (1971) studied a large series of over 500 temporal bones, and in order to avoid confusion with vascular foramina, defined a bony dehiscence as a gap in the canal wall measuring 0·4 mm or larger. Using this criterion, he found that 55 per cent of the Fallopian canals studied had a deshiscence. The majority of these gaps (66 per cent) were found in the oval window region, and approximately 10 per cent were in the vertical segment of the canal. The nerve protruded from roughly one in four of the gaps in the oval window region, and from one in eight of the vertical segment gaps. The bony covering over the geniculate ganglion was studied in 100 temporal bones by Hall *et al.* (1969) and was found to be deficient in 15 per cent. In another 15 per cent, the geniculate ganglion was covered, but no bone extended over the greater petrosal nerve.

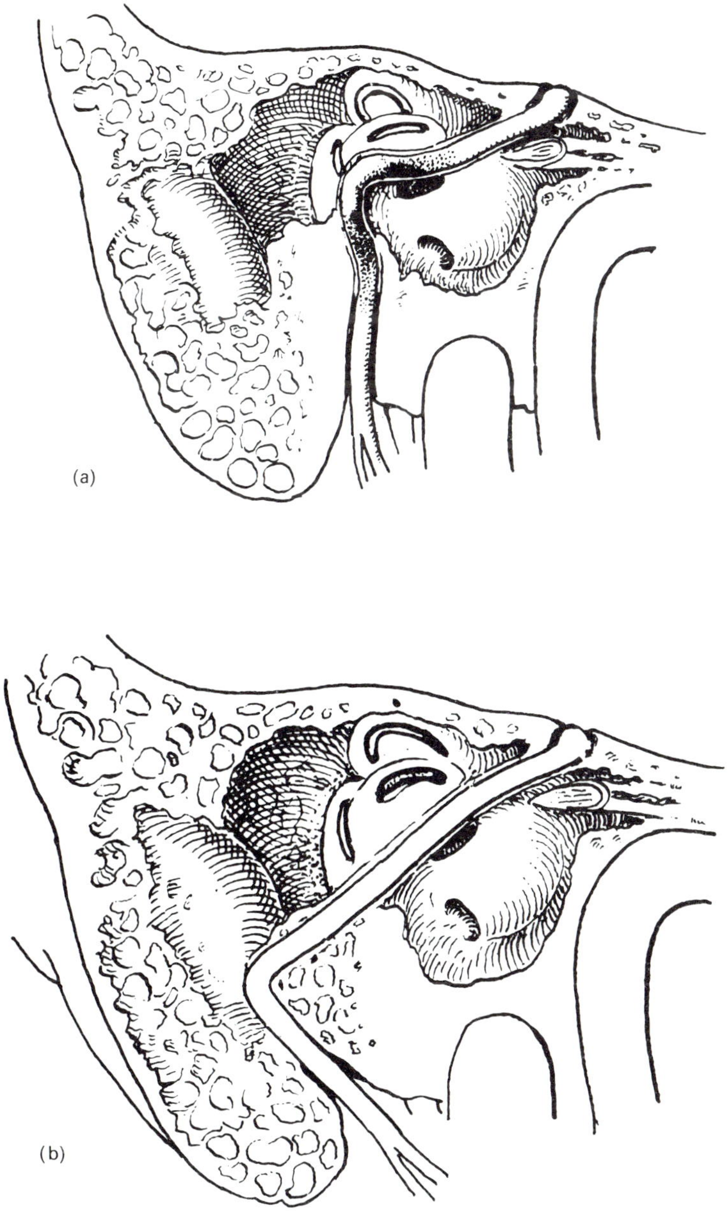

Fig. 1.10. Anatomical variations (Fowler 1961):

(a) a hump posterior and lateral to the prominence of the lateral semicircular canal;

(b) a course markedly posterior to the prominence of the lateral semicircular canal;

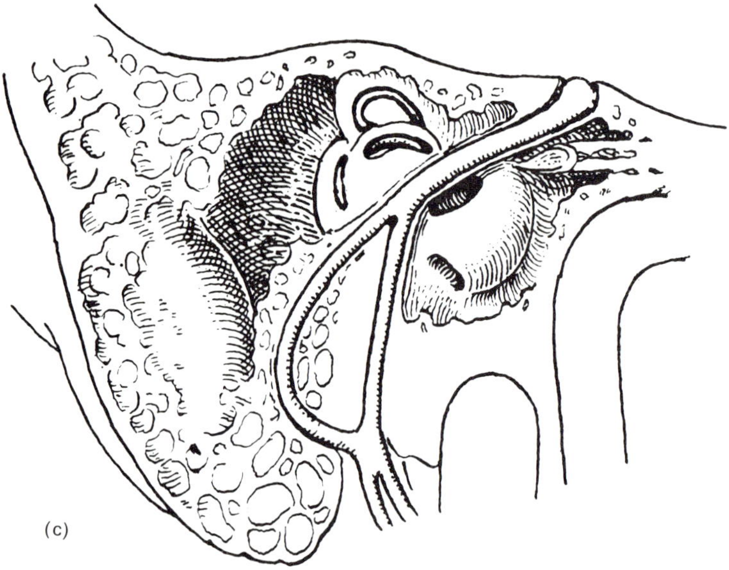

(c)

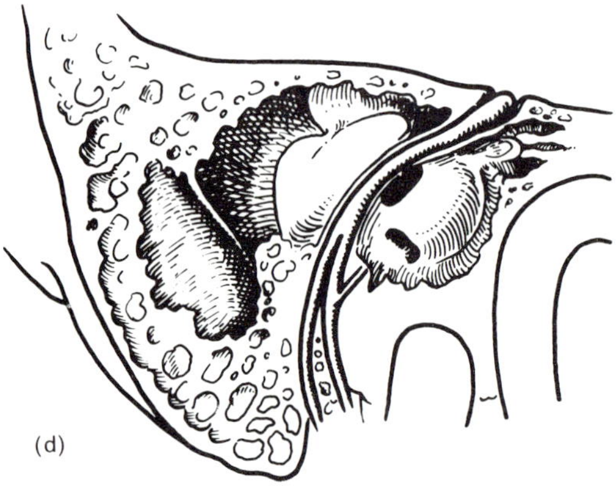

(d)

Fig. 1.10. (continued)

(c) vertical portion of facial nerve in two parts uniting at stylomastoid foramen (after Pierce-Fowler);

(d) bifurcated facial nerve (after Miehlke);

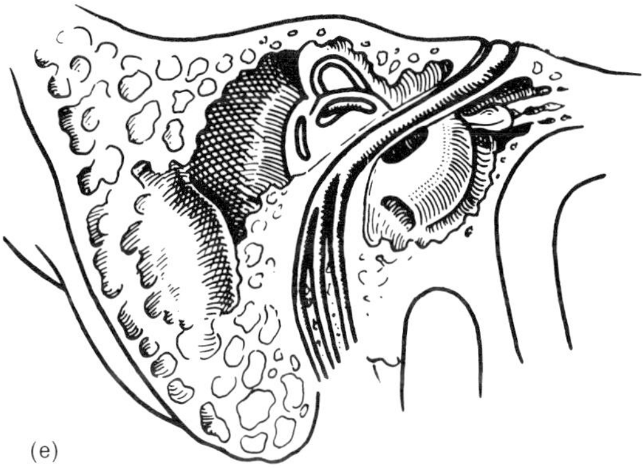

(e)

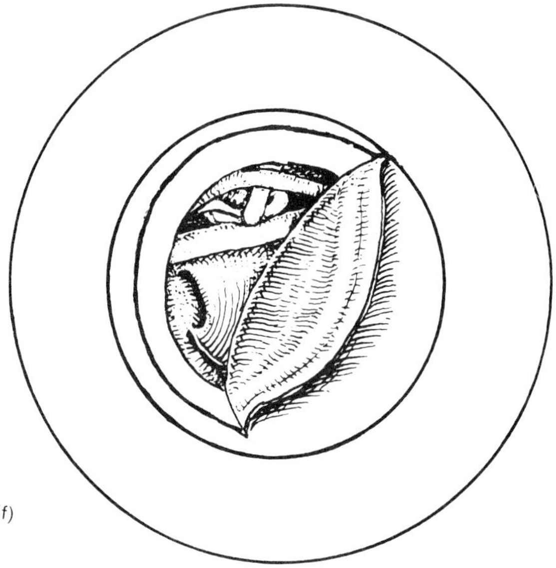

(f)

Fig. 1.10. (continued)
(e) tripartite facial nerve (after Jongkees);
(f) facial nerve coursing between the round and oval windows in patient with persistent stapedial artery.

In a review of the literature, Anson *et al.* (1963) list the findings of several authors and these include cases showing:

(1) the nerve lying free between the geniculate ganglion and the stylomastoid foramen, and bifurcating before leaving the temporal bone;
(2) the free nerve coursing below the oval window;
(3) a persistent stapedial artery which ran through the stapes and penetrated the facial nerve canal;
(4) the nerve lying free, and running with a persistent stapedial artery across the promontary.

Chorda tympani nerve variations

Occasionally the chorda tympani nerve joins the facial nerve at an abnormal level. Cawthorne (1965) referred to temporal bone dissections which demonstrated the junction occurring at different levels between the stylomastoid foramen and the pyramidal bend.

Taste sensation and pathways

Taste receptors or buds are present on the dorsum of the tongue and to a lesser extent on the palate, pharynx, and epiglottis. The taste receptors are modified epithelial cells which undergo a constant process of degeneration and replacement. Four kinds of primary taste sensation are recognized: sweet, bitter, salt, and sour or acid. There is universal agreement that the taste receptors of the anterior two-thirds of the tongue are innervated by the chorda tympani nerve and the receptors in the posterior part of the tongue are innervated by the glossopharyngeal nerve. Whether the taste receptors of the epiglottis are supplied by the glossopharyngeal or vagus nerves is still not certain. The majority of writers state that the palate is innervated by fibres of the greater petrosal nerve whose cell bodies lie in the geniculate ganglion. In the past, no less than nine different pathways have been postulated by which gustatory fibres from the anterior two-thirds of the tongue may reach the central nervous system. Four different trigeminal pathways, four different facial nerve pathways, and a glossopharyngeal route have been proposed as alternative paths from the anterior part of the tongue. None of these paths have been demonstrated anatomically in man. Difficulty in interpreting taste defects in certain patients has been responsible for the construction of these hypothetical pathways. In *Grays Anatomy*, for example, one alternative pathway is said to exist by which taste fibres in the chorda tympani nerve may reach their unipolar cells in the geniculate ganglion. It states that in a few individuals, taste fibres leave the chorda tympani nerve by anastomotic branches connecting it to the otic ganglion, and proceed thence in the greater petrosal nerve to the geniculate ganglion. This is based on deductions made by Schwartz and Weddell (1938) following mastoid surgery. These deductions would not be supported by otologists today who enjoy the immense advantage of the operating microscope which was not available to earlier surgeons.

The nine proposed alternative pathways have been critically reviewed by Rollin (1977) who found no substance in any of them. We would agree with his conclusions that there is only one gustatory pathway from each taste area namely:

(a) from the anterior part of the tongue via the chorda tympani and facial nerve;

(b) from the palate via the nerve of the pterygoid canal, greater petrosal nerve and facial nerve; and,

(c) from the posterior part of the tongue via the glossopharyngeal nerve.
The central processes of the geniculate ganglion cells pass in the nervus intermedius to end in the cephalic part of the nucleus of the tractus solitarius. The central processes from the nodose (glossopharyngeal) ganglion enter the lower part of the nucleus solitarius. After synapse the fibres cross to the

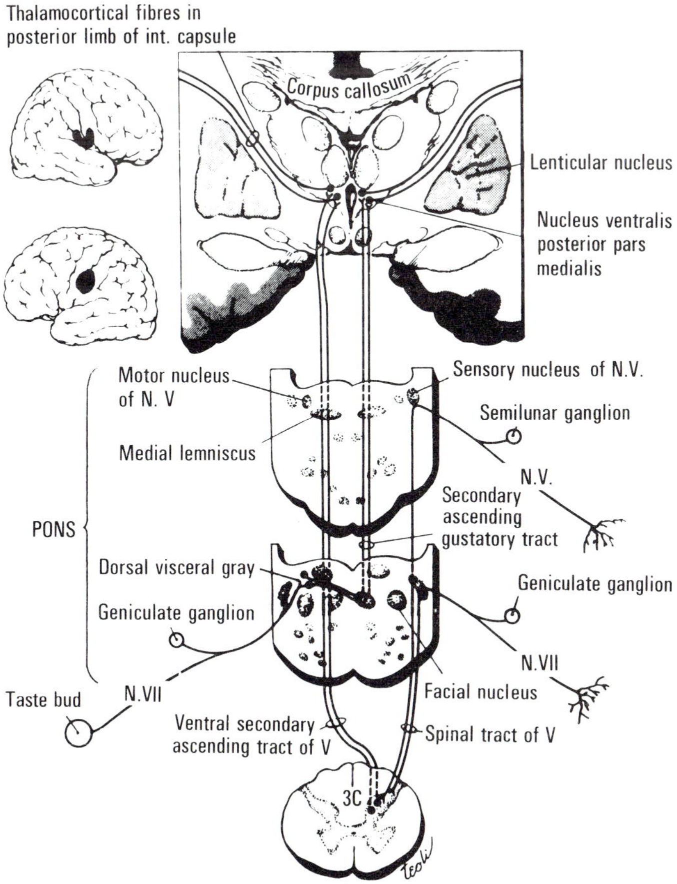

Fig. 1.11. Sensory pathways: This diagram illustrates the pathways by which (i) ordinary sensation (including pain) is projected from the face and external ear to the thalamus and then to the cerebral cortex; and (ii) gustatory impulses from the anterior two thirds of tongue are relayed to their thalamic and cortical terminations.

Two small hemispheres are shown at the top of the figure. The darkened region in the upper one shows the position of the gustatory cortical area. In the lower hemisphere the darkened region illustrates the cortical projection area for cutaneous sensibility of the face. (Crosby and De Jonge 1963) opposite medial lemniscus and reach the thalamus. The third relay arises in the thalamus and ends in the postcentral gyrus (Fig. 1.11).

Chorda tympani nerve section

In microsurgical operations on the middle ear the chorda tympani nerve is frequently divided or displaced to improve access and vision in the small operative field. There has been considerable argument about whether cleanly dividing the nerve, or stretching it to displace it, is the lesser evil. Section of the chorda tympani always produces permanent loss of taste sensation in the anterior two-thirds of the tongue on the same side. No reinnervation of the taste buds takes place either from the chorda tympani of the opposite side or from the posterior third of the tongue supplied by the glossopharyngeal nerve. Permanent loss of chorda tympani innervation results in atrophy of the taste receptors in the anterior two-thirds of the tongue, the dorsum of which becomes smooth and pale. When one chorda tympani nerve is cut, the loss of taste sensation usually passes unnoticed by the patient, because the tongue retains sensation in 66 per cent of its surface.

Stretching the nerve to displace it sometimes produces a persistent abnormal sensation in the tongue, often described as an unpleasant salty or metallic taste. The abnormal sensation is regarded as a paraesthesia of this special sensory nerve. There is a widely held view among otologists that, since the taste loss from cutting the nerve often passes unnoticed by patients, it is better to divide the nerve rather than displace it by stretching, and thereby risk troublesome paraesthesia. This view is misguided. Bull (1965) and Wiberg (1971) have shown that cutting the nerve also produces these unpleasant taste sensations. In a series of 250 cases Bull recorded that division of the nerve produced persistent abnormal taste sensations in 32 per cent of cases whereas displacing the nerve caused persistent symptoms in only 7 per cent of cases. In a smaller series Wiberg showed that 12 (55 per cent) out of 22 patients had persistent symptoms 12 months after the nerve had been sectioned, and in 4 patients (18 per cent) these symptoms were distressing. By contrast, one year after surgery in which the nerve was displaced but not divided, only 4 (24 per cent) out of 17 patients had a mild disturbance of taste.

In addition to the alteration in the sense of taste following loss of the chorda tympani nerve, there is also a loss of the secretomotor supply to the submandibular and sublingual salivary glands of the same side. Fortunately, the majority of patients do not notice a dryness of the mouth as a result of unilateral nerve loss.

Bilateral loss of the chorda tympani, as one would expect, produces more frequent and more persistent symptoms. The majority of patients notice an uncomfortable dryness of the mouth, and they are aware of their reduced sense of taste. Since taste appreciation is confined to the posterior third of the tongue, food may often be tasted only fleetingly, immediately before swallowing. Abnormal taste sensations, e.g. salty, bitter, or metallic tastes, are twice as likely to occur with bilateral loss of the nerve.

The role of copper

The toxic side effects of a drug sometimes provide new information on physiological function. The loss of taste observed in patients treated with penicillamine illustrated the previously unrecognized fact that copper plays an important role in taste function. Henkin *et al.* (1967) showed that patients with Wilson's disease, in which body stores of copper are excessive, rarely suffered taste loss when treated with the chelating agent penicillamine. However, loss of taste occurred in a third of patients treated with this drug for other conditions, e.g. rheumatoid arthritis, in which the body's stores of copper are normal. The drug lowers both the serum copper and the serum concentration of the copper-binding protein, caeruloplasmin. The prophylactic or therapeutic use of copper sulphate 5 mg daily abolishes taste loss due to penicillamine.

Anatomical landmarks

A clear knowledge of the landmarks of the facial nerve is essential for surgeons operating in the posterior fossa, the middle fossa, the temporal bone, the parotid gland, and in the face and neck, and landmarks are summarized here.

Posterior fossa The two facial nerve roots emerge between the olive and the inferior cerebellar peduncle in the cerebellopontine angle, in front of the auditory nerve. The facial nerve lies on the antero-superior surface of the auditory nerve in the internal auditory canal, and it occupies the antero-superior opening in the fundus of the canal (see Fig. 1.6).

Middle fossa The middle meningeal artery is easily identified as it enters the middle fossa through the foramen spinosum. The fibres of the greater petrosal nerve can be seen leaving the middle fossa immediately posterior to this artery. Removal of the bone over the nerve allows one to trace the fibres posteriorly to the geniculate ganglion (see Fig. 1.7).

Geniculate ganglion anatomy Dubozi (1975) has demonstrated that the ganglion cells sit like a cap over the anterior portion of the external genu. Surgical resection of the anterior third of the genu has been shown to remove 90 per cent of the ganglion cells without endangering the motor fibres.

Temporal bone The position of the genu may be located from the middle ear, by the emerging tendon of the tensor tympani muscle. The genu lies immediately deep to the tip of the processus cochleariformis round which the tendon turns to reach the malleus. The horizontal portion of the Fallopian canal is clearly visible above the oval window. The nerve passes underneath the horizontal semicircular canal and immediately posterior to the pyramid. In its vertical course the nerve runs deep to the tympanomastoid suture and all mastoid bone superficial to the suture line may be removed without risk of damage to the facial nerve. Inside the mastoid process the digastric crest or ridge indicates the position of the stylomastoid foramen. The foramen lies at the antero-medial end of the crest.

Landmarks in the neck (a) As it emerges from the stylomastoid foramen, the nerve bisects the angle between the anterior border of the mastoid process and the vaginal process of the tympanic bone which sheathes the styloid process.

(b) Where the posterior belly of the digastric muscle meets the mastoid process, the nerve lies 3 mm above the muscle.

(c) The triangular tip of the tragal cartilage 'points' to the facial nerve 10 mm deep and inferior to the cartilage tip.

(d) The marginal mandibular branch of the nerve descends below the inferior border of the mandible one finger-breadth in front of the angle of the mandible. It loops up after a variable distance to reach the corner of the mouth. Since the nerve branch is always superficial to the deep fascia, it is possible to avoid injuring the nerve by dissecting in the plane underneath the deep fascia. It is safe to incise the deep fascia at the level of the hyoid bone and to reflect it up to the lower border of the mandible to which the fascia is firmly attached.

Facial nerve enigmas

There are a number of observed phenomena which do not fit in with our present-day understanding of the anatomy and physiology of the facial nerve. There is a natural tendency to brush these untidy and uncomfortable facts aside. This is a pity, for they offer us a tantalizing glimpse of the gaps in our knowledge. They lift a corner of the veil of our ignorance and suggest paths of inquiry which may lead to a fuller knowledge of nerve function and nerve recovery after damage. These anomalies should be a source of constant discussion and debate until their mystery has been solved.

Taste anomalies

It has been known for some time that 30 per cent of people with normal taste sensation are unable to detect the bitter taste of phenylthiocarbamide (PTC). Since PTC is not a naturally occurring chemical, the fact that the inability to taste PTC bitter is inherited as a Mendelian recessive character has been regarded as a purely academic curiosity. Henkin and Gillis (1977) have shown that a similar divergence of taste responsiveness to a naturally occurring substance also exists. The fruit of the tree *Antidesma bunius* (popularly called Chinese laurel) is used in making jams, jellies, and syrups. Although it tastes sweet to the majority of normal people, 15 per cent of the 170 subjects tested by Henkin and Gillis found it bitter. Interestingly enough, the 15 per cent were all PTC non-responders. It seemed likely from the family testing carried out that the taste response to Antidesma berries is genetically determined.

It would appear, therefore, that 30 per cent of normal people are unable to detect the bitter taste of PTC and that half of this group find Antidesma berries bitter while the majority of people find them sweet. Are there other undiscovered examples of taste divergence? Clearly our accepted concept of taste is incomplete as it does not account for the divergent taste responses excited by the same substance in normal subjects.

Transitory return of facial nerve function after surgery

A transient recovery of function which lasts for about 12 hours or so before the paralysis returns to its pre-operative level has often been reported to occur immediately after decompression of the nerve in idiopathic facial palsy. Any permanent improvement from the operation becomes evident only weeks or months after surgery. The brief transitory recovery of function post-operatively gives no clue to the degree of permanent recovery that will take place. Our present knowledge of the physiology of nerve function and of nerve recovery is inadequate to explain this (McCabe 1977).

Similar transient recovery of function has also been reported immediately after excision of damaged segment of facial nerve and its replacement with an autogenous nerve graft, or following direct anastomosis. How a nervous impulse can cross the gaps at each end of the graft and travel down the distal degenerated portion of the nerve cannot be explained by current knowledge.

Permanent recovery after excision of segments of the facial nerve

There have been a number of reports of cases where segments of the trunk and branches of the facial nerve have been removed deliberately during tumour surgery and where good, though incomplete, recovery of facial nerve function has taken place 1–2 years later.

No nerve repair during surgery was attempted and in a number of patients whose face required to be re-explored no reunion of the nerve had taken place. It cannot be overemphasized that these exceptions to the normal course of events occur only in isolated cases, but they have been observed and reported by Botman and Jongkees (1955), Martin and Helsper (1957), Miehlke (1973), and Conley (1975).

Hypotheses of the mechanism of facial nerve enigmas

Three hypotheses have been put forward to explain the permanent recovery after surgical excisions.

(a) From the terminal anastomoses between the facial and trigeminal nerves, trigeminal motor fibres extend to take over the function of the lost facial nerve fibres. This would require a relearning process in the cortex.

(b) Facial nerve motor fibres are re-routed through the geniculate ganglion, greater petrosal nerve, and pterygopalatine ganglion and pass into the mandibular division of the trigeminal nerve to reach the facial muscles. This would not require a relearning process in the cortex.

(c) Reinnervation of the facial muscles from the intact facial nerve of the opposite side takes place.

If any or all of these theories are correct, it leaves perhaps a bigger question unanswered. Why does this reinnervation occur so rarely?

No theories have been put forward to explain the taste divergence or the transient recovery of function after surgery.

Summary

The aim of this chapter has been to look critically at the anatomy and physiology of the facial nerve. It may be regarded as unsatisfactory to end the chapter with a riddle, but if the reader will accept these puzzles as a challen e, the purpose of the chapter will have been achieved.

References

Anson, B. J., Donaldson, J. A., Warpeha, R. L., and Rensink, M. J. (1970). The facial nerve sheath and blood supply in relation to the surgery of decompression. *Ann. Otol. Rhinol. Laryngol.* **79**, 710.
——, —— (1973). *Surgical anatomy of the temporal bone and ear*, p. 352. Saunders, Philadelphia.
——, Harper, D. G., and Warpeha, R. L. (1963). Surgical anatomy of the facial canal and facial nerve. *Ann. Otol. Rhinol. Laryngol.* **72**, 713.
Bailey, H. (1941). The treatment of tumours of the parotid gland with special reference to total parotidectomy. *Brit. J. Surg.* **28**, 337.
——. (1947) Parotidectomy: indications and results. *Brit. med. J.* **1**, 404.
Batson, O. U. (1938). Surgical anatomy of the temporal bone. In *Nelson's loose-leaf surgery of the ear.* Thomas Nelson & Sons, New York. Quoted by Kettel (1946).
Baxter, A. (1971). Dehiscence of the Fallopian canal: an anatomical study. *J. Laryngol. Otol.* **85**, 587.
Bell, C. (1821). On the nerves: giving an account of some experiments on their structure and functions which lead to a new arrangement of the system. *Phil. Trans. roy. Soc. Lond.* **111**, 398.
——. (1829). On the nerves of the face. *Phil. Trans. roy. Soc. Lond.* Part 2, p. 317.
Blunt, M. J. (1954). The blood supply of the facial nerve. *J. Anat.* **88**, 520.
——. (1965). Possible role of vascular changes in the aetiology of Bell's palsy. *J. Otol. Laryngol.* **70**, 701.
Botman, J. W. M. and Jongkees, L. B. W. (1955). On transitory recovery immediately after facial nerve grafting and its cause. *Acta Otolaryngol.* **45**, 305.
Bull, T. R. (1965). Taste and the chorda tympani. *J. Laryngol. Otol.* **79**, 479.
Cawthorne, T. (1965). Discussion. *Arch. Otolaryngol.* **81**, 539.
Conley, J. (1975). *Salivary glands and the facial nerve*, p. 349. Georg Thieme, Stuttgart.
Crosby, E. C. and De Jonge, B. R. (1963). Experimental and clinical studies of the central connections and central relations of the facial nerve. *Ann. Otol. Rhinol. Laryngol.* **72**, 735.
Dubozi, M. (1975). Surgical anatomy of the geniculate ganglion. *Acta Otolaryngol.* **80**, 116.
Dunkerley, G. B. (1975). *A basic atlas of the human nervous system.* F. A. Davis, Philadelphia.
Fowler, E. P. (1961). Variations in the temporal bone course of the facial nerve. *Laryngoscope* **71**, 937.
Gasser, R. F. (1970). The early development of the parotid gland around the facial nerve and its branches in man. *Anat. Rec.* **167**, 63.
Gray's anatomy (1973). (ed. R. Warwick and P. L. Williams; 35th edn), p. 1085. Longman.

Hall, G. M., Pulec, J. L., and Rhoton, A. L. (1969). Geniculate ganglion anatomy for the otologist. *Arch. Otolaryngol.* **90**, 568.

Hamilton, W. J., and Harrison, R. J. (1971). In: *Scott-Brown's diseases of the ear, nose and throat* (ed. J. Ballantyne and J. Groves; 3rd edn, Vol. 1, p. 214. Butterworths, London.

Hausman, L. (1971). *Clinical neuroanatomy, neurophysiology and neurology*, p. 118. Charles C. Thomas, Springfield, Illinois.

Henkin, R. I. and Gillis, W. T. (1977). Divergent taste responsiveness to the fruit of the tree *Antidesma bunius. Nature* **265**, 536.

——, Keiser, H. R., Jaffe, I. A., Sternlieb, I., and Scheinberg, I. H. (1967). Decreased taste sensitivity after D-penicillamine reversed by copper administration. *Lancet* **ii**, 1268.

Karnes, W. E. (1975). *Peripheral neuropathy* (ed. P. Dyck, P. K. Thomas, and E. M. Lambert), Vol. 1. p. 573. Saunders, Philadelphia.

Kettel, K. (1946). Abnormal courses of the facial nerve in the Fallopian canal. *Arch. Otolaryngol.* **44**, 406.

McCabe, B. (1977) Decompression for Bell's palsy. Immediate motion post-operative. *Laryngoscope* **87**, 246.

McCormack, L. J., Cauldwell, E. W., and Anson, B. J. (1945). The surgical anatomy of the facial nerve. *Surg. Gynaec. Obstet.* **80**, 620.

McKenzie, J. (1948). The parotid gland in relation to the facial nerve. *J. Anat.* **82**, 183.

Martin, H. and Helsper, J. T. (1957). Spontaneous return of function following surgical incision of VII cranial nerve in the surgery of parotid tumours. *Ann. Surg.* **146**, 715.

Miehlke, A. (1973). *Surgery of the facial nerve*, p. 239. Saunders, Philadelphia, London and Toronto.

Nomina Anatomica (1966) (3rd ed). Excerpta Medica Foundation, Amsterdam.

Patey, D. H. and Ranger, I. (1957). Some points in the surgical anatomy of parotid gland. *Brit. J. Surg.* **45**, 250.

Perlman, H. B. and Lindsay, J. R. (1939). Relation of the internal ear spaces to the meninges. *Arch. Otolaryngol.* **29**, 12.

Rollin, H. (1977). Course of peripheral gustatory nerves. *Ann. Otol.* (*St Louis*) **86**, 251.

Romanes, G. J. (1972). *Cunningham's Textbook of anatomy* (11th edn). Oxford University Press.

——. (1978). *Cunningham's manuals of practical anatomy* (14th edn), Vol. 3. Oxford University Press.

Schwartz, H. G. and Weddell, G. (1938). Observations on the pathways transmitting the sensation of taste. *Brain* **61**, 99.

Shambaugh, G. E. (1967). *Surgery of the ear* (2nd edn), p. 58. Saunders, Philadelphia and London.

Sunderland, S. (1946). The effect of rupture of the perineurium on the contained nerve fibres. *Brain* **69**, 149.

——, (1968). *Nerve and nerve injuries*, Part 1, p. 35. Livingstone, Edinburgh and London.

Wiberg, A. (1971). Function of the chorda tympani before and after operation for clinical otosclerosis. *Thesis*, University of Umea.

Wright, J. W. and Taylor, C. E. (1972). Facial nerve abnormalities revealed by polytomography. *Arch. Otolaryngol.* **95**, 426.

2 Clinical features of facial nerve disorders

2 Clinical features of facial nerve disorders

THE SEVENTH cranial, or facial nerve, is probably the cranial nerve most commonly affected by disease, and its disorders are thus encountered by clinicians of many specialities.

Lesions of the facial nerve are seen in two large, anatomically separate groups. This chapter gives a broad outline of their clinical features. In the first group of disorders the nerve is involved in the facial area of the motor cortex, or in its corticobulbar tract. In the second group lesions occur in the brain-stem nucleus, or the nerve in any portion of its peripheral course. The former group are usually referred to as upper motor neurone lesions, and the latter as lower motor neurone lesions.

Very infrequently a patient with incomplete recovery from facial paralysis due to an upper motor neurone lesion is subsequently stricken by paralysis due to a lower motor neurone lesion. Obviously the permutations and combinations of such double pathology make it both complex, and extremely difficult to diagnose. These cases, however, are fortunately rare in the experience of most clinicians.

Upper motor neurone lesions

A lesion of the face area of the motor cortex, or of the corticobulbar tract, may result in paralysis or stimulation of the opposite side of the face.

Paralysis

Aetiology This condition most commonly occurs as part of a more extensive intracranial disorder, involving the motor cortex or corticobulbar tract. Cerebral haemorrhage, tumour, thrombosis, and trauma are common aetiological factors in producing complete or partial hemiplegia. In addition to these factors other diseases involving the central nervous system may produce upper motor neurone damage to the facial nerve. Some of the recent textbooks on neurology provide useful means of classification (Walton 1977; Merritt 1973; Matthews 1975; Matthews and Miller 1975).

Symptoms The initial 'shock phase', in which there appears to be a sudden depression of all the reflexes served by various areas of the nervous system, may last from a few days to a few weeks. Providing the condition of the patient improves, a lessening of the flaccidity and the appearance of spasticity follows.

The upper portion of the face is bilaterally represented in the cortex. Thus, although facial weakness is obvious on the side affected by established upper motor neurone paralysis, the forehead is quite readily mobile. The lower face may have marked weakness, or indeed no movement at all, depending on the severity of the causative pathology. There is therefore quite definite asymmetry of the face; in particular, loss of the nasolabial fold is noticeable.

The emotional responses are not affected in upper motor neurone facial paralysis, and the patient is still able to smile, cry, and show other types of emotion by facial expression. This is due to such reactions being controlled or mediated through pathways which are not pyramidal. However, it has been reported that in severe unilateral brain damage, facial paralysis can also be associated with loss of emotional expression in the conscious patient. Presumably the lesion or damage is extremely extensive in such cases.

Stimulation

Focal epilepsy and facial dyskinesia are two examples of upper motor neurone lesions which produce stimulation effects on the face. They are discussed in Chapters 3 (p. 105) and 4 (p. 126) together with the other types of abnormal facial movements which occur. Stimulation effects can be produced by irritative lesions, or by lesions which paralyse inhibitory mechanisms.

Lower motor neurone lesions

Lower motor neurone lesions may produce paralysis or stimulation of the same side of the face; occasionally both sides may be affected. They are the commonest cause of facial paralysis.

Paralysis

Motor symptoms Lower motor neurone lesions usually affect the whole of one side of the face (Fig. 2.1). The upper part is as much involved as the lower, unlike the upper motor neurone type of paralysis. The extent of facial involvement depends on the amount of nerve damage. Facial asymmetry is apparent, the nasolabial folds disappear, forehead creases are smoothed, and, depending on the severity, the patient may be unable to close his eye properly. In addition the corner of the mouth droops, and no muscle function is apparent in the face, unless the lesion is partial. Attempts at frowning, smiling, or laughing accentuate the degree of muscle paralysis. Occasionally the protruded tongue may appear to deviate to one side, making the clinician

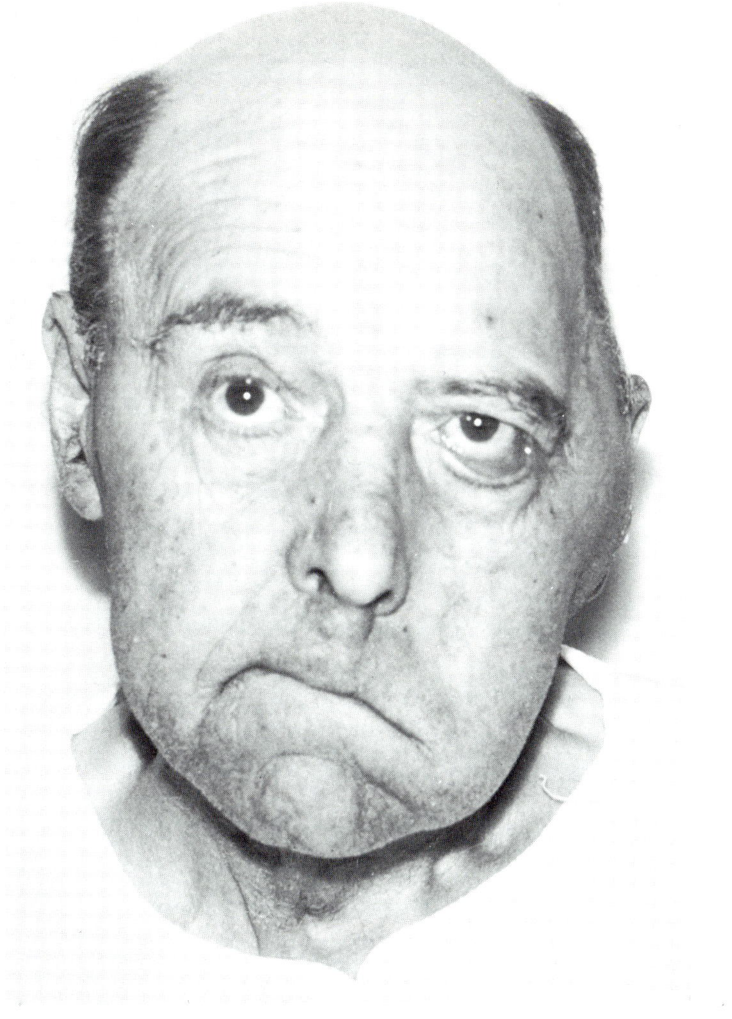

Fig. 2.1. Complete lower motor neurone facial paralysis caused by a middle ear tumour.

suspect an associated hypoglossal nerve involvement. However, the tongue distortion is due to the unilateral mouth weakness, and not to any hypoglossal dysfunction. These patients cannot whistle, or even attempt to do so. (It is wise to remember, however, that not all patients are able to whistle even with intact facial muscles.)

If the patient has a bilateral facial paralysis, then there will be immobility rather than asymmetry of the face. Such patients can escape detection for some time. The Guillain–Barré syndrome, nuclear agenesis, and other possible causes of bilateral paralysis are discussed in Chapter 3.

Bell's phenomenon Probably the best-known facial sign in paralytic conditions is 'Bell's phenomenon', named after the late Sir Charles Bell, who described it in 1829. This sign can be elicited in any type of facial paralysis, provided the nerve supply to the orbicularis oculi muscle has been affected (Fig. 2.2). Bell was apparently the first to document this sign in a patient who had suffered a traumatic facial paralysis, probably resulting from an injury to the nerve as it emerged from the stylomastoid foramen. He noticed that the

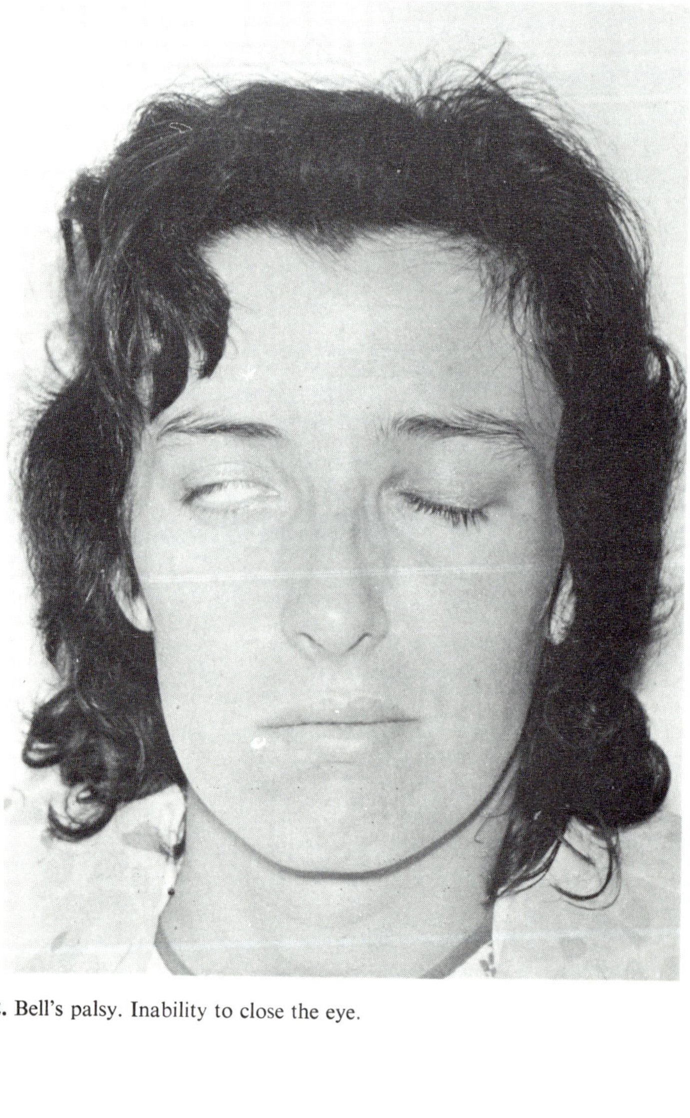

Fig. 2.2. Bell's palsy. Inability to close the eye.

patient could not close the affected eye when requested. The attempt to do so resulted in an upward rolling of the eyeball itself. The eyeball was also turned up in sleep. Upward movement of the eyeball occurs in normal patients when they close their eyes, but it is apparent only in patients with facial paralysis, who cannot close their eyes. The eyeball movement itself is not associated with the seventh nerve damage.

Bell's phenomenon is not always present in paralytic conditions, however, and Fig. 2.3 shows a patient with a very obvious lower motor neurone

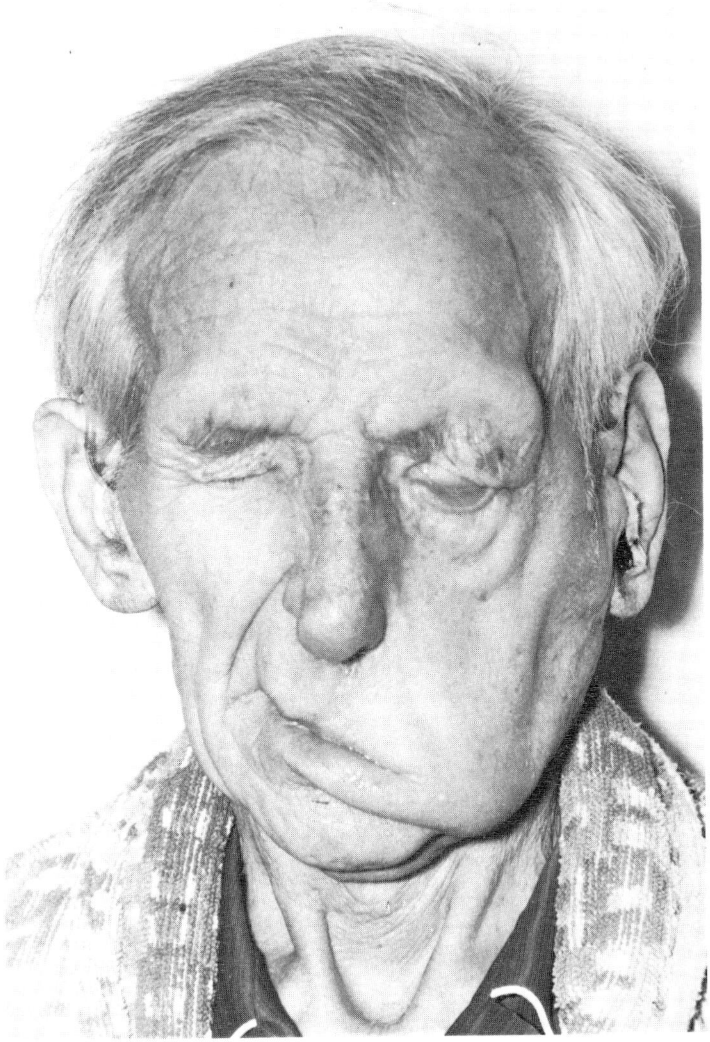

Fig. 2.3. This patient has facial paralysis, but is able to cover the cornea.

paralysis, who was nevertheless able to close his eye. This could be due to the fact that some upper lid movement is innervated via the third nerve, or there could be a partial degree of bilateral representation.

Feeding A complete facial paralysis causes considerable difficulty with eating and drinking. Food tends to collect between teeth or dentures and the cheek and there is overspilling of fluid and food out of the side of the mouth during meals.

Negro's sign This is sometimes seen in lower motor neurone paralysis. When the patient looks upward, the eyball on the paralysed side goes up higher than on the normal side. It is suggested that the sign is caused by excessive contraction of the ocular and palpebral levators to compensate for the defective contractility of the frontalis muscle.

Dupuy–Dutemps sign The patient is first asked to look downwards. Usually he can follow this instruction and both eyelids and eyeballs move down. The patient is then told to close his eyes tightly. The eye on the normal side remains closed, whereas that on the paralysed side shows a gradual upward lift of the eyelid to expose the eyeball.

These clinical features are seen when the orbicularis oculi muscle is involved.

Sensory symptoms The facial nerve is said to have some somatic sensory function, although there is not total agreement about this. It is reputed to carry proprioceptive impulses from the facial muscles, and cutaneous sensation from a small strip of skin on the postero-medical surface of the pinna and from around the entrance of the external auditory canal. However, it is seldom possible to detect any sensory loss in patients with lesions of the facial nerve.

Undoubtedly many patients complain of stiffness in the affected side of the face, but they rarely complain of pain. Transient facial weakness in migraine can be associated with a sensation of 'pins and needles', and, in herpes zoster lesions pain occurs in the external canal area, and less commonly behind the ear.

Taste The seventh nerve conveys the taste fibres of the chorda tympani nerve from the anterior two-thirds of the tongue. Any damage occurring to the facial nerve above the level of the chorda tympani branch will result in partial or complete loss of taste in this area of the tongue. Damage to the chorda tympani nerve itself, as in permeatal myringoplasty, or stapedectomy, can of course produce loss of taste without involving any motor components of the facial nerve.

Patients are able to localize very accurately the area of the tongue from which taste has been lost. They may find this a persistent and obtrusive symptom, especially if permanent damage has occurred. According to May *et al.* (1975) taste symptoms may precede the onset of facial paralysis in some patients. The lesion in multiple sclerosis often produces severe facial paralysis, but spares the sense of taste (Oppenheim 1911).

Reflex symptoms In addition to motor and sensory symptoms, certain reflex deficiencies can be associated with lower motor neurone facial paralysis.

Hyperacusis or phonophobia Paralysis of the stapedius muscle in the middle ear results in a loss of the protective mechanism against unduly loud noises. The symptom of hearing excessively loud noises is called hyperacusis or phonophobia. When present, this complaint is a reasonable indication of stapedial muscle paralysis and will help to localize the level of the seventh nerve damage. It is important to remember that hyperacusis can also occur in patients who have a recruiting sensori-neural deafness. Tests to investigate middle ear reflexes are discussed in Chapter 6.
The blink reflex This can be stimulated in normal people in a variety of ways. The reflex may be absent or delayed in patients with facial paralysis involving the orbicularis oculi muscle.

Bergara–Wartenburg sign If a normal person is asked to close his eyes tightly, the orbicularis oculi can be felt vibrating when the upper lid is pressed lightly with one finger. This effect disappears at a very early stage in cases of facial paralysis, and this reflex deficiency is therefore an early indication of the possible spread of paralysis to the eye region.

Associated conditions

Headache This is a symptom most commonly found in those patients who have facial nerve lesions associated with chronic ear disease. Usually it indicates the start of intracranial complications caused by spread of the infection. Neoplasms of the middle ear can give rise to headaches at the stage at which dural involvement occurs (Fig. 2.4). Headache can also be present in some intracranial tumours which involve the seventh nerve. The pain is apparently due to initial dilation of pain-sensitive structures such as the meninges, venous sinuses, and major arteries. It varies from comparatively mild to extremely severe and incapacitating episodes of pain.

In posterior fossa tumours, such as acoustic neuromas, metastatic lesions, meningiomas, or cerebellar neoplasms, the headache is usually occipital in the early stages. For many patients the position of the pain in the head usually overlies the pathology. The long-standing belief that headache is necessarily associated with increased intracranial pressure in the early stages is now known to be false.

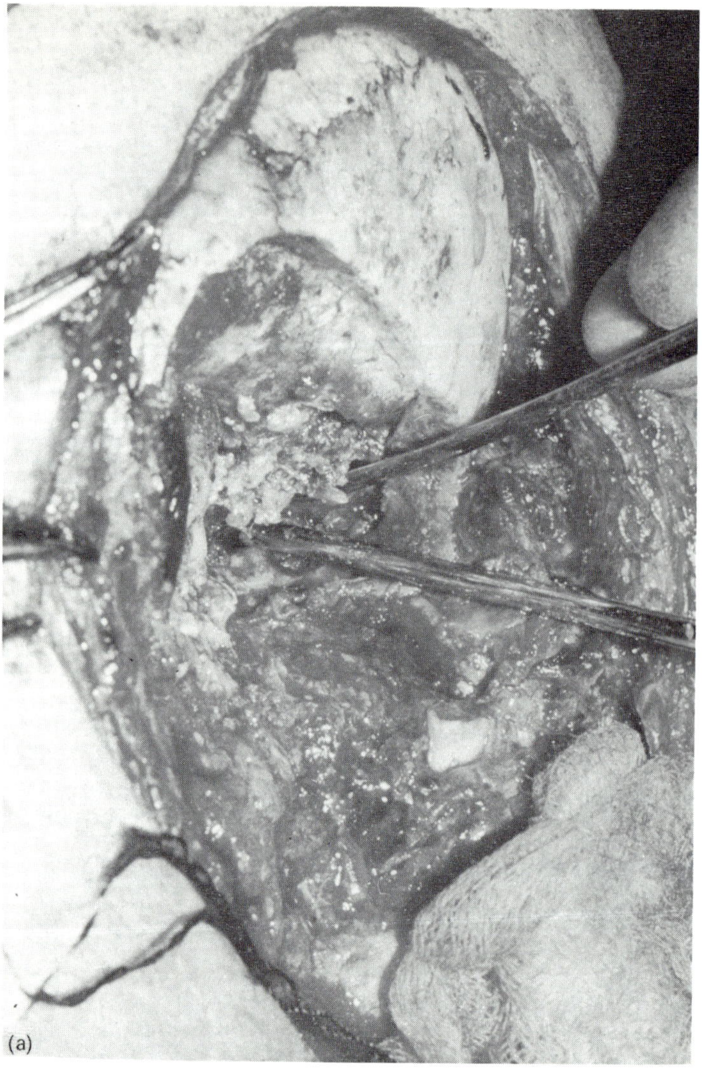

Fig. 2.4. (a) Dural involvement by squamous carcinoma from the middle ear. (b) Repair of dura after excision of the neoplasm.

Migraine This type of headache can be associated with various transient neurological lesions. These vary from hemiplegia to individual arm, leg, or face lesions. The latter may be a motor paralysis, usually unilateral and often associated with a feeling of facial 'pins and needles'. This is well discussed by Pearce (1975). Prodromal symptoms, visual or other, may well be present. The headache is often extremely severe, and can be associated with nausea and vomiting.

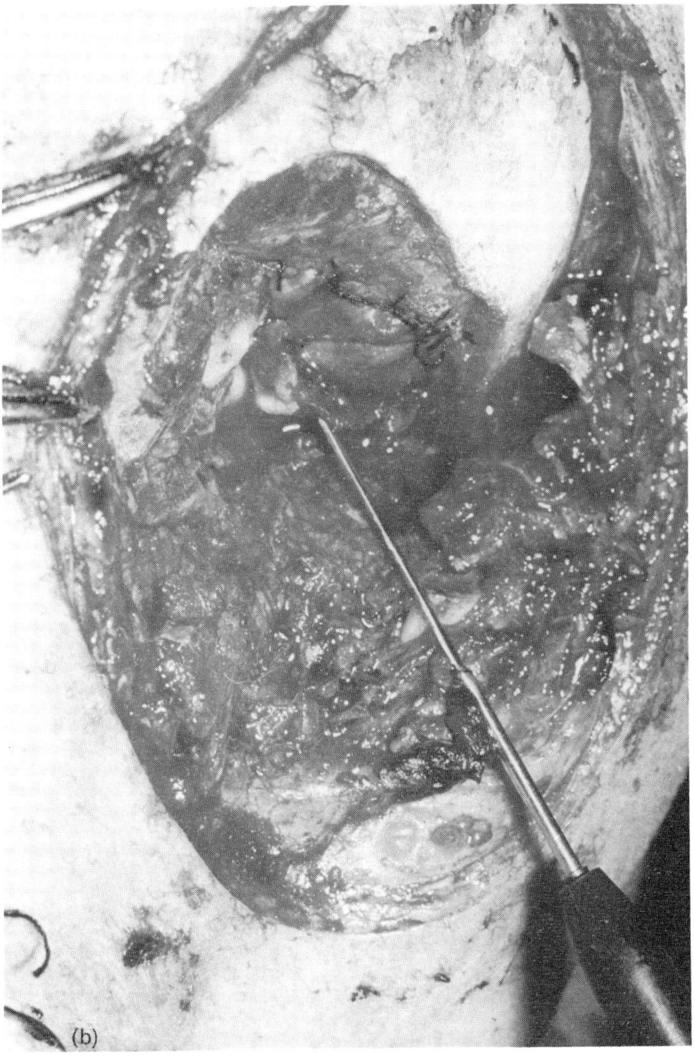

Fig. 2.4. (continued)

Virus infections Severe preliminary headache is sometimes noticed by patients with herpes zoster oticus. Just how many patients with virus involvement of the central nervous system show clinical evidence of infection is not known. However, the clinical features when they are present vary from headache and malaise to facial palsy, meningitis, and encephalitis. It is not uncommon for patients with idiopathic lower motor neurone facial paralysis to complain of a preliminary headache and some general malaise.

Infection with arboviruses may cause transient lesions of cranial nerves, including the seventh nerve. These lesions occur after the initial phase of the illness, in which there is a febrile upset with tender glands, occasional gastrointestinal symptoms, and headache. Careful virology studies are required when these symptoms occur, and for details the reader is recommended to read the excellent chapter in Webb (1975).

In these days of rapid intercontinental travel, the possibility of transmissible diseases of a virus nature from abroad should not be forgotten. It must be borne in mind that such infections may also produce the mild headache and lower motor neurone cranial nerve involvement. A concise and up-to-date book on virology of the nervous system is edited by Illis (1975).

Facial asymmetry In congenital facial paralysis, there may be an associated lack of growth of the damaged side of the face. It must be remembered that in progressive facial hemiatrophy the appearances at rest are similar, but facial movements are normal since there is no damage to the facial nerve.

Pinna deformity The most common types of ear deformity are usually associated with deafness, either conductive or sensori-neural. The Treacher–Collins deformity (Collins 1900) is probably the syndrome most familiar to clinicians. Deafness with bilateral or unilateral facial paralysis is also well documented, first by Michel (1863). In addition to various forms of malformations of the inner and middle ears, there are also reports of varying involvement of the external ear and seventh nerve. Other parts of the body may also be damaged. Iatrogenesis, especially with thalidomide, should be remembered when investigating such patients (Krucke *et al.* 1971; Scheibe 1892).

It is fortunate that among all these patients, involvement of the external ear with seventh nerve paralysis is rare. Destructive diseases involving the pinna and the facial nerve are rarely seen in this country. Neoplasms are the most common; and, rarely, granulomas are also seen. Destructive diseases such as leprosy, and the noma following measles, occur more commonly in tropical countries (Martinson 1975; Yassin *et al.* 1975).

Palatal lesions In lower motor neurone facial paralysis, palatal function is not affected. However, painful ulcers may appear in patients with the Ramsay Hunt syndrome. They appear simultaneously with the vesicles on the pinna, and can be seen just above the tonsillar area (Fig. 2.5). Both ear and palate are involved on the same side.

Vertigo Among the numerous features associated with lower motor neurone seventh nerve paralysis, vertigo is most important. It may be elicited as a symptom only by questioning the patient closely. Other symptoms, such as

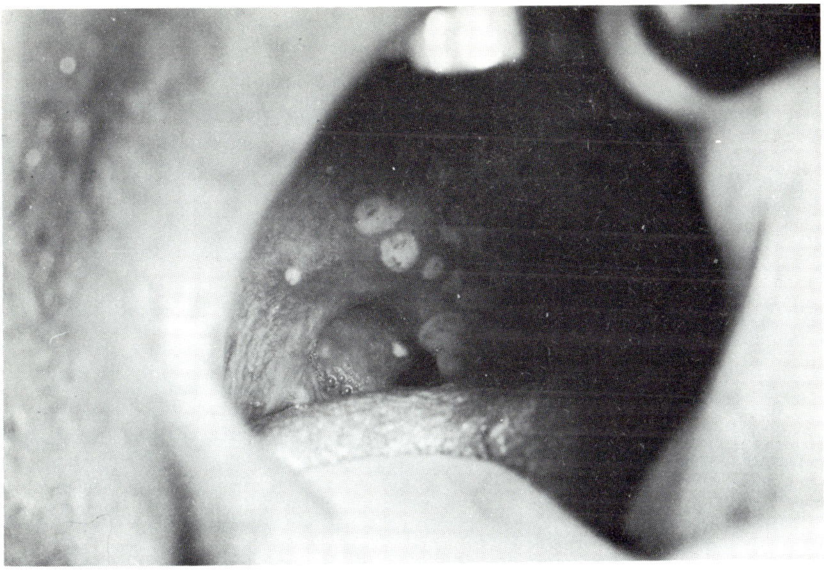

Fig. 2.5. Herpes of soft palate in Ramsay Hunt syndrome.

facial paralysis, take precedence in his mind. Occasionally it is only when spontaneous nystagmus is noted that patients will admit to vertigo (or perhaps only 'dizziness') and sometimes nausea.

Vertigo may well be manifest in cases where facial paralysis is associated with middle ear disease. Tumours in the internal auditory meatus or cerebellopontine angle can involve both seventh and eighth nerves. Facial paralysis with vertigo requires full neuro-otological investigation (Chapter 6). Vertigo is often experienced by patients with herpes zoster lesions involving the facial nerve.

The vertigo is usually rotational, and occasionally positional, the latter especially in cases of acoustic neuroma. In multiple sclerosis facial paralysis and vertigo may occur together. This probably indicates a plaque in the floor of the fourth ventricle. Occasionally, the sixth nerve will be involved, being in such close proximity. Bladder symptoms of retention with lower motor neurone lesions as mentioned above should indicate multiple sclerosis as a possible diagnosis.

Staggering, or actual drop attacks, preceded by momentary rotational sensations can occur with lesions in the cerebellopontine angle. Typical cerebellar signs, including spontaneous nystagmus, usually indicate a large tumour if the seventh nerve is also involved. Loss of the corneal reflex, and changes of sensation in the face will be present if there is damage to the fifth nerve. Vestibular symptoms have been described in patients with Bell's paralysis (Rauchbach *et al.* 1975).

Multiple sclerosis This disease is associated with seventh nerve paralysis. In such an unpredictable disease, mainifestations of many conditions may be seen in patients, either together, or separately. As mentioned previously, Oppenheim (1911) believed that a lower motor neurone facial paralysis could pre-date the other symptoms of multiple sclerosis. He also described the distinctive clinical features which distinguish this particular type of seventh nerve involvement.

(a) Depending on the exact site of the lesion in the brain-stem, there may be sixth nerve paralysis.
(b) The sense of taste is spared in the majority of cases.
(c) Rapid recovery with no residual neurological deficit is the general outcome.
(d) Vertigo, commonly rotational, may also occur. It usually resolves spontaneously.

In one series 5 per cent of multiple sclerosis patients presented with a lower motor neurone seventh nerve paralysis (Müller 1949).

Similar types of facial paralysis can occur in established cases of multiple sclerosis. A full discussion of the varied clinical features of multiple sclerosis, including facial paralysis, is given in McAlpine *et al.* (1975). These authors also discuss genetic factors.

Pregnancy It has not been our experience that facial paralysis is more common during pregnancy (see also Faris 1955). We have, of course, seen facial paralysis during a pregnancy, but there is no reason why such patients should be any more or less susceptible than the rest of the female population of a similar age group. However, more recent statistical work by Robinson and Pou (1972) has suggested that there may well be a connection. The association between pregnancy and deafness is discussed by Story (1958).

Sixth nerve paralysis This can be found in association with lower motor neurone facial paralysis. Congenital facial nerve lesions are sometimes seen with involvement of the sixth cranial nerve, for example in the Moebius syndrome. Fig. 1.1 shows that the facial nerve and sixth nerve nuclei are in close proximity in the brain-stem. Pathology in this region may well involve either or both nerves.

Corneal damage A patient with paralysis of the orbicularis oculi is unable to blink properly. This inability to move the lids and close the eye leaves the cornea unprotected. Dust and other foreign bodies gain easy access and may produce severe and permanent damage (Fig. 2.6).

Lacrimation Much of the excessive watering of the involved eye in lower motor neurone paralysis is due to a mechanical failure of the tear duct.

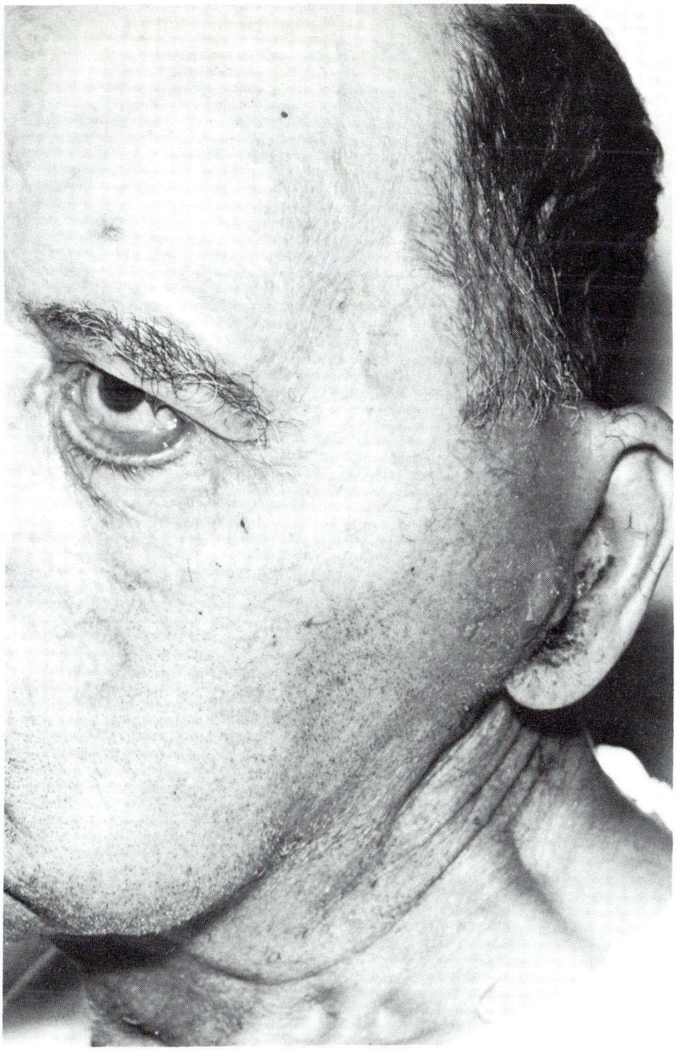

Fig. 2.6. Sagging of lower lid.

Sagging of the lower lid means that the punctum is unable to accept and drain the usual lacrimation. Tests to measure lacrimation will be discussed in Chapter 6.

Regeneration changes Many patients recover completely from facial paralysis with no residual after-effects. However, some patients show evidence of

changes which have taken place during the regeneration of the seventh nerve.
1. *Synkinesis.* This syndrome has been observed by many authors. It can be seen in some patients who appear to have recovered completely after suffering a lower motor neurone facial paralysis. If the patient is asked to blink his eyes rapidly, small contractions of the orbicularis oris on the previously damaged side will occur. Conversely, contraction of the orbicularis oris can produce movements of the orbicularis oculi. These areas appear to have been incorrectly re-innervated. More simply, nerves have extended from their own field of activity and provided function to other parts of the face as well. Such uncontrollable movements can be embarrassing to patients. Treatment will be discussed in Chapter 7.
2. *Crocodile tears* The unusual name was coined by a comment attributed to Pliny, who is reputed to have said that crocodiles produced tears when eating their prey. It is a condition which may occur a considerable time after complete recovery from facial paralysis. The previously damaged side is always the one subsequently affected. As the name implies, tears appear for the wrong reason (Chorobsky 1951). Quite suddenly, for example during a meal, the patients experience a profuse and uncontrollable secretion of tears. Although not very common, the condition is extremely distressing to the patient. The mechanism is obscure, but the condition is thought to result from the erroneous re-routing of parasympathetic fibres, intended for the salivary glands. At present accurate knowledge of the pathology is lacking. Results of operative attempts at cure by tympanic neurectomy are not always successful, confirming doubts about the aetiology.
3. *Gustatory sweating: Frey's syndrome* This was first described by Frey (1923) and was subsequently discussed by Spiro and Martin (1967). In both cases this symptom presented following wounds to the parotid gland. In Frey's syndrome eating or drinking results in sweating on the affected side of the face (Fig. 2.7). Usually it follows parotid surgery, but injury to the facial nerve in other forms of surgery or trauma may also produce the symptoms. The onset can vary from several months to a year or more after the trauma. In many patients, the condition appears to subside quite spontaneously.

Rauch (1959) recommends that when the facial nerve is dissected the fine autonomic filaments should be preserved as a prophylaxis against development of this syndrome. Laage-Hellman (1958) has written an authoritative article on the subject. He maintains that the aetiology is the misdirection, after injury, of severed salivary nerve fibres. He describes this as a regular sequel to parotidectomy, but many surgeons would not agree. His series of 57 adult patients did show a latent period of about 5 weeks before developing symptoms, thus allowing time for the re-growing fibres to reach the skin.

It is now accepted that gustatory sweating will always occur where the nerves which carry secretory and vasodilator impulses are injured. These include the greater auricular, lesser occipital, or indeed any branch of the

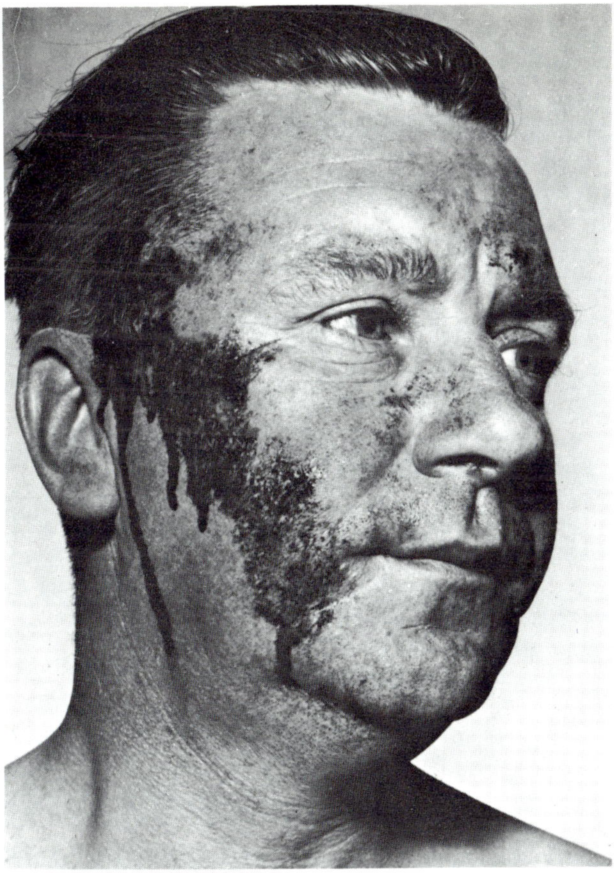

Fig. 2.7. Gustatory sweating. From Spillane (1975). By courtesy of the author and publisher.

cervical plexus. The following features are reasonably constant in this syndrome.

1. Post-ganglionic parasympathetic fibres to the large salivary glands are always involved.
2. There appears to be a latent period before the symptoms appear (Laage-Hellman 1958).
3. A cervical sympathetic block is ineffective.
4. The affected skin will react to the injection of acetylcholine locally.

We agree with Spiro and Martin, and other surgeons, that it is a rare syndrome, and usually subsides spontaneously. Their article is of great interest. Fortunately, we have never seen any patient who had to be submitted to surgery for relief of gustatory sweating.

4. *Contracture* Following incomplete recovery from a lower motor neurone paralysis, the affected side of the face may show a drawn appearance. There is still some argument as to the precise pathology involved in these cases. Gradual shortening of the muscle fibres was shown by Spiller (1919). Other workers have found that this could be associated with low-frequency activity of motor units (Taverner 1955). Bratslavsky and Eecken (1978) suggest that associated movements and contracture are partly due to changes in the motor nucleus, i.e. enhanced excitability of facial motor neurones. In long-standing cases some muscle fibrosis must inevitably add to the clinical picture.

Stimulation

Facial tic This is sometimes called a habit spasm. This affliction is much more variable than in any other condition involving the seventh nerve. It very commonly affects the outer canthus area, but can include the whole of one side of the face. Often the tic is increased by emotion. Some tics may disappear when some form of distraction is provided. Movements of the neck may also be apparent in some cases. In children, the tics usually disappear spontaneously as the patient matures, and treatment is seldom effective. Adults tend to be even more resistant to suggestion or other types of therapy.

Hemifacial spasm This alarming condition may involve part or the whole of one side of the face. It is possible to classify the patients into groups.

1. *Irritative lesions along the peripheral nerve* Tumours in the pontine angle, such as acoustic neuromas or congenital temporal bone cholesteatomas, serve as examples. Very often the earliest indication of these lesions is involvement of the seventh nerve, either in the angle, or in the bone itself. Spasm of the corresponding side of the face is the presenting symptom. Facial spasm is discussed in Chapter 4.

2. *Clonic facial spasm* (*tic convulsif*) This uncommon disorder was first described by Gowers (1888). It appears to be limited to adult patients, and is more common in women. The patient has intermittent attacks of clonic twitching. Initially the spasm occurs around the eye, and then it spreads, to a varying extent in each patient. As mentioned, clonic facial spasm is said occasionally to affect patients who have recovered from a facial paralysis of lower motor neurone type.

3 *Post-traumatic* The authors have seen some patients in whom an intermittent hemifacial spasm has followed trauma. One patient had recurrent spasm affecting the outer aspect of one eye following an accident which fractured the malar bone on the same side. Treatment is discussed in Chapter 7.

Trigeminal neuralgia Trigeminal neuralgia has been reported in association with both clonic facial spasm and post-traumatic spasm. It need not necessarily occur on the same side as the facial nerve involvement, and the aetiology is obscure. Kumagumi (1974) discusses a possible reason for the connection between trigeminal neuralgia and hemifacial spasm.

The genetics of facial nerve lesions

Patients often ask whether their condition is hereditary but, with the exception of a few well known conditions, we cannot yet answer this question (see Rosek 1976). History-taking in patients with facial nerve lesions should include questions as to whether the patient's symptoms have ever occurred in other members of his family, as diagnosis and subsequent prognosis can be substantially influenced by the known genetic factors of certain conditions.

Bell's palsy An excellent attempt to produce some significant genetic correlation in the occurrence of this condition has been reported by Alter (1963). He studied 105 patients with presumed Bell's palsy, and found that 30 of their relatives had also had the same disease at some time. In a group of 105 control patients, only 4 relatives had been previously affected. This is one of the few controlled series we can find. Alter stated that the rate of occurrence of Bell's palsy in first-degree relatives of affected patients was 3 per cent. He hypothesized a dominant inheritance with reduced manifestation for this condition. More recent work is by Willbrand *et al.* (1974). This is discussed in Chapter 4.

Melkersson's syndrome This disease is most common in the Scandinavian countries and is reputed to be inherited. It has been described (Scott 1964) as a dominant over two generations. The syndrome is rarely encountered in Great Britain.

Congenital facial paralysis This had been described as a dominant gene in 40 people over six generations (Rosin 1963). This author also reported an occasional bilateral incidence in 46 persons over six generations. Further discussions are by Thomas (1898) and Van der Wiel (1957).

Congenital facial diplegia with other cranial nerve palsies (the Moebius syndrome) is not generally thought to be genetically determined. One author, however, found it a dominant factor over two generations (Scott 1964).

Hemifacial spasm Genetic factors here are less well documented. Hellsing (1930) described the occurrence of hemifacial spasm in six members of a family. There appeared to be a dominant transmission over four generations.

However, some of these patients apparently showed evidence of other neurological deficits, especially alterations in tendon and muscle reflexes. The presence of similar abnormalities in family members who were unaffected by spasm has meant there is now some loss of credence in this genetic study. Apart from this curious group, most examples of hemifacial spasm appear to be quite isolated.

Multiple neurofibromatosis The genetic study of this disease is beyond the scope of this book. Readers are referred to the studies by Cockayne (1933), Borberg (1951), and Crowe *et al.* (1956). There is a summary in the book by Pratt (1968).

Discussion

We hope that our description of the clinical features of facial nerve disorders illustrates that not all lesions which affect the facial nerve need be paralytic; spasms and tics may be equally distressing symptoms.

We are all vain to some extent, and damage to the function of the face is therefore distressing to us. When there is loss of ability to speak clearly a patient's employment may be jeopardized also. Some patients adapt to the disabling clinical features without much anxiety. They accept reassurance, and pursue their daily tasks. Others remain extremely worried until some signs of recovery appear. There is no particular group who can be assessed as either good, or difficult patients. Young, middle-aged, or old, they will all react differently to their affliction.

Many patients are considerably handicapped not only by their facial condition, but also by the basic pathology with which it is associated. Partial facial afflictions are obviously easier to manage, but partial loss does not necessarily indicate better prognosis of full recovery, or of non-recurrence. This applies to both paralytic and stimulation afflictions.

It is the duty of the doctor to try to minimize the effects of facial afflictions, and provide encouragement. An increased awareness amongst general practitioners of the possible advantages to be gained from early hospital referral for diagnostic purposes is now, in this country at least, well established. Curiously enough, the delay is very often on the part of the patient before seeking advice.

Depending on the site and nature of the causative pathology, all or some of the clinical features described in this chapter will be manifest. The differential diagnosis in these conditions has to be made between pathology due to a cortical or tract lesion, and that from damage to the nucleus or the actual peripheral nerve. Should only a mild degree of weakness exist, then it may not be possible always to arrive at a satisfactory answer.

References

Alter, M. (1963). Familial aggregation of Bell's palsy. *Arch. Neurol.* (*Chic*). **8**, 557.

Bell, C. (1829). On the nerves of the face. *Phil. Trans. roy. Soc. Lond.*, Part 2, 317.

Borberg, A. (1951). Clinical and genetic investigations into tuberous sclerosis and Recklinghausen's neuro-fibromatosis. *Acta Psychiat.* (*Scand.*) *Suppl.* **71**, 1–239.

Bratslavsky, M. and Eecken, H. van (1978). Altered synaptic organization in facial nucleus following facial nerve regeneration. An electrophysiological study in man. *Ann. Neurol.* **2**, 71.

Chorobski, J. (1951). The syndrome of crocodile tears. *Arch. Neurol. Psychiat.* (*Chic.*) **65**, 299.

Cockayne, E. A. (1933). *Inherited abnormalities of the skin and its appendages.* Oxford University Press, New York.

Collins, E. (1900) Case with symmetrical notches in the outer part of each lower lid and defective development of the malar bones. *Trans. Ophthalm. Soc. U.K.* **20**, 90.

Critchley, M., O'Leary, J. L. and Jennet, B. (1972). *Scientific foundations of neurology.* Heinemann, London.

Crowe, F. W., Schule, W. J., and Neel, J. V. (1956). *A clinical, pathological and genetic study of multiple neurofibromatosis.* Charles Thomas, Springfield, Ill.

Faris, B. D. (1955). Facial paralysis during pregnancy. *Med. Times* (*N.Y.*) **83**, 185.

Frey, L. (1923). Le syndrome du N. auriculo-temporal. *Rev. Neurol.* **39**, 97.

Gowers, W. R. (1888). *A manual of diseases of the nervous system.* Blakiston, Philadelphia.

Hellsing, G. (1930). Hereditärer Facialiskrampf. *Acta Med.* (*Scand.*) **73**, 526.

Illis, L. S., ed. (1975). *Viral diseases of the nervous system.* Baillière Tindall, London.

Krucke, W., von Hartrott, H. H., and Schröder, J. M. (1971) Licht und electronmikroskopische Untersuchungen züm Spatstadium der Thalidomid-polyneuropathy, *Fortschr. Neurol. Psychiat.* **39**, 17.

Kumagumi, H. (1974). Neuropathic findings of hemi-facial spasm and trigeminal neuralgia. *Arch. Otolaryngol.* **99**, 160.

Laage-Hellman, J. E. (1958). Gustatory sweating and flushing, aetiological implications of latent period, and mode of development after parotidectomy. *Acta oto-laryngol.* (Stockh.) **49**, 306.

Lenz, W. (1962). Thalidomide and congenital abnormalities. *Lancet* **i**, 45.

Martinson, F. S. (1975). Measles: oto-laryngological complications of in West Africa. *J. Laryng.* **89**, 631.

Matthews, W. B. (1975). *Recent advances in clinical neurology.* Churchill Livingstone, Edinburgh.

—— and Miller, H. G. (1975). *Diseases of the nervous system*, 2nd edn. Blackwell Scientific Publications, Oxford.

May, M., Wetts, R., Hardin, W. B., and Sullivan, J. (1975). The chorda tympani and Bell's palsy. *Laryngoscope* **85**, 1957.

McAlpine, D., Lumsden, C. E., and Acheson, E. S. (1975). *Multiple sclerosis. A re-appraisal.* Churchill Livingstone, Edinburgh.

Merritt, H. H., ed. (1973). *A textbook of neurology.* Lea and Febiger, Philadelphia.

Michel, E. M. (1863). Memoire sur les anomolies congénitales de l'oreille interne. *Gaz. Med. Strasburg.*

Müller, R. (1949). Studies in disseminated sclerosis. *Acta Med.* (*Scand.*), *Suppl.* **222**.

Oppenheim, H. (1911). *Textbook of nervous diseases for physicians and students.* (trans. A. Bruce); 5th edn. Vol. I, Foulis, London.

Pearce, J. (1975). *Modern topics in migraine.* Heinemann, London.

Pratt, R. T. C. (1968). *The genetics of neurological disorders.* Oxford University Press, London.

Rauch, S. (1959). Das Salivo-idostpare syndrome. *Z. Leprosy U.S.W.* **38**, 259.

Rauchbach, E., May, M., and Stroud, M. H. (1975). Vestibular involvement in Bell's palsy. *Laryngoscope* **88**, 1396.

Robinson, J. R. and Pou, J. W. (1972). Bell's palsy. A predisposition of pregnant women. *Arch. Otolaryng.* **95**, 125.

Rosek, M. (1976). *Medical genetics. Medical diagnosis and treatment.* Longe, Calif.

Rosin, V. S. (1963). Hereditary facial paralysis (in Russian), *Z.R. Nevropat. Psikhiat.* **63**, 1320.

Scheibe, A. (1892). A case of deaf–mutism with auditory atrophy and anomalies of development in the membranous labyrinth of both ears. *Arch. Otolaryng.* **21**, 12.

Scott, G. A. (1964). Melkersson's syndrome. *Brit. J. Clin. Pract.* **18**, 415.

Spillane, J. D. (1975). *An atlas of clinical neurology*, 2nd edn. Oxford University Press.

Spiller, W. G. (1919). Contracture occurring in partial recovery from paralysis of the facial nerve and other nerves. *Arch. Neurol. Psychiat.* (*Chic.*) **1**, 564.

Spiro, R. H., and Martin, H. (1967). Gustatory sweating following parotid surgery and neck dissection. *Ann. Surg.* **165**, 118.

Story, S. R. (1958). Conductive deafness, seventh nerve paralysis, and absence of vestibular response during pregnancy. *Arch. Otolaryng.* **68**, 632.

Taverner, D. L. (1955). Bell's palsy. *Brain* **78**, 209.

Thomas, H. M. (1898). Congenital facial paralysis. *J. Nerv. Ment. Dis.* **25**, 571.

Van Der Weil, H. J. (1957). Hereditary congenital facia lparalysis. *Acta Genet.* (*Basel*) **7**, 348.

Walton, J. N. (1977). *Brain's diseases of the nervous system.* 8th edn. Oxford University Press.

Webb, H. E. (1975). The arbovirus encephalitides. In: *Viral diseases of the nervous system.* (ed. L. S. Illis). Baillière Tindall, London.

Willbrand, J. W., Blumhagen, J. S., and May, M. (1974). Inherited Bell's palsy. *Ann. Otolaryyng.* (*St. Louis*) **83**, 343.

Yassin, A., El-Shennawy, M., El-Eamy, G., Wassef, N. *et al.* (1975). Leprosy of the upper respiratory tract. *J. Laryng.* **89**, 505.

3 Disorders that affect the facial nerve and are of known aetiology

3 Disorders that affect the facial nerve and are of known aetiology

'Classification is Ariadne's clue through the labyrinth of nature'.
(George Sand)

Introduction

WE HAVE taken the unusual course of classifying disorders involving the facial nerve into two principal groups, namely those of known aetiology and those of unknown aetiology, reserving a separate chapter for facial nerve trauma. The reader will be able to think of other classifications which would be at least equally good, but we hope that a careful study of what is known will help our understanding of what is unknown, and that from established causes we may find clues to causes which remain mysterious. We trust that by holding firmly to the thread of knowledge, we will not become lost in a maze of fruitless speculation.

This does not mean that everything is known about the aetiology of the disorders that are described in this chapter. Rather it is intended to group together here those diseases whose basic pathology is fairly well understood, and in which a facial nerve disorder is a well recognized feature. A great deal remains to be discovered about the inadequate supply of insulin in diabetes, for example, and the mechanism of diabetic neuropathy is not fully understood. Nonetheless, facial paralysis in diabetic neuropathy is a well known occurrence and is, therefore, described in this chapter.

Congenital facial paralysis

The Moebius syndrome

The unusual syndrome of congenital bilateral facial paralysis with loss of lateral movement of the eyes was first described in the late nineteenth century (von Graefe 1880; Harlan 1881; Chisholm 1882). Moebius (1888, 1892) compared his own cases of congenital facial paralysis with those reported by von Graefe and Chisholm and suggested that congenital bilateral abducens/facial paralysis might be an independent pathological entity due to nuclear degeneration. The syndrome has been described under several titles, namely congenital paralysis of sixth and seventh nerves, congenital facial diplegia, and oculofacial paralysis, but now it is most frequently called the Moebius syndrome.

As early as 1898, Thomas described congenital facial paralysis in two brothers who also had congenital deafness and malformation of the ears. It is of great interest that over 60 years later Miehlke (1965) reported thalidomide-damaged children with bilateral severe aural malformations and bilateral facial and abducens paralysis.

Clinical features Congenital facial paralysis is a constant feature and the paralysis is usually bilateral and complete. Sometimes the lower part of the face is spared and the paralysis is occasionally unilateral. There is an inability to abduct the eyes beyond the mid-point but vertical movements of the eyes are normal. It is well recognized that other deformities of the head, trunk, and limbs may accompany the sixth and seventh nerve lesions in some patients. Partial atrophy of the tongue is common and there is often a loss of some of the muscles of mastication. Deformities seen in the trunk and limbs include defects of the pectoral muscles, syndactylism, and club foot deformities. In some cases the lacrimal glands and caruncles are absent with the result that no tears are produced when the child cries. Mental deficiency is occasionally present but the majority of the children have a normal I.Q. However, affected infants are often mistakenly thought to be retarded, because oral paralysis results in constant drooling of saliva and feeding difficulties, and the lack of facial animation gives them a dull and vacant appearance. The congenital muscular deficiency does not increase after birth and this distinguishes the Moebius syndrome from other conditions such as dystrophia myotonica in which there is progressive weakness. There may in fact be some improvement in muscle function as the child grows, through the normal development of the unaffected muscle tissue in the area.

Congenital facial paralysis is unlike acquired facial paralysis in one major feature, and that is that the face does not sag in the congenital lesion. The skin is drawn smoothly over the face and, as a rule, there are no wrinkles. The skin does not move easily over the subcutaneous tissues and there is replacement of some of the muscle tissue by connective tissue. Sometimes the lower part of the face is spared, and this contrasts with the preservation of movement of the upper part of the face which characterizes acquired upper motor neurone lesions. Since the condition is usually bilateral, the face is symmetrically involved and the deformity is not grotesque. Indeed the paralysis may not be immediately obvious. Bell's phenomenon is present in the congenital paralysis, however, and is a helpful diagnostic sign. It is difficult to improve upon Harlan's description (1881) of his 18 year old patient: 'The immobility of this man's face is very striking; it is as smooth and expressionless as if carved out of wood. The passions and emotions of 18 years have left no trace upon it, and time has altered only its size.'

Aetiology A family history of congenital facial paralysis has only occasionally been traced in the Moebius syndrome. Danis (1945) found a familial history in 5 out of 81 cases. Ford (1973) quotes the history of a family where five children (three girls and two boys) over three generations were afflicted, and it would appear from the small number of such reports that genetic factors play little part in the aetiology of this disease.

Since Moebius first described the syndrome there has been great speculation about the primary defect responsible for the condition. Moebius suggested that it was due to a degeneration of the fifth and sixth cranial nerve nuclei. The lack of morphological evidence of degeneration in unequivocal cases of the syndrome has led most authors to the view that the defect is due to primary dysplasia rather than degeneration. The main debate now centres round the question whether the dysplasia is primarily neuronal (ectodermal) or muscular (mesodermal). Rainy and Fowler (1903) considered the primary pathology to be in the muscles with secondary atrophic changes in the nucleus. There are a number of points in favour of the theory of primary mesodermal dysplasia. First, the frequent association of musculoskeletal defects such as absent pectoral muscles, syndactylism, and club-foot deformities are suggestive. Evans (1955) pointed out that the major defects all involve structures which are differentiated at the end of the second month of intrauterine life. Second, the presence of a normal facial nerve and nucleus has been demonstrated in some well-documented cases. Wallis (1960) reported marked creatinuria in two infants with the Moebius syndrome. Creatinuria, which is found in myasthenia and muscular dystrophy, suggests the presence of a myopathic disorder. In the one infant who died Wallis could find no macroscopic evidence of abnormality in the central nervous system at post mortem examination. A very detailed microscopic examination of the nervous system was carried out by Pitner *et al.* (1965) in an infant with the Moebius syndrome who died at the age of seven weeks. They found normally developed facial nuclei and nerves. The facial muscles showed a marked decrease in the number of myofibres but no changes suggestive of a neurogenic muscle atrophy. In their opinion the histological examination suggested a probable primary dysplasia of muscle.

The third point in favour of the mesodermal dysplasia theory is that some children with muscular dystrophy have presented at birth with congenital facial diplegia without abducens paralysis and have later proceeded to show the progressive nature of their myopathy (Parker 1963; Hanson and Rowland 1971). This illustrates that the facial palsy component of the Moebius syndrome at least, could have a myopathic basis.

However, the majority of undisputed and well-documented cases tend to support the theory that the syndrome is due to an aplasia or hypoplasia of the motor nuclei. Heubner (1900) recorded the pathological findings in a child with the Moebius syndrome who died at the age of 20 months. There was an absence of neurones in the left hypoglossal nucleus and a severe reduction in the number of neurones in the left facial nucleus and both abducens nuclei. The tongue was examined and was considered to show neurogenic atrophy on the left side. Henderson (1939) reviewed 61 cases of congenital facial diplegia, 43 of whom also had bilateral abducens paralysis. The pathological reports available showed nuclear hypoplasia, and the nerve roots were either absent or incompletely developed, depending on the degree of neuronal cell deficiency. Richter (1958) reported the autopsy findings on a one-month-old infant with right-sided facial paralysis and numerous other congenital anomalies involving the musculoskeletal system, heart, and urinary tract. The right facial nucleus was almost non-existent except for a few neurones in the caudal portion, which were mature and normal. Only a few fibres of the ascending limb and internal genu were present and no emergent root was identified. No evidence of degeneration, of neuroglial reaction, pigment accumulation, or perivascular infiltration was found, and Richter concluded that it was a developmental hypoplasia rather than an acquired atrophy. The electromyographic studies of Van Allen and Blodi (1960) support the view of normal muscles with defective innervation. They pointed out that no autopsy reports before 1960 had demonstrated a normal brain stem in an undisputed case of the Moebius syndrome.

Although nearly all the reports since 1960 record nuclear hypoplasia, proponents of the mesodermal theory argue that changes in the motor nuclei could be secondary to a failure of their associated muscles to develop in the first few months of embryonic life.

The interrelationships in the embryo between the developing neurone, nerve fibre, and muscle which form the adult motor unit remain obscure. Indeed the relationship between muscle and its nerve supply in the adult is not fully understood. It is of interest in this respect that McComas *et al.* (1970) suggested that muscular dystrophy itself may be a primarily neurogenic lesion with secondary changes in the muscle. In addition Bradley (1971) states that 'Hallowed concepts in muscular dystrophy are being attacked, not only by those believing it to be due to a primary disorder of the motor nerves, but also by those suggesting that it is a primary disorder of blood vessels'. In the writer's view, therefore, argument on whether the Moebius syndrome is primarily a myogenic or neurogenic lesion may turn out to be a sterile debate, which leads us no nearer to finding the cause. Until the cause is found it might be simpler to regard the lesion as a defective development of the motor unit.

There has been a tendency in recent years to apply the term Moebius syndrome to cases of congenital facial paralysis without abducens paralysis (Rubinstein *et al.* 1975; Ziter *et al.* 1977), and thereby include disorders of widely different aetiology and pathogenesis. Ziter *et al.* record an interesting family which over three generations, produced seven members with congenital facial diplegia and finger contractures. Each affected member had an identical chromosomal abnormality, namely, translocation between chromosome 1 and 13. The concurrence of the clinical and the cytogenetic abnormality suggested a direct and possibly aetiologic relationship. In all seven individuals, however, the ocular muscles were normal. There is probably an advantage to be gained by restricting the term Moebius syndrome to cases of congenital abducens/facial paralysis with or without associated defects.

Thalidomide embryopathy

The deformity of phocomelia (seal-like limbs) was described by Ballantyne (1904) and apparently has been known since Babylonian times. It was the sudden increased incidence of this known, but hitherto rare, deformity between 1958 and 1962 that led observers to search for an environmental cause, and to finally prove that the recently introduced central nervous system sedative, thalidomide, was responsible. Genetic factors appear to play no part in the development of thalidomide deformities, although some unknown constitutional factor may be responsible for the unusually high susceptibility of certain patients to the drug.

It is generally believed that the embryo is most susceptible to thalidomide damage between the 28th and 42nd day of the pregnancy (counting from the first day of the last menstrual period). Gordon (1966) has proposed an interesting theory on the mechanism of thalidomide-induced damage. He suggests that the drug acts in the embryo as a central nervous system inhibitor because it acts as a nervous system sedative in the adult. Thalidomide may prevent the initial nerve impulses reaching the muscle and thus prevent the functional junction between nerve and muscle from taking place. Deprived of effective neurotrophic stimulation, the muscles fail to develop, and according to Gordon's hypothesis, this leads to the affected part of the limb becoming resorbed.

We cannot know how often thalidomide caused foetal death, but among survivors deformities extend from the eyes down to the lower limbs. Anencephaly is not seen and normal mental development is characteristic. Facial paralysis in thalidomide embryopathy is associated with the arrested development of the ear known as microtia, and with abducens paralysis. The otitic deformity can involve the inner, middle, and external ear so that deafness and vestibular inexcitability may add to the victim's numerous disabilities. The facial paralysis is of the peripheral type and is usually unilateral. It occurs on the side of the more severely deformed ear. Bilateral facial paralysis occurs only in cases of severe bilateral otitic malformation. In a series of 21 children with thalidomide-induced otitic malformation and facial paralysis, Miehlke (1965) found 18 cases with paralysis of the abducens nerve. In his opinion, abducens paralysis is often overlooked because young children

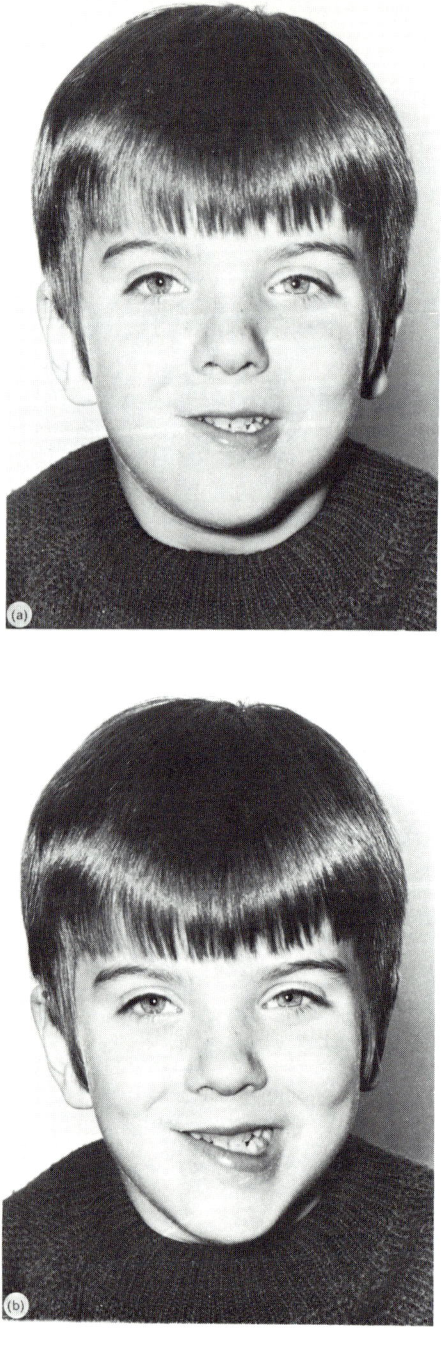
(a)
(b)

readily compensate for the deficient ocular movements by rotating the head. In Great Britain, Livingstone (1965) recorded that 5 of his 14 cases of thalidomide-induced microtia had congenital facial palsy, whereas only 4 out of his 110 cases of non-thalidomide otitic malformations had congenital facial paralysis. In Japan Takemori *et al.* (1976) reported their findings in 18 young people of 12–16 years of age who had sustained thalidomide embryopathy. Three patients had limb deformities only, while the remaining 15 suffered some degree of cochlear and vestibular loss. Of these 15 children, 11 had bilateral abducens paralysis, 7 had the crocodile-tear syndrome, 3 had bilateral facial palsy, and a further 3 had unilateral facial paralysis. The very high percentage of patients with otitic malformations in this thalidomide group is presumably the result of selection inevitable in a series of patients from an otolaryngology department.

The thalidomide disaster has shown that an external toxic agent can produce congenital facial and abducens paralysis. Since genetic factors are seldom involved in the pathogenesis of the Moebius syndrome we should, therefore, perhaps seek an environmental cause.

Marginal mandibular paralysis

Congenital unilateral partial facial paralysis confined to the lower lip depressor muscles (mentalis, depressor anguli oris, and depressor labii inferioris) has been described by a number of writers (Marino 1953; Hoefnagel and Penry 1960). These muscles are innervated by the marginal mandibular branch of the facial nerve and, in the cases described, all the other branches of the facial nerve functioned normally. The paralysis has usually been attributed to birth trauma although it occurs in children born by Caesarian section and it does not tend to recover spontaneously. In those children delivered by Caesarian section, the nerve has been believed to be damaged as it crossed the ramus of the mandible, by pressure of the shoulder due to an unfavourable 'lie' or position of the child in the womb (Fig. 3.1).

In 1967 Caylor drew attention to the association of this marginal mandibular paralysis and congenital heart disease. He found both conditions present in eight children examined during the first 12 weeks of life. Caylor commented that he had not previously seen these two lesions associated and that all the affected children were born within a 100-mile radius of his hospital during an 18-month period. This clustering of cases prompted him

---

Fig. 3.1. Right marginal mandibular paralysis
(a) Aged 7 years. Born by elective Caesarian section (maternal diabetes). Mild asymmetry of lips on gentle smiling.
(b) Note (i) failure of right lower lip to descend; and (ii) normal right nasolabial fold.

to speculate that a common environmental agent, operating during the first trimester of pregnancy, caused both the facial paralysis and the cardiac malformations.

Marginal mandibular paralysis is also described in the literature as 'asymmetric crying facies' and Pape and Pickering (1972) listed a variety of other congenital anomalies that are sometimes found in affected children. Nelson and Eng (1972) believe that the lesion is a congenital hypoplasia of the depressor anguli oris muscle rather than a nerve paralysis and this is reminiscent of the debate on the Moebius syndrome.

Viral infections

It has been known for many years that viruses can cause lower motor neurone facial paralysis, and pride of place in this respect must go to the neurotropic viruses of herpes zoster and poliomyelitis. However, it has been fully established that several other viruses cause facial paralysis, and many people speculate that the majority of cases of Bell's palsy will eventually be shown to have a viral basis.

Ramsay Hunt syndrome

(synonyms: geniculate herpes, herpes zoster oticus, and cephalic zoster)

Lower motor neurone weakness is uncommon with herpes zoster infections and since Ramsay Hunt (1907) described the post mortem findings in a patient who had herpetic vesicles around the pinna and an ipsilateral facial paralysis, this syndrome has been called by his name. Head and Campbell (1900) had demonstrated the changes which occurred in the Gasserian ganglion in ophthalmic herpes zoster. Hunt reasoned that similar changes occurred in the geniculate ganglion and accounted for both the herpetic rash around the ear and the facial paralysis. If one accepts that the geniculate ganglion is the equivalent of a dorsal root ganglion, and that peri-auricular cutaneous nerves synapse in the geniculate ganglion, then it does seem reasonable to attribute the circumaural vesicles to geniculate herpes. What is no longer accepted is the theory that a lesion in the ganglion can cause the facial palsy and the other features of the syndrome. Hunt (1915) later extended his concept of the 'sensory field of the facial nerve' and attributed herpetiform eruptions in the face and head beyond the peri-auricular region to geniculate herpes. On clinical grounds he divided his cases into three groups:

(a) those with a vesicular rash only,
(b) those with a vesicular rash and a facial palsy,
(c) those with a vesicular rash, a facial palsy, and impairment of eighth nerve function also.

Unfortunately, in the one autopsy described in Hunt's first paper, the geniculate ganglion was lost, and he did not demonstrate a histological lesion in the ganglion in any of his subsequent papers.

Aitken and Brain (1933) provided some pathological support for the viral aetiology. Using complement fixation tests, they demonstrated the presence of antibodies to herpes zoster virus in all cases in a series of nine patients with facial paralysis and a herpetiform eruption around the ear.

There have been few reports in the literature detailing the histological findings in the facial nerve in the Ramsay Hunt syndrome. Denny-Brown *et al.* (1944) rejected Hunt's theory. They showed that in the spinal form of herpes zoster, the dorsal root ganglion suffers severe inflammatory changes with pannecrosis. In their autopsy on a patient with herpes zoster oticus and facial palsy they found an intense neuritis of the facial nerve with patchy lymphocytic infiltrations, but the geniculate ganglion was normal. Although other pathological studies of the ganglion have produced other varying results, no autopsy study yet has shown that the ganglion suffers more damage than any other part of the nerve. Most of the studies reveal that cranial herpes zoster usually involves two or more segments of the neuroaxis. Paralysis of the third, fourth, and sixth cranial nerves with ophthalmic zoster have been described but are rare, and Engström and Wohlfart (1949) reported herpes zoster involving the seventh, eighth, ninth, and tenth cranial nerves. Blackley *et al.* (1967) demonstrated perivascular cuffing and lymphocytic infiltration of the seventh and eighth cranial nerves in a post-mortem study of a woman who died seven months after developing the Ramsay Hunt syndrome. Since their report once more confirmed that the syndrome is due to a more generalized infection and not simply a viral lesion of the geniculate ganglion, they recommended that the disease be regarded as a 'cephalic zoster'. Aleksic *et al.* (1973) showed some pathological changes in the geniculate ganglion in their autopsy study. The ganglion was moderately depleted of neurones and small collections of lymphocytes and macrophages were seen in its stroma. The facial nerve showed an intense neuritis occurring both proximal and distal to the ganglion. These authors reflect the modern view of a cephalic zoster, with viral neuritis of the seventh and eighth nerves being responsible for the facial palsy and the cochlear and vestibular loss, while involvement of the geniculate ganglion can probably account for the circumaural herpes.

Clinical features The same virus causes varicella and herpes zoster, and it is now believed that varicella is the primary infection, and zoster is a secondary, or reactivation, infection in one who is partially immune. Varicella is seen in epidemic form in children while zoster tends to occur sporadically in people in the sixth to the eighth decades of life. The Ramsay Hunt syndrome, therefore, occurs in middle-aged and elderly patients without any seasonal variation in incidence and without a history of person-to-person spread. The disease usually begins as a systemic upset with malaise, headache, and earache which is frequently severe. This is followed after a day or two by the sudden appearance of a herpetiform rash behind the ear and on the pinna and in the external auditory canal. The vesicles are sometimes seen in the face, mouth, palate, tongue, or neck. The rash is accompanied or followed by the abrupt onset of a lower motor neurone facial paralysis, which is usually a dense,

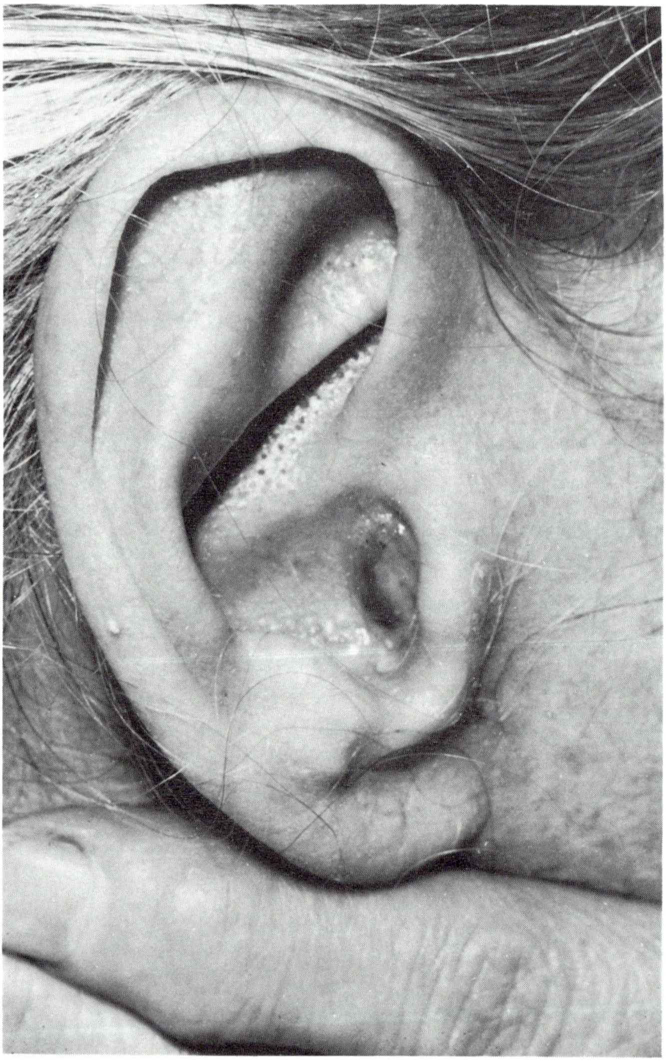

Fig. 3.2. Ramsay Hunt syndrome. Vesicles around external auditory canal.

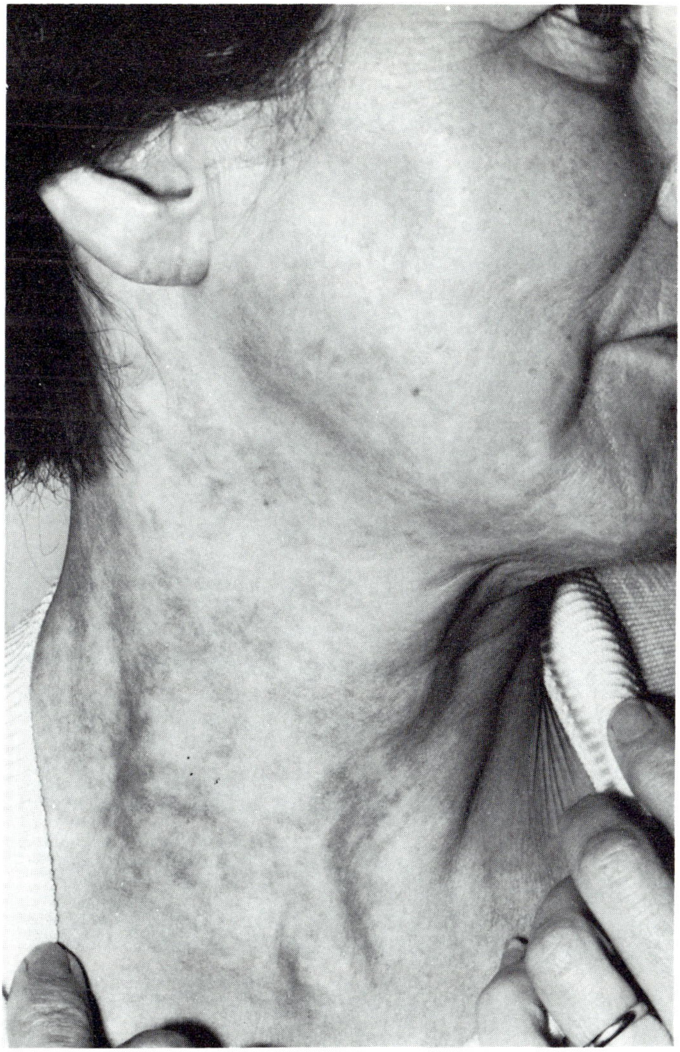

Fig. 3.3. Aged 52 years. Patient had right-sided Ramsay Hunt syndrome two years previously. Note residual scarring of skin of face and neck.

total paralysis. The paralysis may be delayed and appear shortly after the rash has cleared. Occasionally the paralysis develops before the rash (Fig. 3.2).

The vesicles become turbid and dry up leaving crusted secretion in their place. Years later the presence of clusters of small, round white scars bear witness to the eruption (Fig. 3.3). The facial palsy always improves, but

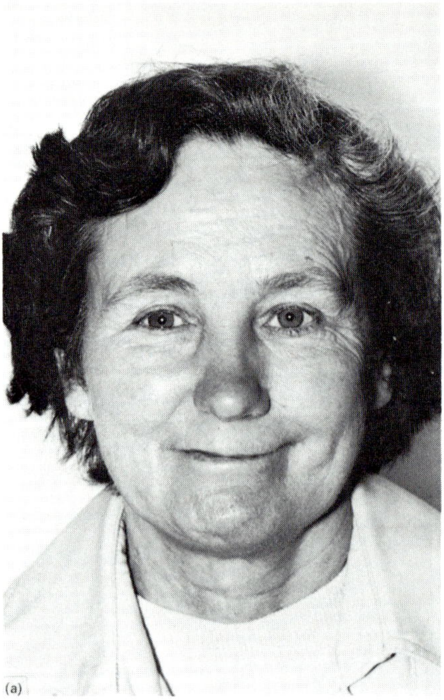

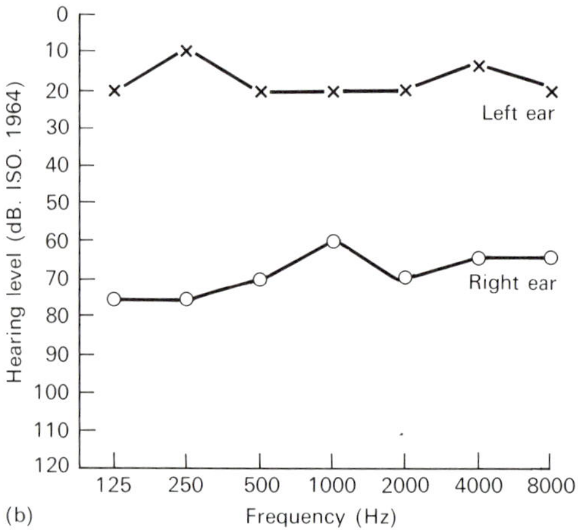

Fig. 3.4. (a) Same patient as in Fig. 3.3. Good recovery of right facial nerve function.
(b) Same patient as in Fig. 3.3. Persistent deafness right ear.

because the disease usually produces some degree of degeneration in the nerve, recovery is often delayed and incomplete. Residual facial weakness, crocodile tears, and synkinesis are seen in a number of patients. The rash and the palsy are often accompanied by a severe sensori-neural deafness and tinnitus on the affected side, together with vertigo and nystagmus. The eighth nerve lesion can be disabling as well as distressing and is slow to recover. Permanent partial deafness is the expected result, while the vertigo and nystagmus usually diminish slowly, but ultimately disappear completely. Fortunately, post-herpetic neuralgia is not a common feature of this syndrome (Fig. 3.4).

Poliomyelitis

Poliomyelitis provides another clear-cut example of a viral cause of peripheral facial paralysis. In the past, the bulbar form of poliomyelitis was frequently accompanied by damage to the motor neurones of the facial nucleus. The resultant facial palsy was often completely overshadowed by the life-threatening respiratory paralysis, but sometimes the facial lesion was the only paralytic sign of the disease. In a review of 500 cases of poliomyelitis Engler and Missal (1955) recorded the presence of facial palsy in 100 patients (20 per cent). It occurred in the bulbar forms of the disease which constituted 22·4 per cent of the 500 cases. The ninth and tenth cranial nerves are the most frequently involved in bulbar poliomyelitis and the facial nerve is the next most commonly affected. Of the 100 cases of facial palsy reported by Engler and Missal, 55 had isolated facial paralysis, without any other cranial nerve deficit. In a larger series of 5784 patients quoted by Menkes (1974) there was a 40 per cent incidence of facial paralysis.

The pathological changes, unlike those seen in the Ramsay Hunt syndrome, are centred in the motor neurones. Polio viruses contain RNA as their genetic material and when they infect neurones they render messenger RNA incapable of attaching new ribosomes. As a result, the production of cellular RNA and protein by the host cell is impaired. Cell necrosis is accompanied by a marked inflammatory reaction in poliomyelitis. Degenerated neurones are removed by macrophages (neuronophages) which persist for a time as small clusters of microglia. The axons of irreversibly damaged motor neurone cells degenerate and their associated muscles suffer a severe denervation atrophy. Less severely damaged neurones show chromatolysis and are capable of some degree of recovery. Weakness or paralysis develops quickly and, once begun, it achieves its maximum severity within 48 hours in most cases. Recovery of muscle function may continue over a period of years, partly by recovery of reversibly damaged neurones, partly by reinnervation of denervated muscle through sprouting of surviving axons, and partly by hypertrophy of surviving muscle.

The dramatic success of vaccination has abolished the frightening epidemics of this crippling disease in temperate climates and we now tend to speak about poliomyelitis in the past tense. However, outbreaks of the disease will inevitably recur if the population becomes apathetic towards immunization. Nicholas *et al.* (1977) remind us that the disease is still endemic in some tropical countries. They point out the high price paid for acquired immunity in tropical countries without an immunization programme. In their part of Ghana the observed prevalence of lameness attributable to poliomyelitis was 7 per 1000 in school-age children and they estimate the annual incidence to be 28 per 100 000 population.

Viral meningitis and encephalitis

Facial paralysis is encountered in viral meningitis and encephalitis but it does not form a characteristic feature of these infections as it does in bulbar poliomyelitis and the Ramsay Hunt syndrome. Facial paralysis is seen quite commonly in brain-stem encephalitis but this is an unusual form of the disease. Its clinical features are those of infection within the midbrain, pons, and medulla with multiple cranial nerve defects, ataxia, and long tract signs. In viral encephalitis it is principally the grey matter that is involved. Post-vaccinial and post-infectious encephalomyelitis, in which the white matter is predominantly affected, will be discussed separately.

The mumps virus is widely recognized to be one of the most common causes of aseptic meningitis. Mumps encephalitis is much less common, but when it occurs the cranial nerves are frequently affected. The eighth cranial nerve is the one most often involved. One or both facial nerves may be paralysed. The oculomotor, trigeminal, glossopharyngeal, and hypoglossal nerves may also be affected. Facial paralysis is occasionally seen in arbovirus encephalitis (Illis 1975), herpes simplex encephalitis (Bell and McCormick 1975), and in the encephalitis sometimes encountered in lymphocytic choriomeningitis (Menkes 1974).

Infectious mononucleosis

Most authorities are of the opinion that this disease is probably caused by the Epstein–Barr virus, which often attacks the nervous system as well as the haemopoietic system. In addition to causing aseptic meningitis and encephalitis the virus can also cause mononeuritis and polyradiculoneuritis (Guillain–Barré syndrome). The cranial nerves are more often affected by mononeuritis multiplex than the spinal nerves. Optic neuritis, facial palsy, and oculomotor palsies are the most frequent cranial nerve lesions. Facial paralysis may be unilateral but it is usually bilateral. The Guillain–Barré syndrome is the most widely recognized peripheral nerve disorder which may develop during the course of infectious mononucleosis. Bilateral facial paralysis is a frequent feature of this syndrome. Seventh nerve paralysis is reputed to be present in 14 per cent of the neurological forms of mononucleosis (Boudouresques *et al.* 1970).

The Guillain–Barré syndrome
(synonyms: acute inflammatory polyradiculoneuropathy; post-infectious polyneuritis; acute polyneuritis with facial diplegia)

Bilateral facial paralysis is such a common feature of this syndrome that it is incorporated into one of the many alternative titles given to this disease. It is frequently stated that facial diplegia can be detected in at least half of the patients. It is characteristic in this condition to find a symmetrical distribution of the motor weakness. The facial paralysis is an exception to the rule, however, because one side is often affected before, and to a greater degree than, the other. Sometimes facial paralysis remains unilateral. All degrees of severity from mild weakness to total paralysis of the face can be encountered. Less often, lower cranial nerve dysfunction gives rise to dysphagia or dysarthria. Other cranial nerves may be affected but much less frequently than the facial and the lower cranial nerves. The disease develops subacutely and usually presents with symmetrical motor weakness in the limbs accompanied by paraesthesia and pain.

The cerebrospinal fluid has a raised protein content with a normal cell count (protein-cell dissociation). The natural history of the disease shows a strong tendency to spontaneous recovery, and regression usually begins before the end of the seventh week. Satisfactory recovery occurs in 85 per cent of cases within six months. A small proportion of patients show permanent deficits, e.g. mild motor loss in the limbs, mild residual facial asymmetry, and synkinesis.

Recurrent forms of the disease have been described but are rare (Thomas *et al.* 1969). They occur more often in adults than in children. Austin (1958) recorded the case of an adult who had 20 attacks or relapses of the Guillain–Barré syndrome during a five-year period. There are striking similarities between the natural history of the paralysis in this disease and the paralysis in Bell's palsy. These have led some clinicians to the belief that Bell's palsy is a '*forme fruste*' of the Guillain–Barré syndrome.

Pathology and pathogenesis The pathological changes are clear cut and well defined. The peripheral nervous system is primarily involved. There is infiltration with lymphocytes and glial cells around the small veins and this is accompanied by patchy destruction of the myelin sheaths. The pathological changes in the central nervous system are secondary in nature due to retrograde involvement of the motor neurones of the anterior horn cells and cranial nerve nuclei. Various degrees of swelling and chromatolysis are seen in the motor neurones. When axonal interruption occurs close to the cell body the motor neurone may die.

The syndrome may follow a number of viral, bacterial, and mycoplasmal infections, immunization procedures, and surgical operations. The time interval between these and the onset of the disease is usually one to three weeks. Approximately half of the patients give no history of such an antecedent event. There are two rival theories of pathogenesis, the infective or viral, and the immunological. In favour of the viral theory, neurotropic viruses have been isolated from the cerebrospinal fluid and specific antibodies have been identified in the blood of some patients. Against the viral theory is the fact that a uniform clinical picture is unlikely to be caused by many different viruses (see Table 3.1). Supporters of the immunological theory point to the time interval between the 'prodromal event' and the onset of the disease, the uniform clinical picture, the protein-cell dissociation, and the increase of gammaglobulins in the cerebrospinal fluid.

Table 3.1
Viral infections associated with the Guillain–Barré syndrome

Coxsacki	Influenza
Cytomegalovirus	Measles
Echo	Mumps
Epstein–Barr	Rubella
Herpes Zoster virus	Vaccinia
Infectious hepatitis virus	Variola

In addition to the viruses listed in Table 3.1 it should be mentioned that the syndrome can follow antirabies vaccination. When this vaccine was obtained from rabbit spinal cord it was not infrequently associated with the development of the Guillain–Barré syndrome. Since an attenuated rabies vaccine free from animal nerve protein has been introduced, it is claimed that pure forms of the vaccine are virtually free from this complication. This lends further support to the immunological theory of pathogenesis. The Guillain–Barré syndrome has also been described following the administration of tetanus antitoxin and typhoid paratyphoid vaccine.

Acute disseminated encephalomyelitis
(synonyms: post-infectious or post-vaccinial encephalitis)

This disease is an inflammatory reaction within the central nervous system, predominantly affecting the white matter of the brain and spinal cord. It is characterized by multifocal perivenous lymphocytic and microglial infiltration, and is frequently accompanied by patchy demyelination. It is often preceded by a variety of infections or vaccinations. The pathological changes in the central nervous system are similar to those seen in the peripheral nervous system in the Guillain–Barré syndrome. Most of the infections which produce acute disseminated encephalomyelitis are viral. Measles, chickenpox, and smallpox are the best known examples, and the disease sometimes follows vaccination against smallpox and rabies. In general the pathological changes are most prominent in the white matter of the cerebrum, brain-stem, and spinal cord. The facial paralysis occasionally seen in measles encephalomyelitis is, therefore, most commonly an upper motor neurone lesion. The grey matter is seldom involved and neuronal degenerative changes are usually slight. The central nervous system involvement occurs between 4 and 21 days after the appearance of the measles rash. It can occur before the rash appears, however, and it occasionally occurs in measles contacts who do not develop the rash.

The pathogenesis is attributed by some to viral infection and by others to an immunological reaction on similar grounds to those advocated in the pathogenesis of the Guillain–Barré syndrome. Recent studies have proved that the measles virus does invade the brain in measles encephalomyelitis. It is still not clear whether the damage is due to the direct action of the virus or whether the virus acts indirectly by triggering an immunological reaction.

Facial paralysis is seen in the encephalomyelitis following other viral infections and vaccinations, but it is reported more frequently with measles, which serves as a useful example to represent the whole group.

Bacterial infections

Facial paralysis can be produced by a great variety of bacterial infections. Since historically it has been so frequently linked with otitis media, we may begin by looking at facial paralysis in ear infections.

Malignant otitis externa

This term is applied to a severe necrotizing infection originating in the external auditory canal. Although it is destructive it is not a neoplastic process, and the term can therefore be misleading.

The destructive otitis externa is seen almost exclusively in elderly diabetic patients and it is caused by *Pseudomonas aeruginosa*. A characteristic feature of the disease is the presence of active granulation tissue in the external auditory canal at the junction of the osseous and cartilagenous portions. The ear is extremely painful and movement of the temporomandibular joint aggravates the pain.

Cellulitis, chondritis, and osteomyelitis of the temporal bone and base of skull may result in multiple cranial nerve palsies. Facial palsy can result from infection in and around the facial nerve distal to the stylomastoid foramen, or within the Fallopian canal itself. In a series of 38 patients with this virulent form of external otitis described by Chandler (1972), 16 patients developed facial paralysis. Eight of these died, 2 had permanent paralysis, 3 had a partial recovery, and 3 had complete recovery. The high mortality and morbidity produced by this pyocyaneous osteomyelitis in elderly diabetics has been reduced in recent years by the advent of the effective antibiotics gentamicin, colistin, and carbenicillin.

Joachims (1976) drew attention to the fact that pyocyaneous osteomyelitis also occurs in non-diabetic children suffering from malnutrition and anaemia. Both the children he reported suffered a peripheral facial palsy also. It would appear that some degree of debility and weakening of the natural defence mechanism must exist, before the pseudomonas organism can produce a malignant or necrotizing type of infection. In non-debilitated patients mundane otitis externa due to pseudomonas infection occurs quite commonly and is not a cause of anxiety.

Otitis media

A sharp distinction has to be made between facial paralysis occurring in *acute* otitis media and its presence in *chronic* otitis media. In the former it is a relatively unimportant sign, whereas in the latter it is a serious matter with a practical bearing on diagnosis, prognosis, and treatment. Basically the presence of facial palsy in otitis media means one thing only: there is a defect in the bony Fallopian canal. If the Fallopian canal is intact the nerve is completely protected from middle ear suppuration.

Acute otitis media, by definition, is an acute infection confined to the mucosa or mucoperiosteum of the middle ear cleft. The mucosal infection can involve the facial nerve only if there is a pre-existing defect in its protective canal which, in practice, means a congenital dehiscence. Such a congenital dehiscence does not influence the severity or the progress of the otitis media and does not necessitate any modification in treatment. When the acute otitis media yields to systemic antibiotic therapy, the facial nerve paralysis quickly recovers. In short, facial paralysis in acute otitis media simply reveals a hitherto unsuspected congenital dehiscence of the Fallopian canal.

By contrast the development of facial paralysis in chronic otitis media indicates that a pathological process is eroding bone, that a previously intact Fallopian canal has been breached, and that unchecked erosion will permit the spread of infection to the inner ear and to the intracranial cavity. In industrially developed countries, where antibiotics are readily available and are routinely used in otitis media, the pathological process which erodes bone is almost always a cholesteatoma. Medical therapy has no place in the management of cholesteatoma. The development of facial palsy in chronic otitis media therefore is an absolute indication for surgical treatment. The operation is directed towards the removal of the cholesteatoma and nothing is to be gained by removing more of the protective bony Fallopian canal. Any attempt to 'decompress' the nerve by slitting the nerve sheath, which thereby exposes the nerve bundles to the middle ear suppuration, is unwise.

In pre-antibiotic days, facial paralysis in acute otitis media was classified as 'early' or 'late'. Early paralysis was attributed to Fallopian canal dehiscence and late paralysis to osteomyelitis (mastoiditis or petrositis). In the absence of antibiotics, osteomyelitis was treated surgically by cortical mastoidectomy without exploration of the Fallopian canal.

Chronic tuberculous otitis media is now very rare but when it does occur it still has a high incidence of facial paralysis. The management of patients with incomplete recovery of facial nerve function after treatment of middle ear infection will be discussed in Chapter 7.

Meningitis

Cranial nerve palsies are found in a number of cases of bacterial meningitis but the pathogenesis of the neuropathy is not fully understood. Perineural inflammation that extends into the substance of the cranial nerve is sometimes seen in purulent meningitis due to the meningococcus, the pneumococcus, or *Haemophilus influenzae*. The perineural inflammation gives rise to vascular changes also, which may be partly responsible for the nerve paralysis. It is not known why the eighth cranial nerve is more often involved than the seventh in this type of meningitis; the eighth nerve loss tends to be permanent. The third and fourth cranial nerves are also more frequently involved than the seventh, but fortunately the ocular palsies tend to disappear soon after the meningitis has been successfully treated.

In tuberculous meningitis the disease starts at the base of the brain (basal meningitis) and is much more marked there than in the vertex. An abundant exudate is formed in the loose arachnoid around the optic chiasma and anterior surfaces of the pons. The exudate may be copious and yellowish with a considerable amount of fibrin present, or the principal change may be more an inflammatory oedema with greyish opacity and thickening of the membranes. This inflammatory exudate involves the oculomotor nerve more frequently than any other cranial nerve. The eighth nerve too sometimes shows tuberculous infiltration of its sheath. Facial nerve paralysis is much less common. Damage to the nerve roots by endarteritis and infarction also occurs in chronic tuberculous meningitis in addition to the damage done by inflammatory infiltration. Spillane (1973) recorded an unusual case where a tuberculoma produced an upper motor neurone paralysis of the right side of the face. The carotid angiogram demonstrated a shift of the left anterior cerebral artery towards the right side.

Leprosy

Leprosy is a most interesting disease, which produces a unique type of facial paralysis. Descriptions of a disease resembling leprosy have been recorded in Chinese manuscripts dating back to 500 B.C. (Cochrane 1964) and ancient Indian, Hebrew, Greek, and Roman physicians were familiar with the disease. It is estimated that 10–20 million people suffer from the disease in the world today.

Pathology Leprosy results from infection by the *Mycobacterium leprae* which is the only bacterium which consistently invades peripheral nerves. Although it is customary to classify the disease into high-resistance tuberculoid leprosy and low-resistance lepromatous leprosy, bacillary invasion of the peripheral nerves occurs in all cases, and facial paralysis is found in patients exhibiting both forms of the disease. The main portal of entry of infection is the skin and the disease usually presents with a variety of rashes and skin lesions. Infection through the upper respiratory tract also occurs.

The skin lesions extend into the subcutaneous plane and involve the cutaneous and subcutaneous nerves. The major mixed nerves that are most commonly affected are the ulnar, median, peroneal, and facial nerves because of their superficial or subcutaneous course. The histological appearance of the damaged nerve is different in the tuberculoid and lepromatous forms of the disease. In tuberculoid leprosy there is severe destruction of the neural elements by an epithelioid granuloma and few bacilli are present in the nerve. In lepromatous leprosy great numbers of bacilli are present in the nerves which are also infiltrated with foamy histiocytes. It is now accepted that the bacilli are concentrated in the Schwann cells and not within the axons. Schwann cell involvement leads to segmental demyelination. Some remyelination does take place but does not keep pace with the demyelination.

Clinical features Leprosy produces a unique type of patchy bilateral facial paralysis due to selective infection of multiple small branches of the facial nerve. The branches are affected where they assume a superficial course. Weakness of eyelid closure results from damage to the temporal and zygomatic branches of the facial nerve which run superficially over the zygomatic arch and orbital rim to supply the orbicularis oculi and frontalis muscles. The medial segments of the frontalis muscle are paralysed before the lateral, and on attempted wrinkling of the brow, only the sides of the forehead rise. The superficial fibres of the buccal branch of the facial nerve, which run between the skin and the superficial muscles, become involved causing flattening of the nasolabial fold and weakness of the corner of the mouth. However, the deep fibres of the buccal branch, which pass beneath the superficial muscles to innervate the buccinator and orbicularis oris, are spared.

The action of the intact buccinator, combined with paralysis of the more superficial muscles, produces a series of concentric creases around the corner of the mouth forming the so-called 'buccinator smile'. In leprosy the upper half of the face tends to be symmetrically affected while asymmetric involvement of the lower half of the face is the rule. Although Sabin and Swift (1975) say that 'total facial paralysis is not present even in the most advanced cases of lepromatous leprosy', Spillane (1973) states that leprosy can produce a

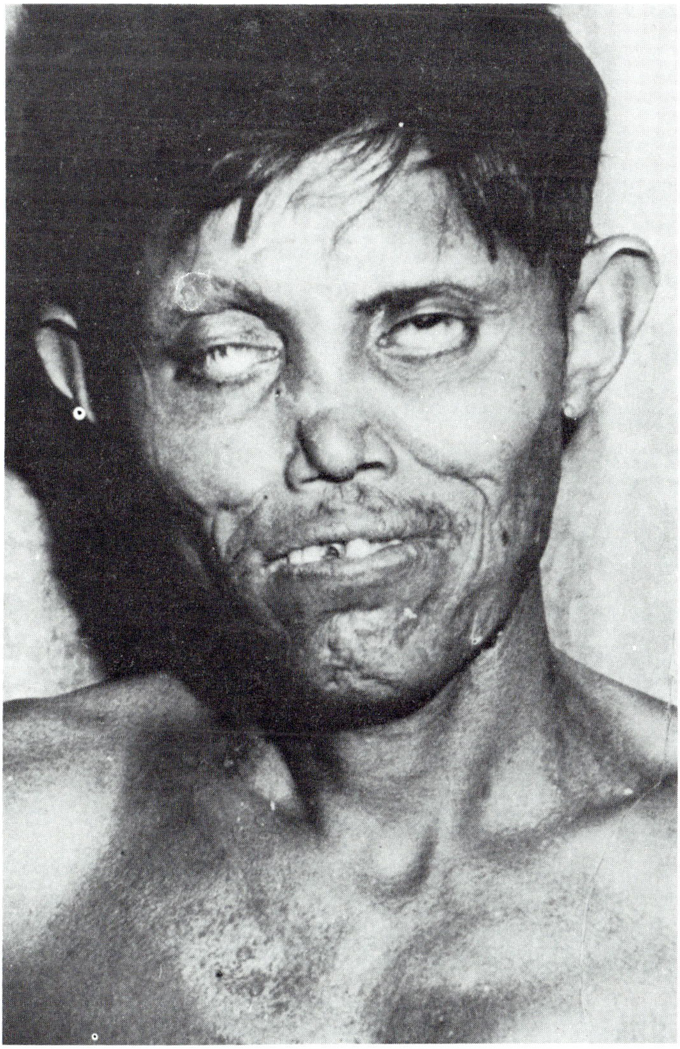

Fig. 3.5. Leprosy. Note bilateral facial paralysis, Bell's phenomenon, and buccinator smile.

sudden-onset total facial paralysis. It would appear that Cochrane (1964) is also familiar with cases of total facial paralysis in leprosy and he discusses the possible site of the lesion in these cases. Reichart (1976) quotes that during lepra reactions 'acute Bell's palsy may develop', and this has been attributed to an allergic or immunological response. Tuberculoid and dimorphous leprosy involve the seventh cranial nerve earlier and more often than does lepromatous leprosy (Fig. 3.5).

Sarcoidosis

Sarcoidosis is a systemic disease of unknown aetiology but many authorities suspect that tubercle bacilli are implicated in its causation. Although, strictly speaking, it cannot be classified as a 'bacterial infection' it seems reasonable to consider it here along with the other two chronic granulomatous diseases, tuberculosis and leprosy. When sarcoidosis involves the nervous system the clinical picture is usually either that of a peripheral neuropathy or of a chronic meningitis with multiple cranial nerves palsies. In the latter event, the cerebrospinal fluid often shows an increase in number of lymphocytes and a raised protein level. One of the most bizarre features of the nervous system involvement is the occurrence of multiple, intermittent, and fluctuating cranial nerve palsies. The seventh nerve is the one most frequently involved, and facial paralysis is found in over one-third of patients with sarcoidosis of the nervous system. Bilateral facial nerve involvement is common but the two sides are not usually affected at the same time. In manner of onset, duration, and recovery, the facial nerve paralysis in sarcoidosis is identical to that seen in Bell's palsy. The paralysis begins abruptly and, interestingly enough, is often preceded by pain behind the ear. After a variable number of weeks spontaneous recovery of the paralysis takes place. Some degeneration of the facial nerve occurs so that recovery becomes less complete following each episode of paralysis. In Heerfordt's syndrome of uveo–parotid fever (uveitis and bilateral parotid swelling due to sarcoidosis) the facial paralysis has been wrongly attributed to damage to the nerve in the swollen parotid gland. The parotitis probably plays no part at all, since the facial paralysis may include loss of taste sensation and it occurs in patients without overt parotitis (Lambert and Richards 1964).

There is, however, no general agreement on the mechanism of sarcoid neuropathy and three theories are currently debated (Mathews 1975). The first is that granulomatous meningitis results in inflammatory infiltration of the nerve roots like that found in tuberculous meningitis. However, autopsy evidence for this is lacking and the clinical pattern of sarcoid neuropathy, with its frequent involvement of the seventh cranial nerve and its rare involvement of the third nerve, is quite unlike tuberculous meningitis. The second theory holds that the neuropathy is due to the presence of sarcoid tissue within the nerve itself, and indeed a number of autopsies have shown that this does sometimes occur. However, it has not been demonstrated sufficiently often to account for the myriad neuropathies of the disease. The third theory is based on the concept of demyelination of the nerve similar to that encountered in post-infectious polyneuropathy. There is no autopsy evidence for this and very few nerve conduction velocity tests have been carried out in sufferers from this disease. A reduced conduction velocity compatible with segmental demyelination has been shown to occur in only a few isolated reports. One of the attractions of this theory is that episodes of demyelination followed by repair could explain the recurring relapses and spontaneous recovery which are such a characteristic feature of sarcoid neuropathy.

Diphtheria

Fortunately, this disease has practically disappeared in industrially developed countries as a result of widespread immunization programmes. The disease is caused by the *Corynebacterium diphtheriae* (Klebs–Löffler bacillus) which produces an extremely powerful, soluble exotoxin which damages cells at the site of infection. The toxin is carried by the blood stream and damages distant organs particularly the myocardium and the kidneys. Degenerative changes in the central nervous system occur in most of the severe cases, and their extent is directly proportional to the duration of infection before antitoxin is given. In cases where the diagnosis has been missed and when patients survive without antitoxin, the incidence of nerve damage is particularly high. Paley and Truelove (1948) reported a series of 245 treated cases of whom approximately 15 per cent had palatal palsies and 0·4 per cent had facial paralysis. The paralyses are due to nerve damage by the diphtheria toxin.

It has been established by autopsy studies and by animal experiments that the outstanding feature of the diphtheritic neuropathy is segmental demyelination with preservation of axonal continuity. Although some axons may show abnormalities only a few undergo complete degeneration.

Tetanus

This acute infectious disease, caused by *Clostridium tetani*, resembles diphtheria in its production of a most virulent exotoxin. The distribution of peripheral nerve lesions in 757 cases collected by Starzecka (1960) was as follows:

facial paralysis	3·57 per cent
oculomotor paralysis	0·53 per cent
lower limb paralysis	0·39 per cent

Cephalic tetanus with facial palsy is a well-recognized form of the disease. It occurs as a result of a wound in the region of the branches of the facial nerve. The palsy is always on the same side as the wound and when the wound is in the mid-line there is usually a facial diplegia. The paralysis is usually total but may be partial and confined to the upper or lower branches of the nerve. The prognosis depends mainly on the rapidity of onset of paralysis. If the onset is delayed the prognosis is good. In most fatal cases the paralysis develops between the second and eighth days.

There is considerable debate about the site of the facial nerve lesion in cephalic tetanus. Watkins (1939) suggested that the lesion was in the peripheral nerve because he noted a loss of taste on the same side as the facial paralysis. Park (1970) described the EMG findings in one of his 7 cases and came to the conclusion that the paralysis was compatible with a nuclear lesion. Both these views were rejected by Vakil *et al.* (1973). They reported 22 cases and concluded from their electrophysiological studies that no denervation lesion or true paralysis occurred in cephalic tetanus. A clinical and electrophysiological study of 15 cases by Dastur *et al.* (1977) led to a completely different conclusion however. These authors have put forward the hypothesis that there is a dual lesion in cephalic tetanus. They noted that muscle paralysis is maximal close to the site of injury, while spasm is evident at more distant sites. As muscle paralysis improved with time, they observed that it was succeeded by muscle spasm. They postulated that paralysis is due to a high local concentration of toxin in the brain stem, while lesser concentrations cause spasm by abolishing inhibition. They concluded from their investigations that the paralysis is of the lower motor neurone type. The main features noted in their electrophysiological tests were denervation potentials, hyperirritability, loss of motor units, and marginally increased distal latencies.

Spirochaetal infections

Leptospirosis

In this disease the spirochaetes seldom breach the meninges to invade the nervous system although they do attack the meningeal barrier, and leptospiral meningitis is a common enough complication. Mononeuritis multiplex has been recorded and Boudouresques *et al.* (1970) quote a thesis in which the details of 11 patients were reported. The majority of these patients had a unilateral peripheral facial palsy and 2 had bilateral facial paralysis. The paralysis was a late development which appeared abruptly 20–30 days after the first signs of infection. These authors suggest that the late paralyses are best explained in terms of an immunological process.

Syphilis

In this disease not only does the spirochaete *Treponema pallidum* attack the meningeal barrier but it breaches it readily and produces the enormous variety of lesions associated with neurosyphilis. The facial nerve is involved in two of the three main forms of neurosyphilis, meningovascular syphilis and general paresis, usually by a lower motor neurone involvement in the former, and an upper motor neurone involvement in the latter.

Meningovascular neurosyphilis The primary vascular lesion is an endarteritis obliterans with cellular infiltration of the perivascular space. This causes impairment of the blood supply to the nervous tissue by reduction of the lumen of the blood vessel, and by actual thrombosis in some instances. An area of necrosis or caseation is thus formed, and a granuloma arises in this site and is surrounded by a zone of fibrous tissue reaction. The clinical manifestations of meningovascular syphilis depend on the locations of this granuloma formation.

Syphilitic meningitis may involve the dura or the leptomeninges, although not infrequently both are involved and adhesions are present. Syphilitic leptomeningitis is most common at the base of the brain where it causes a diffuse thickening of the membranes with, as a rule, some superficial involvement of the brain substance. Various cranial nerves may become implicated and a lower motor neurone facial paralysis may result. A large gumma arising from the meninges is now rare. On the other hand, as a consequence of obliterative endarteritis, a focal cerebral lesion may result. Such a focal lesion can produce a hemiplegia or a single cranial nerve palsy.

General paresis In this late form of the disease the pathology is essentially a chronic syphilitic meningo-encephalitis with thickening of the meninges and cerebral cortical atrophy. The facial expression is often vacant or mask-like suggesting involvement of the emotional upper motor neurone facial pathways. Weakness of voluntary muscle power, frequently associated with tremor, is often seen in the face, suggesting involvement of the neurones of the motor cortex in the pre-central gyrus.

Fungal and parasitic infections

Fungal infections

Fungal infections of the nervous system are fortunately uncommon. The infection may be primary or, more usually, secondary to diabetes, chronic debilitating illness, or infection elsewhere in the body. The incidence of fungal infections is however, increasing as a result of the increased use of antibiotics and immunosuppressive drugs which have been so helpful in the treatment of malignant disease and in organ transplantation.

Although occasional reports of partial and complete facial paralysis in fungal infections are found, the paralysis is usually a very minor feature of the illness and may often be due to the primary disease rather than to the complication of fungal infection.

Chronic granulomatous meningitis and abscess formation are the two characteristic features of fungal infection of the nervous system and a great variety of general and focal nervous lesions may thus be produced. Actinomycosis and blastomycosis are two of the more common varieties of fungal infections encountered today.

Parasitic infections

Polyneuritis is a well recognized feature of malaria and toxoplasmosis. However, the literature also contains scattered reports of mononeuritis involving the seventh nerve in these diseases, and cases of facial diplegia have been recorded. In trichinosis cranial nerve palsies are rare and Boudouresques *et al.* (1970) found two recorded cases of peripheral facial palsy in the literature.

Spillane (1973) has pointed out that a cerebral hydatid cyst sometimes produces a supranuclear facial paralysis.

In congenital toxoplasmosis chorioretinitis, intracerebral calcification, hydrocephaly, and convulsions are common complications.

Postnatally acquired toxoplasmosis is often asymptomatic. When clinical manifestations become obvious patients may develop lymphadenopathy, pneumonia, hepatomegaly, and sometimes a mild encephalitis. Occasionally an isolated facial palsy is encountered (Francois 1963; Fondu and De Meuter 1969).

Apart from toxoplasmosis, none of these diseases is common in North America or Western Europe.

Tumours

Peripheral facial nerve paralysis can be produced by primary tumours of the nerve, or by secondary involvement of the nerve by adjacent tumours in the brain, in the temporal bone, and in the face and neck. Facial palsy occurring in the reticuloses will be discussed separately. It is frequently stated that neoplasms account for 5 per cent of peripheral facial paralysis.

Facial nerve tumours

Facial nerve tumours are uncommon and the majority of them are neurinomas. Pulec (1969, 1972) carried out a thorough search of the literature and found a total of 98 neurinomas. Neely and Alford (1974) added 4 further cases of their own. Conley and Janecka (1974) drew attention to the fact that neurilemomas do not always occur singly. They found 23 tumours in 17 facial nerves. Two of these tumours were malignant schwannomas.

A neurinoma can arise in any part of the facial nerve or its branches from the posterior fossa to the parotid gland. It may arise in the Fallopian canal and grow into the internal auditory canal or middle fossa. Similarly a neurinoma can erode into the middle ear cavity, the mastoid process, and the external auditory canal.

A report by Saito and Baxter (1972) makes one speculate about the possibility of there being a large number of asymptomatic facial neurinomas despite the small number of recorded cases. In their study of 600 temporal bones they found 5 facial neurinomas, 4 of which had produced no facial dysfunction during life.

Other tumours of the facial nerve are extraordinarily rare. Three sarcomas arising from the mesodermal sheath of the facial nerve have been reported by Figi and Hempstead (1943), Kettel (1950), and Guttman and Simon (1951). Very surprisingly two intratympanic meningiomas of the facial nerve have been recorded, one by Cawthorne (quoted by Kettel 1959) and one by Debain *et al.* (1966).

It was mentioned in Chapter 1 that the meninges may penetrate deeply into the Fallopian canal, and that the bone covering the superior aspect of the geniculate ganglion may be absent. One wonders if either of these anomalies could account for an intratympanic facial nerve meningioma.

Pathology A neurinoma or schwannoma is a benign encapsulated tumour arising from the Schwann cells of the nerve trunk. It contains few, if any, nerve fibres and consists of areas of dense connective tissue with characteristic pallisading of the nuclei (Antoni type A tissue). Areas of loose reticular or myxomatous connective tissue (Antoni type B) are intermingled with the dense connective tissue bundles. In malignant schwannomas the histological picture is characterized by an increase in cellularity, pleomorphism, and mitotic figures.

Clinical features The commonest age of onset is 10–40 years of age and females are more often affected than males. It usually presents as a slowly progressive facial paralysis. Abrupt onset of paralysis sometimes occurs and may lead to a mistaken diagnosis of Bell's palsy. Occasionally the paralysis fluctuates in severity. Facial twitching sometimes appears before any facial weakness can be detected. If the neurinoma extends into the middle ear cleft conductive deafness will be present. The tumour may extend into the external canal from the middle ear or the mastoid process. Secondary infection, aural discharge, and pain in the ear may then develop. If the neurinoma erodes the petrous part of the temporal bone sensori-neural deafness will occur. Extension of the tumour into the middle and posterior fossae will produce the signs and symptoms of an intracranial space-occupying lesion. A decrease in lacrimation and a loss of taste sensation on the affected side is to be expected in tumours proximal to the geniculate ganglion. Tumours arising from the terminal branches of the nerve usually present clinically as parotid tumours, and may not have an associated facial paralysis.

Tumours of the pons and medulla

The pontine astrocytoma of childhood is the commonest tumour of the brain stem, and tumours in this region give rise to localizing signs before producing increased intracranial pressure.

Crossed paralysis is usually present at an early stage, weakness of the facial muscles and jaw on one side, being frequently accompanied by weakness of the soft palate tongue and limbs on the other side. Later bilateral paralysis of the facial, palatal, lingual, and limb muscles usually develops. Sensory paralysis may be predominantly unilateral or bilateral and anaesthesia in the region of the trigeminal nerve distribution together with loss of auditory function is commonly found.

By contrast fourth ventricle tumours present with signs of increased intracranial pressure as their first manifestation. Headache, vomiting, papilloedema, and other features of hydrocephalus usually develop rapidly. Nystagmus and vertigo aggravated by changes in head position are characteristic features. Disturbance of cranial nerve function is usually slight. In young patients ependymoma is the commonest fourth ventricle tumour, but in patients over 50 years of age the tumour is usually a metastasis. Bronchial and breast carcinomas are the commonest source of origin.

Cerebellopontine angle tumours Tumours in this site frequently involve the facial nerve and produce both irritative and later paralytic features.

Approximately 80 per cent of cerebellopontine angle tumours are acoustic neurinomas and indeed this neoplasm accounts for 8 per cent of all intracranial tumours. Revilla (1948) reported the following distribution of the tumours found in the cerebellopontine angle in a series of 205 cases: 78 per cent neurinomas; 6 per cent meningiomas; 6 per cent epidermoid cysts (congenital cholesteatoma); 6 per cent glomus tumours (paragangliomas); 4 per cent miscellaneous tumours of unspecified type. Schuknecht *et al.* (1977) recorded the presence of several cases of metastasis from primary neoplasms of the lung and breast to the cerebellopontine angle in his unique collection of temporal bones.

Acoustic neurinomas usually occur as isolated or single tumours but bilateral tumours are seen in patients with von Recklinghausen's familial neurofibromatosis. In the latter case, the family history, the presence of *café au lait* skin pigmentation and of cutaneous neurofibromas may help to establish the diagnosis (Fig. 3.6).

Patients usually present with symptoms in middle life though it is often possible to extract a history of unilateral deafness or tinnitus of many years'

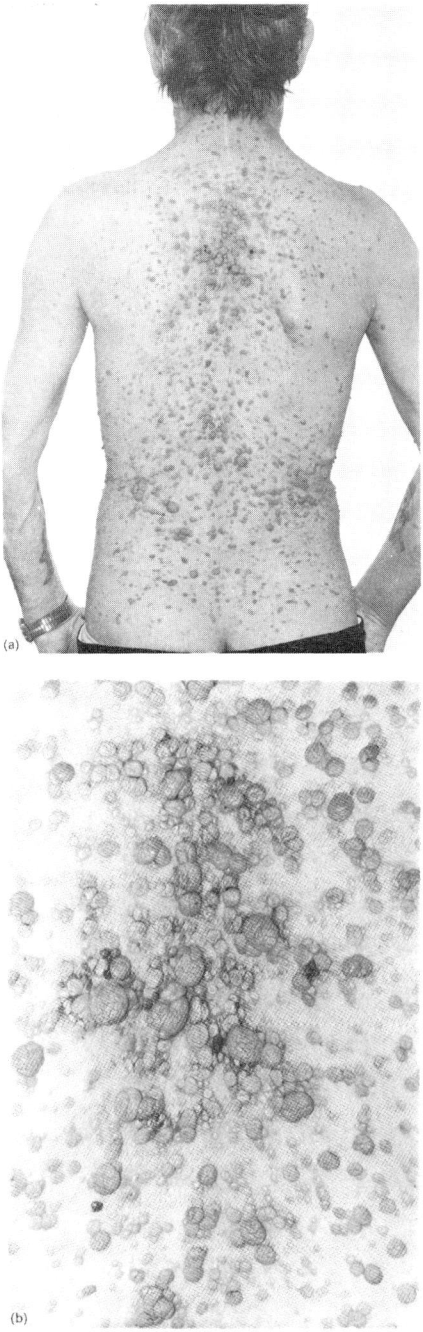

Fig. 3.6. Von Recklinghausen's disease. (a) cutaneous neuromas; (b) close-up view.

duration. This is because the tumour grows slowly and auditory symptoms usually exist for years before there is increased intracranial pressure. Mild chronic vertigo may also be present for many years because the tumour more commonly arises from the vestibular than the cochlear nerve. As the tumour encroaches on the facial nerve it causes facial twitching and/or facial weakness. It is surprising at operation how often the facial nerve is found to be stretched by the acoustic tumour without loss of facial nerve function. Further growth of the tumour may involve the more anteriorly placed trigeminal nerve, with loss of the corneal reflex and facial sensation. Sixth nerve involvement produces weakness of the lateral rectus muscle and compression of the cerebellar hemisphere causes symptoms of cerebellar deficiency on the side of the tumour.

The cerebrospinal fluid has a raised protein concentration in cases with large tumours but in small tumours the protein level is normal. The diagnosis is usually made radiologically by plain x-rays or tomography which demonstrate the eroded internal auditory canal, or by contrast radiography with myodil (Pantopaque) or metrizamide (Fig. 6.4; p. 201). Audiometry and vestibulometry are invaluable aids to early diagnosis of small tumours.

Tumours of the ear and temporal bone

In addition to the tumours already described, other tumours occur in the middle ear and temporal bone and cause facial paralysis, other cranial nerve palsies, and deafness. Fortunately, they are rare.

The commonest malignant tumour encountered is a squamous carcinoma of the ear and the commonest benign neoplasm is a glomus jugulare tumour.

Malignant tumours of the ear *Carcinoma of middle and external ear* Chronic middle ear suppuration appears to be a predisposing factor and many of the patients have a long history of otorrhoea. A change in the nature of the aural discharge, e.g. the presence of blood-staining or the onset of pain raises the suspicion of the development of malignant change. Pain is a characteristic feature of carcinoma of the ear. It is deep-seated and boring or throbbing in nature and tends to persist relentlessly. It is quite unlike the relatively milder and shorter-lived pain of acute otitis media. Chronic middle ear suppuration usually causes a painless aural discharge. The tumour tends to spread within the natural cavities of the middle ear cleft and then erodes through to the intracranial cavity (Figs 3.7 and 3.8). Vertigo and lower cranial nerve palsies indicate that the tumour has eroded extensively and the prospect of complete eradication is poor. Metastases to the lymph nodes of the neck are late and only occur after the tumour has extended into the skin and soft tissues beyond the temporal bone. The tumour therefore can involve the facial nerve in its infratemporal course as well as in the temporal bone. Carcinoma occurs in the over-40 age group.

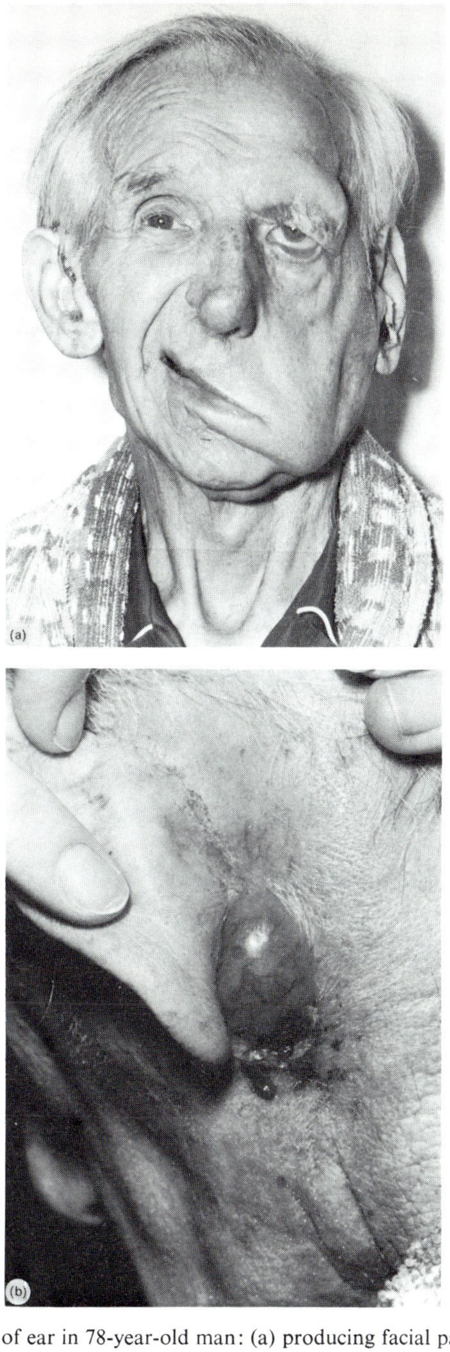

Fig. 3.7. Carcinoma of ear in 78-year-old man: (a) producing facial palsy; (b) post-auricular extension.

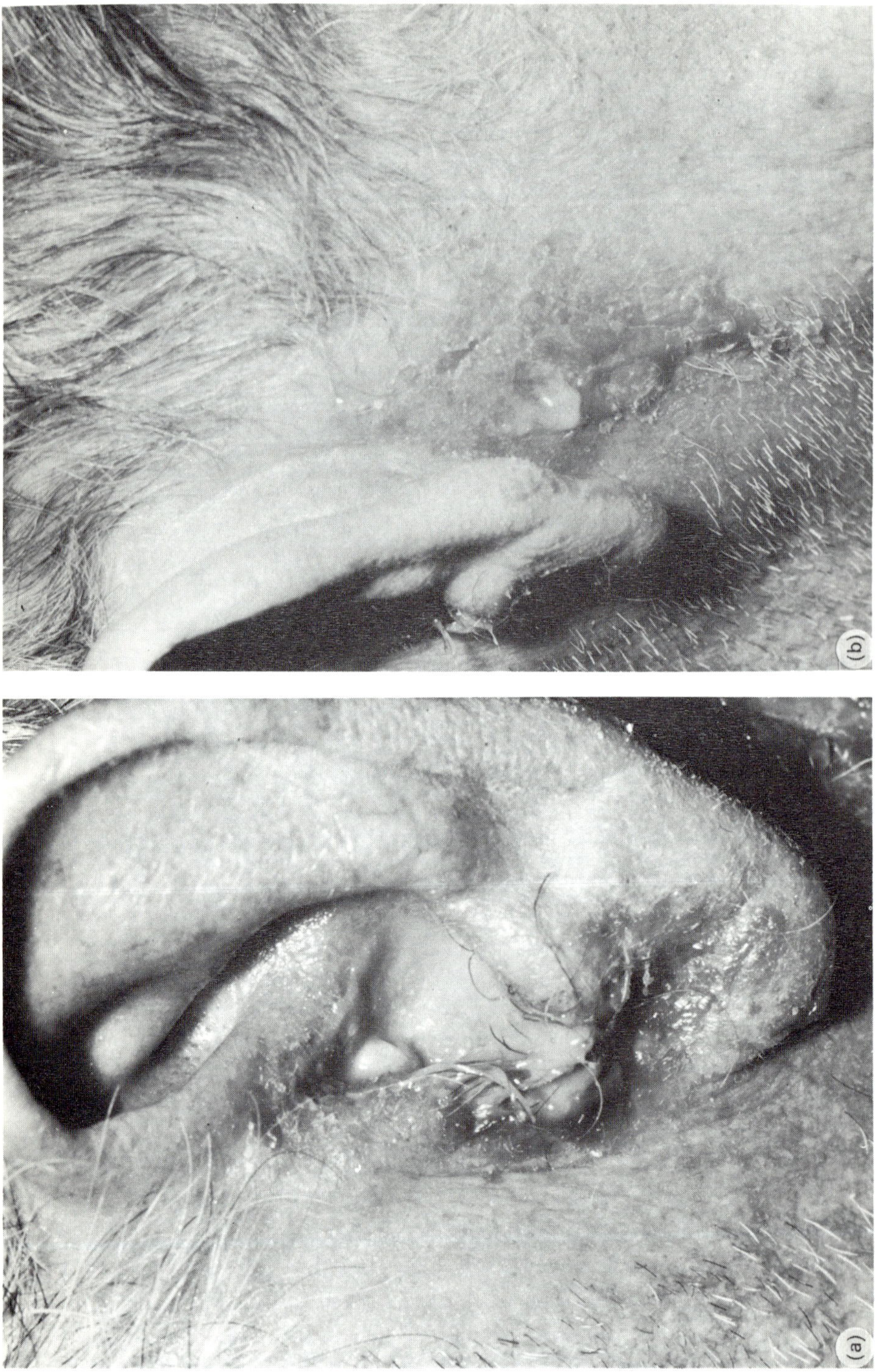

Fig. 3.8. Carcinoma of ear in 65-year-old man: (a) presenting at external auditory canal; (b) eroding mastoid process.

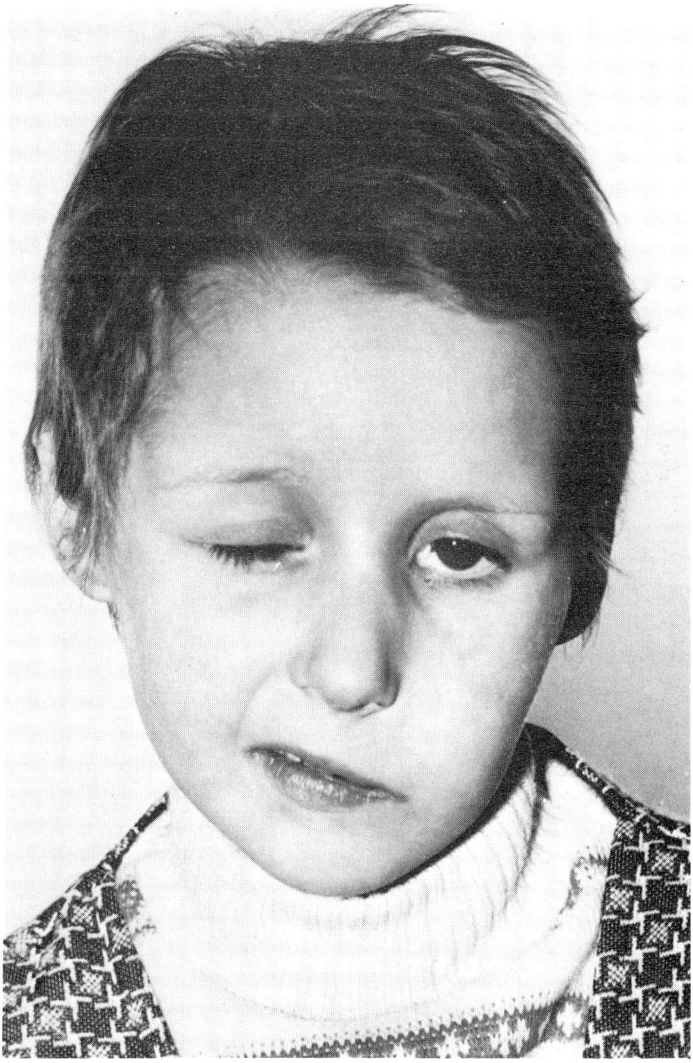

Fig. 3.9. Left peripheral facial paralysis produced by a rhabdomyosarcoma in a 7-year-old girl. Patient treated by radiotherapy and cytotoxic drugs.

Sarcoma This is 10 times less common than carcinoma of the tempora bone but it occurs mainly in the under-40 age group and it is the more common tumour in children. Rhabdomyosarcoma, spindle cell sarcoma, and neurofibrosarcoma are the varieties most frequently recorded (Fig. 3.9). Naufal (1973) searched the world literature for the previous 100 years and found 211 recorded cases to which he added 4 further cases from his own hospital. These 4 patients all had peripheral facial palsy. Other symptoms of primary sarcoma of the temporal bone include aural discharge, bleeding, and deafness. These tumours are highly aggressive and destroy the middle ear, mastoid process, petrous apex, and bony labyrinth by local infiltration.

Facial nerve involvement usually occurs early in the disease and extension of the tumour into the middle fossa and posterior fossa commonly takes place. Dissemination of the tumour by the lymphatics and the blood-stream produces widespread metastases in the lungs and bony skeleton.

Benign tumours of the ear *Glomus jugulare tumours* These tumours arise from chemoreceptor tissue in the adventitia of the jugular bulb. These and similar tumours arising from chemoreceptor tissue in the adventitia of other major blood-vessels are known by the generic name of chemodectomas, or the somewhat more unwieldy term of non-chromaffin paragangliomas.

Glomus jugulare tumours are often multicentric in origin and consist of clumps of large polyhedral epithelioid cells in an alveolar pattern with a vascular stroma which contains unmyelinated nerve fibrils. The tumour is slow-growing and locally invasive with a tendency to recur. Malignant glomus tumours with metastases have been reported but are much less common than the benign tumours. Very occasionally a glomus jugulare tumour secretes catecholamines and behaves like a phaeochromocytoma.

If the tumour arises in the tympanum, pulsatile tinnitus may be the earliest symptom, followed by deafness. The tumour may be seen through an intact tympanic membrane as a red mass or it may perforate the tympanic membrane and present as an aural 'polyp'. In many cases the facial nerve is involved either before or after the tumour has appeared in the external auditory canal (Fig. 3.10). Tumours originating from the jugular bulb produce a jugular foramen syndrome with lower cranial nerve palsies before invasion of the tympanum produces aural symptoms.

Diagnosis is greatly helped by temporal bone tomography and particularly by contrast radiography. Retrograde jugular venograms and subtraction films are most useful (Fig. 3.11). Because the tumours are very slow-growing and have a multicentric origin, recurrence years after apparently successful treatment is not uncommon. The patient whose picture and radiographs are shown (in Fig. 3.11) first presented with an 'aural polyp' in 1948. She has had two courses of radiotherapy using different portals of entry in the past, and at present she has no disability apart from facial palsy and unilateral deafness, although the tumour has been progressing very slowly for more than 30 years.

Epidermoid cysts (congenital cholesteatomas) occur in the temporal bone more often than in the cerebellopontine angle and it is generally agreed that at least 3 per cent of all cholesteatomas of the ear are of the congenital type. When they expand it is the site of origin which determines whether erosion

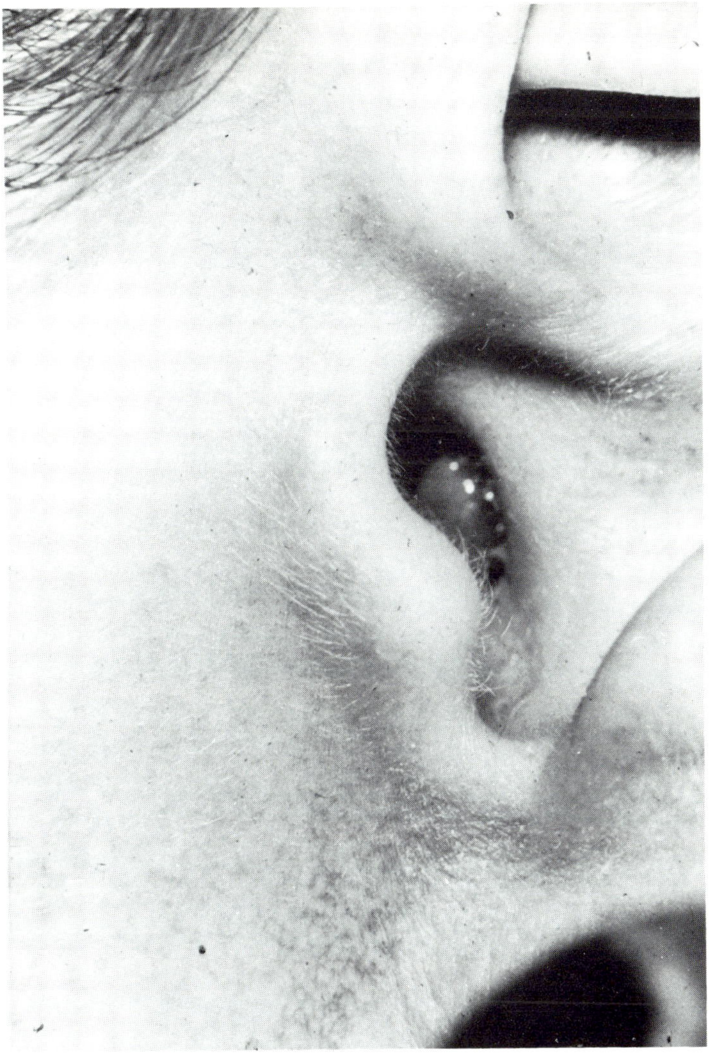

Fig. 3.10. Glomus jugulare tumour presenting as an 'aural polyp'.

into the Fallopian canal with facial twitching and weakness will occur before (a) erosion into the middle ear or inner ear produces deafness, or (b) erosion into the external ear allows secondary infection with aural discharge to develop.

In the patient shown in Fig. 6.5 (p. 204) left-sided facial twitching and weakness was the presenting symptom, and the cholesteatoma was found to have eroded the tegmen tympani, and the horizontal part of the left Fallopian

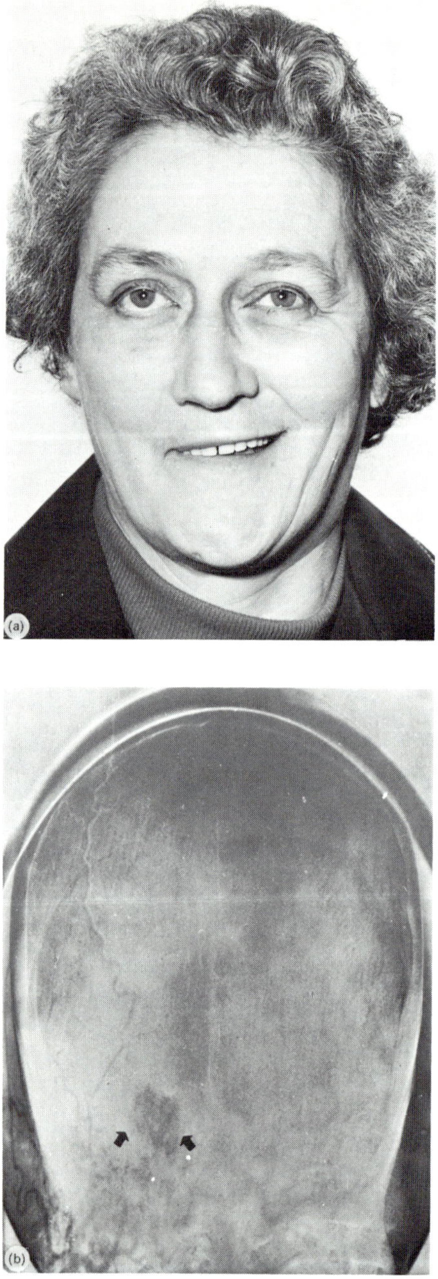

Fig. 3.11. Glomus jugulare tumour (52 years): (a) producing right facial palsy; (b) angiogram (subtraction film) showing the pathological circulation.

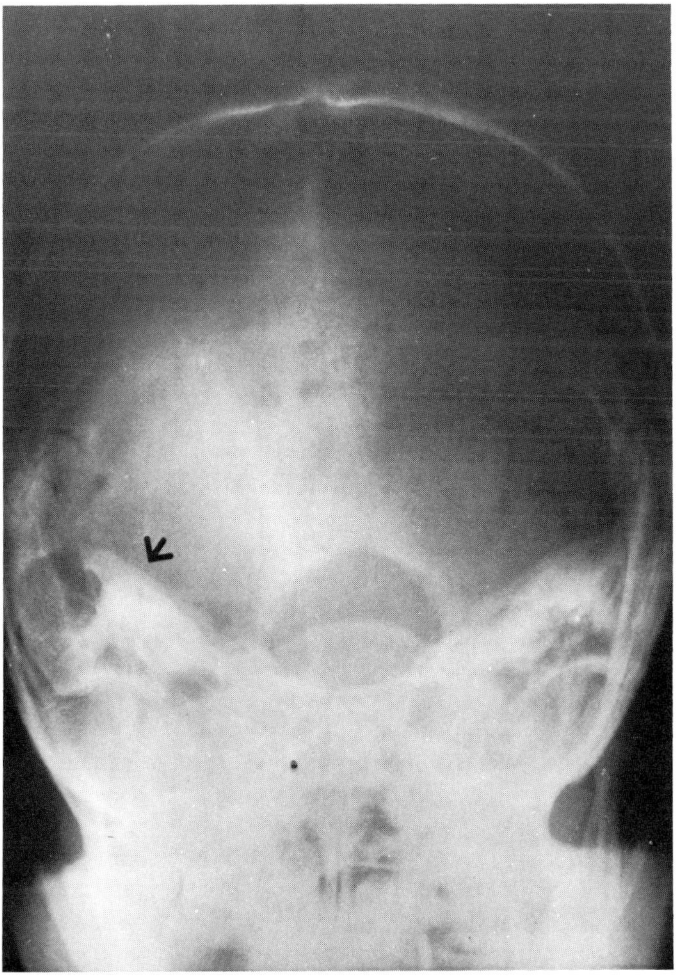

Fig. 3.12. Congenital cholesteatoma (epidermoid cyst) punched-out circular lesion in temporal bone lateral to the arrow.

canal. A symptomless right-sided cholesteatoma was also noted radiologically. It eventually eroded into the attic region without ever involving the facial nerve (Fig. 3.12).

Meningioma en-plaque involves the temporal bone and the facial nerve very rarely (Fig. 6.1, p. 197). Multiple myelomas are sometimes seen in the temporal bone but this is usually an insignificant feature in advanced disease. Neurinomas of the ninth and tenth cranial nerves involving the temporal bone are also very rare.

Metastatic tumours of temporal bone

Secondary malignant tumours in the temporal bone are less frequent than primary malignancies and a search of the world literature reveals fewer than 100 recorded cases.

In 1968 Schuknecht *et al.* found a total of 63 metastases to the temporal bone recorded in the literature and to this number they added 6 cases of their own. Fifteen of these 69 (21·7 per cent) metastases arose from primary neoplasms of the breast. Primary tumours of the kidney accounted for the second largest group of temporal bone metastases.

Adams *et al.* (1971) searched the records of their hospital for the preceding 15 years and found 10 cases of metastases to the temporal bone.

The majority of all these patients suffered from otalgia, otorrhoea, hearing loss, and peri-auricular swelling. Facial palsy was never either the first or the only manifestation of their disease. Indeed many of these patients had known metastases in other parts of the body before facial palsy developed.

Breadon *et al.* (1977), however, reported a case of breast cancer in which facial paralysis from temporal bone metastasis was the presenting sign. The breast tumour had not been noticed and no other metastases were present. They reported another temporal bone metastases from a breast cancer in a second patient and pointed out that both these patients had pain in the mastoid region and brief episodes of temporary facial paralysis before permanent paralysis occurred.

The reticuloses *Acute leukaemia* While cerebral haemorrhage and leukaemic infiltration of brain are the most common neurological complications of leukaemia, cranial nerve palsies also sometimes occur. The facial and abducent nerves are the most often affected and this can arise either directly from haemorrhage or leukaemic infiltration of the brain-stem or cranial nerves, or indirectly from meningeal involvement. Leukaemic infiltration appears to arise from intravascular thrombi of leukaemic cells and more extensive lesions lead to the infiltration of the perivascular space with leukaemic cells. Chronic lymphatic and chronic myeloid leukaemia have a lesser incidence of cellular infiltration of cranial nerves.

Lymphoma (term includes Hodgkin's disease, reticulum cell sarcoma, lymphosarcoma, and follicular lymphoma) It is estimated that the nervous system is involved in 10–25 per cent of patients with lymphoma. Direct involvement by local deposits on the brain, spinal cord, and cranial and spinal nerves are easy to understand. In addition, however, non-metastatic involvement by encephalomyelitis, cerebellar degeneration, or peripheral neuropathy occur and are incapable of complete explanation as yet.

Cranial nerves are affected by compression, meningeal involvement, or by direct invasion. The third, fifth, sixth, and seventh nerves are the most frequently involved; the optic nerve is usually spared. The fifth and seventh nerves are often affected extracranially also.

Paparella and El Fiky (1972) described in detail the pathological changes in 16 temporal bones of patients with malignant lymphoma. Facial palsy occurred in one patient in whom gross infiltration of the facial nerve in the temporal bone was found. Lesser degrees of infiltration of the facial nerve were seen in 3 other patients (6 temporal bones) in whom there was no loss of facial nerve function.

Uncommon granulomatous disease of temporal bone *Histiocytosis X* Eosinophilic granuloma of bone, Hand–Schuller–Christian disease, and Letterer–Siwe disease constitute a complex of diseases of unknown aetiology and of variable histology. Many authorities (Farber 1941; Lichtenstein 1953; Oberman 1961) believe that the three diseases represent variations in degree, stage of involvement, and localization of the same disease process. Lichtenstein grouped the three conditions under the name 'Histiocytosis X' to emphasize the proliferation of histiocytes in all three, and the enigmatic aetiology. This classification is adopted in *Conybeare's textbook of medicine* (Mann 1975) but is strongly opposed by Lieberman in Beeson and McDermott (1975). In this group of diseases, granulomatous tumours are formed by histiocytic proliferation of unknown cause. The facial nerve may be compromised by such tumours in the temporal bone or posterior fossa.

Letterer–Siwe disease is the most severe of the three and often pursues a rapidly fatal course. Next in order of severity is Hand–Schuller–Christian disease, of which Tos (1969) was able to collect 500 cases from the literature. The temporal bone was involved in 284 cases (61 per cent) and bilateral temporal bone involvement occurred in 144 (31 per cent). Lower motor neurone facial nerve paralysis occurred in only 14 of the 500 cases (2·8 per cent) but it was the initial sign of the disease in 2 patients. Four of the facial palsies were presumed to be nuclear because the midbrain and cerebellum were extensively involved. Granulomas in the middle and posterior cranial fossae involved the facial and other cranial nerves in 2 cases. In the remaining 8 cases, the facial nerve was involved by granulomas in the temporal bone. Tos was struck by the fact that although 472 temporal bones were eroded, often very extensively, by this disease only 8 patients had intratemporal facial paralysis and only one had bilateral facial paralysis. Although the bony Fallopian canal is often destroyed the nerve sheath is extremely resistant to invasion or compression by these soft granulomas. Tos attributed the facial paralysis to interference with the blood-supply of the nerve. All the reported intratemporal facial palsies improved quickly, either spontaneously or after radiotherapy. This is quite contrary to what is found with cholesteatomas (epidermoids) which are also soft osteolytic masses. When they produce intratemporal facial palsy, spontaneous improvement does not occur.

Eosinophilic granulomas are the least severe of these granulomatous diseases and the long-term survival of these patients is good. There are not many recorded cases of temporal bone involvement in this disease. Toothill *et al.* (1973) were able to find only 13 cases of eosinophilic granuloma of the temporal bone recorded in the literature during the 20 years from 1952–72. Otorrhoea, post-auricular swelling, and pain were the most common presenting symptoms. Erosion of the bony facial canal was reported in 8 of the temporal bones with actual facial paralysis in 2 patients. Toothill described 3 further cases of his own none of whom suffered from facial palsy, although in the two cases whose temporal bone he explored, erosion of the Fallopian canal was found.

Wegener's granuloma and periarteritis nodosa Wegener's granulomatosis is classified as one of the collagen diseases and it is considered to be a variant of periarteritis nodosa.

Three types of lesions occur:

(1) necrotizing granulomas of the respiratory tract including the nose, sinuses, orbit, and middle ear;
(2) focal necrotizing vasculitis of arteries and veins;
(3) glomerulonephritis with granulomatous changes in the kidney.

The aetiology is unknown but an allergic hypersensitivity mechanism is suspected.

When Wegener's granuloma affects the middle ear the clinical and radiological appearances are indistinguishable from those of malignant neoplasms of the temporal bone.

The cranial nerves can be involved by invasion from granulomas in the adjacent paranasal sinuses, by granulomatous lesions along the lower brain stem, and by vasculitis of the vasa nervorum. A mononeuritis multiplex often results. Drachman (1963) found involvement of the cranial and peripheral nerves in at least 28 per cent of cases. If the facial nerve is involved by a granulomatous lesion the paralysis is likely to be progressive. The neuropathy produced by vasculitis of the vasa nervorum may be transitory but more often it is progressive.

It may be worth mentioning at this point that facial paralysis is sometimes found in the other collagen diseases, e.g. rheumatoid arthritis, systemic lupus erythematosis, cranial arteritis, and Sjogren's syndrome. In the latter disease the facial paralysis is independent of the parotid enlargement. A mononeuritis multiplex may be seen in these connective tissue diseases and is responsible for the facial palsy which sometimes occurs.

Other diseases involving the temporal bone Some of the other diseases which can involve the temporal bone and produce occasional facial paralysis may be briefly considered here.

Osteopetrosis (synonyms: marble bone disease; Albers Schonberg's disease) This disease is characterized by excessive density of all the bones. Involvement of the skull leads to narrowing of the foramina with compression of cranial nerves causing impairment of vision, facial paralysis, and deafness.

Von Recklinghausen's disease of bone In generalized osteitis fibrosa there is a great disturbance of calcium metabolism due to parathyroid hyperfunction. The bones become softened and are often enlarged. In addition tumour-like swellings may occur in them. Page *et al.* (1975) described a remarkable case with facial and auditory nerve palsies due to bony changes in the internal auditory canal. When the offending parathyroid adenoma was removed by Page, the radiological changes of the petrous apex improved markedly and both the facial paralysis and the neural deafness also improved. Facial paralysis was the presenting symptom and Bell's palsy was the initial diagnosis before the patient was referred to these authors.

Paget's disease (synonym: osteitis deformans) This disease is also characterized by enlargement of the bones and a certain degree of softening. The parathyroid function and the serum calcium and phosphorus levels are all normal, but the alkaline phosphatase is greatly increased. The aetiology remains completely unknown. Narrowing of skull foramina has produced deafness and facial paralysis in some patients. The facial nerve may also be involved throughout its course in the Fallopian canal. Nager (1975) has demonstrated quite marked narrowing of the Fallopian canal by new bone in his excellent description of Paget's disease of the temporal bone.

Parotid tumours

Neoplasms of salivary glands constitute approximately 5 per cent of all head and neck tumours. About 70 per cent of salivary gland tumours occur in the parotid glands and approximately 70 per cent of this group are benign (Edgerton and Williams 1972). Conley (1975) recorded that 13 per cent of his series of 280 malignant parotid tumours had pre-operative facial paralysis and he quotes that in other published series the incidence varies between 8 and 33 per cent. Facial paralysis in benign and inflammatory conditions of the parotid gland is extremely rare and is usually due to coincidental pathology unrelated to the benign lesion of the gland. In Conley's view, 'facial nerve paresis in the presence of a parotid tumour is almost pathognomic of cancer'. The more aggressive or the more undifferentiated the tumour, the more likely it is to invade the facial nerve and its branches. Many clinicians have come to regard the involvement of the facial nerve as an indication of a highly malignant tumour with a poor prognosis. Within certain limits this is true, although it should be remembered that the development of facial paralysis is influenced by the site and size of the cancer as well as by its degree of malignancy. Eneroth (1972) reviewed the cases of parotid tumours seen at the Karolinska Otolaryngology Department, Stockholm, during the 50 years 1919–69. 2158 true salivary gland tumours were recorded, 378 of which were malignant. Forty-six (12 per cent) of the malignant tumours produced facial palsy, an incidence very similar to that recorded by Conley.

Interestingly enough 6 of Eneroth's 46 malignant parotid cases had facial palsy as the first and only symptom or sign of their disease. The interval between the onset of the paralysis and the diagnosis of the tumour in these 6 patients varied from one month to 2 years. Eneroth emphasized that in a patient with a spontaneously developing facial palsy of unknown cause, an occult malignant tumour of the parotid must be considered, especially if topographic tests suggest an infraforaminal lesion.

Diseases of the nervous system

Multiple sclerosis

This interesting disease produces a great variety of focal lesions in the central nervous system. The essential pathological process is a patch of demyelination in the white matter of the brain and spinal cord. After the damaged myelin has been removed remyelination can occur. After several attacks of demyelination, the healing process of gliosis prevents further remyelination taking place and permanent sclerosis and loss of function results.

Although the lesions do not involve peripheral nerves, multiple sclerosis produces supranuclear, nuclear, and infranuclear lesions of the facial nerve. Plaques of disease can involve the white matter of the corticonuclear tracts and produce weakness and spasticity of the facial muscles. Hemifacial spasm is sometimes seen in multiple sclerosis and is considered by some to be due to a supranuclear irritative lesion. The spasm may exist without an associated facial paralysis or it may precede or follow a facial palsy.

Facial myokymia also occurs in multiple sclerosis and it does not progress to a palsy. Myokymia is considered to be due to a plaque impinging on the facial nucleus in the pons. Andermann *et al.* (1961) believed that myokymia usually occurs early in the disease and that it can be a useful diagnostic sign.

Lower motor facial paralysis is not uncommon in multiple sclerosis. It is frequently stated that a characteristic feature of this paralysis is the retention of normal taste sensation, and there appear to be only a few exceptions to this general rule. The reason for this feature is that the plaque or patch of sclerosis involves the infranuclear motor fibres which run through the pons. Afferent taste fibres in the nervus intermedius, on the other hand, pass to the nucleus solitarius in the medulla. Oppenheim (1911) pointed out that facial paralysis can herald the onset of the disease. In Muller's (1949) series 5 per cent of his cases had facial paralysis as the first sign of multiple sclerosis.

Unlike Bell's palsy and herpes zoster oticus the onset of facial palsy in multiple sclerosis is painless and this may help in the differential diagnosis. Like all the other focal lesions in multiple sclerosis, the three types of facial nerve lesions tend to recover quickly and completely although they may recur during the long course of the disease.

Motor neurone disease

The basic pathological feature of this disease is a loss of neurones in the ventral horns of the spinal cord and in the motor nuclei of the lower brain stem. The sixth, fourth, and third cranial nerve nuclei are very rarely affected so that ocular movements remain normal while limb, trunk, and facial muscles become progressively weaker. In addition to the steady degeneration of lower motor neurones, many patients have loss of myelin in the anterior lateral white columns and loss of upper motor neurones in the cortex.

The clinical picture of the disease is of an asymmetric progressive muscular atrophy with fasciculations and weakness. The disease may start in the muscles of a limb but sometimes weakness in the face, mouth, and tongue is the initial sign. The weakness of the facial muscles may be accompanied by weakness of the muscles of mastication supplied by the trigeminal nerve. In these circumstances the patient has difficulty in chewing food and in keeping it from collecting in the buccal space between teeth and cheek. In addition, atrophy of the tongue muscles makes it difficult to move the food into the pharynx to initiate swallowing. Classic motor neurone disease usually begins in the seventh decade and has a well marked familial incidence.

Juvenile motor neurone disease In South India a special subgroup of motor neurone disease is recognized by its frequent occurrence in the first and second decades of life. A high incidence of involvement of the facial and bulbar nuclei is found. The facial muscles are often asymmetrically affected and the condition is not considered to be familial (Spillane 1973).

Epilepsy

An upper motor facial paresis is sometimes seen in temporal lobe epilepsy but it does not seem to be a particularly important feature of the disease. Its occurrence suggests a spread of the seizure discharge across the sylvian fissure. One would expect the facial weakness to be of brief duration.

Remillard *et al.* (1977) have recently drawn attention to the presence of prolonged and presumably permanent facial weakness in their series of 50 consecutive patients with temporal lobe seizures. Thirty-seven patients (74 per cent) had a unilateral temporal focus and 13 (26 per cent) had bitemporal foci. In the unilateral group of 37 patients 13 per cent had a symmetrical face, 13 per cent had an ipsilateral facial weakness, and 73 per cent had contra-lateral facial weakness. The weakness was usually more striking on emotional movement. In the group of 13 patients with bitemporal independent discharges, 61 per cent had facial asymmetry. These authors felt that facial weakness could be employed as a useful though not absolute lateralizing sign.

Cerebrovascular disease

Vascular causes of upper motor neurone lesions are widely recognized and haemorrhage embolism and thrombosis can produce cerebrovascular accidents of varying severity. Upper motor facial paralysis is usually a fairly obvious feature of hemiplegia from a vascular lesion of the internal capsule.

Brain-stem vascular accidents produce a characteristic crossed paralysis. In pontine haemorrhage, for example, the early clinical features are an ipsilateral lower motor facial palsy with a flaccid paralysis of the limbs of the opposite side. Extension of the haemorrhage soon involves the other side of the pons and quite often the signs are bilateral from the beginning. When both sides of the pons are thus involved, a bilateral lower facial palsy is accompanied by a bilateral upper motor paralysis of the arms and legs.

Focal vascular lesions causing facial paralysis are occasionally seen in rare aneurysms, in migraine, in Moschcowitz's disease, and in hypertension.

Aneurysm of the internal auditory artery has occasionally mimicked a cerebellopontine angle tumour and been diagnosed only at operation. Transient hemiplegia with upper motor neurone facial paralysis may occur in migraine. The diagnosis is usually obvious because it is accompanied by the familiar features of migraine and is followed by rapid and complete recovery.

Moschcowitz's disease In this condition of unknown aetiology, a thrombocytopenic micro-angiothrombosis produces neurological signs in roughly half of the patients. A great variety of general and focal signs are encountered including headache, vomiting, convulsions, hemiplegia, monoplegia, and cranial nerve palsies. Facial paralysis has been reported on a number of occasions. Like the other neurological signs in this disease the facial paralysis tends to appear abruptly and regress spontaneously (d'Eramo and Levi 1972).

Hypertension One of the earliest reports of facial paralysis due to hypertension is to be found in an article by Moxon (1869). He recorded the development of a facial palsy, shortly before death, in a 48-year-old man with Bright's disease. Autopsy revealed a haemorrhage into the Fallopian canal. The level of the blood-pressure was not stated but hypertension was inferred. Keith *et al.* (1928) noted two patients with facial palsy in their series of 81 patients with malignant hypertension. One was a 37-year-old lady with severe hypertension and visual disturbances and the other was a 15-year-old girl with hypertension and albuminuria. Amberg (1929) gave further details of this 15-year-old girl and also described two younger children with facial paralysis. All three children had malignant hypertension. Further autopsy evidence that facial paralysis in hypertensive subjects can be caused by haemorrhage into the Fallopian canal was provided by Monier-Vinard and Puech (1930). Their patient was a 21-year-old man with chronic nephritis, hypertension, and severe papilloedema who developed a right facial paralysis shortly before death. The post-mortem examination revealed a recent haemorrhage into the right Fallopian canal.

In a review of the neurological complications of malignant hypertension Clarke and Murphy (1956) found that in a series of 190 patients with malignant hypertension, 73 patients (38 per cent) had nervous system involvement, and 7 patients (3·7 per cent) had peripheral facial paralysis. More recently, Lloyd *et al.* (1966) reported the occurrence of lower motor facial paralysis in 7 (20 per cent) of the 35 children with severe hypertension seen at the Great Ormond Street Hospital in the preceding 10 years. The facial paralysis recovered in all patients, but 2 had a second episode of paralysis coinciding with an exacerbation of their hypertension. The causal relationship between severe hypertension and peripheral facial paralysis, particularly in young people, seems to be well established by these reports. The differential diagnosis between hypertensive facial paralysis and idiopathic facial paralysis is more difficult in the middle-aged and elderly who have a greater incidence of hypertension. This diagnostic problem was discussed by Merwarth (1942), who suggested that hypertensive facial paralysis can be distinguished by its abrupt onset, the absence of associated pain around the ear, and by the absence of taste disturbance. It is difficult to accept his claim that taste sensation is preserved in hypertensive facial paralysis, particularly in view of Moxon's (1869) autopsy finding of haemorrhage which was maximal at the geniculate ganglion level.

It seems reasonable to conclude that in a patient with peripheral facial paralysis and malignant hypertension, the hypertension is likely to be a causative factor if the onset of paralysis is abrupt and not accompanied by peri-auricular pain, and if there is a history of other hypertensive haemorrhages, e.g. repeated epistaxes, retinal haemorrhages, etc. In a patient with facial palsy and the benign form of hypertension, the hypertension is likely to be a coincidental factor.

Toxic neuropathy

Toxic neuropathies can result from exposure to certain drugs, metals, and industrial chemicals. Although the toxic substances are of a very diverse nature, the clinical features they produce have many similarities since they result from peripheral nerve damage.

The peripheral neuropathy is usually symmetrically distributed but mononeuropathy multiplex is sometimes seen. Facial paralysis never occurs as an isolated feature in toxic neuropathies and it is usually seen as one of several nervous system signs in a multisystem disorder. It would serve no useful purpose to list all those neuropathies in which facial nerve lesions have been recorded, even if it was possible to do so. The following examples have been selected because of their general interest and their well-recognized association with facial paralysis.

Trichloroethylene (trilene, $CHCl \cdot CCl_2$)

This substance is used medically as an anaesthetic agent and industrially as a de-greasing agent and solvent. In its pure form the substance appears to be safe, but impurities or breakdown products in it cause cranial nerve damage. Decomposition of trilene occurs when it is used as an anaesthetic agent in a closed circuit with soda lime. Dichloroacetylene is the breakdown product that is thought to be responsible for the neuropathy. Now that soda lime is no longer used with trilene in anaesthesia, neuropathy does not occur in these circumstances today.

However, scattered reports of cranial nerve damage following industrial exposure still appear (Buxton and Hayward 1967). The trigeminal nerve is the most frequently affected but damage to cranial nerves 2–7 and to cranial nerves, 9, 10, and 12 have been reported, and bulbar palsy is sometimes the principal clinical feature. Buxton and Hayward suggest that the toxic effect of trilene is exerted on the nerve cells directly rather than on the peripheral nerve. Cranial nerve palsies commence 8–48 hours after exposure and progress over several days. Partial recovery may take place over the ensuing 18 months.

Metals

Arsenic Arsenical neuropathy usually takes the form of a mixed sensory and motor symmetrical involvement of the lower limbs. More severe intoxication leads to involvement of the upper limbs also, but usually of a much milder degree. Cranial nerve paralysis is uncommon in arsenic poisoning but both unilateral and bilateral facial paralysis have been recorded. Mercury poisoning produces a somewhat similar picture.

In arsenic neuropathy the neurones appear to suffer principally, and Wallerian degeneration of the axons is the usual finding in the peripheral nerve.

Lead Neuropathy due to lead poisoning differs from arsenical neuropathy in some interesting and unexplained ways. For example, the peripheral neuropathy produced in adults is not always symmetrical and it involves the upper limbs more often than the lower limbs. In children lead poisoning may cause an encephalopathy more frequently than a peripheral neuropathy.

Monoplegia, diplegia, hemiplegia, and upper motor neurone facial paralysis are seen in patients with severe central nervous system involvement.

When lead intoxication produces a peripheral neuropathy, segmental demyelination and some axonal degeneration are found.

Aluminium Aluminium poisoning is a rarity. It has been the subject of considerable interest, however, since McLaughlin *et al.* (1962) described an encephalopathy similar to lead encephalopathy with upper motor facial paresis in a man who was exposed to high concentrations of aluminium at work. In 1972, Alfrey *et al.* described a new syndrome of unknown aetiology in patients undergoing renal dialysis, which has come to be known as progressive dialysis encephalopathy. Some patients have focal neurological deficits, most commonly a facial weakness, and some have convulsions. The encephalopathy is similar to that described by McLaughlin *et al.* In 1976 Alfrey *et al.* reported an increased aluminium content in the brain, bone, and muscle in dialysis patients with and without the encephalopathy syndrome. Further evidence is required to prove a causal relationship between aluminium and dialysis encephalopathy.

Gold Toxic complications following the use of gold salts in the treatment of rheumatoid arthritis are not uncommon, and fever and skin rashes are the two most frequent manifestations. Occasional cases of cranial nerve damage in which facial weakness was a feature have been recorded. However, it is well recognized that peripheral neuropathy is a complication of rheumatoid arthritis and it seems impossible to be certain whether the facial paralysis should be attributed to the disease or the treatment.

Drug-induced dyskinesia

The toxic neuropathies we have described have all produced paralysis of function. It is worth remembering that certain drugs will produce stimulation of movement with facial and oral dyskinesias. The phenothiazines are particularly liable to produce this effect. Some patients appear to have a personal idiosyncrasy, for symptoms begin in the early stages of treatment, and usually subside when the drug is withdrawn. The dyskinesia may be delayed in onset and associated with the features of drug-induced Parkinsonism. The patient may then have irregular spasms affecting the muscles of the mouth and lips with an otherwise expressionless facies. (See Chapter 4, p. 126.)

Peripheral neuropathy can be caused by many other drugs, especially antibacterial drugs such as sulphonamides, isoniazid, and the nitrofurans, sedative drugs such as thalidomide, and anticancer drugs such as vincristine.

In the majority of these cases the neuropathy is primarily sensory and affects the limbs. Cranial nerve abnormalities do not seem to occur to any significant extent and there are few reports in the literature. Hussain and Koilpillai (1960) and Lee (1960) have recorded cranial nerve lesions following treatment with the nitrofuran derivative furaltadone (Altafur) but no cases of facial palsy were recorded.

Metabolic neuropathy

Diabetes mellitus

Diabetes mellitus is a generalized metabolic disorder characterized by an inappropriate elevation of the blood glucose level. A relative or absolute deficiency of insulin is responsible for the hyperglycaemia, but the fundamental mechanism causing the insulin lack is unknown. The disease is prone to damage the vascular system by causing atherosclerosis and micro-angiopathy. Diabetes mellitus also seems to have a special tendency to produce central and peripheral nervous system disorders.

The peripheral nervous system disorders are more common and have been classified as follows:

(1) symmetric peripheral neuropathy;
(2) asymmetric peripheral neuropathy (a mononeuropathy or mononeuropathy multiplex);
(3) radiculopathy;
(4) autonomic visceral neuropathy;
(5) cranial neuropathy and retinopathy.

Our particular interest is in the fourth and fifth groups and it is widely accepted that cranial nerve palsies occur much more often in diabetics than in non-diabetic subjects.

Interestingly enough, multiple symmetrical bilateral cranial nerve palsies, including bilateral facial palsy, have been recorded (Larson and Auchincloss 1950). The clinical picture resembled that of the Guillain–Barré syndrome. However, asymmetric involvement of the cranial nerves is more usually seen. The external ocular muscles supplied by the third, fourth, and sixth cranial nerves are the most frequently affected. The facial nerve is the next most commonly involved. The onset of facial palsy in diabetic neuropathy is usually abrupt, like that seen in Bell's palsy and is often accompanied by pain behind the ear.

The presence of a unilateral peripheral facial paralysis in a diabetic presents a diagnostic dilemma. One might reasonably argue that the presence of diabetes renders the diagnosis of idiopathic facial paralysis untenable, and many clinicians would attribute all such paralyses to diabetic neuropathy. However, if this line of reasoning is followed to its logical conclusion, one is left in the indefensible position of maintaining that Bell's palsy never occurs in diabetics and therefore diabetes must in some way confer total immunity from Bell's paralysis.

We believe that in a diabetic patient it is impossible to distinguish a Bell's palsy from a diabetic neuropathy of the facial nerve with any degree of certainty. Diabetic neuropathy is particularly associated with uncontrolled diabetic states. The presence of uncontrolled diabetes, and the co-existence of other diabetic neuropathies in a patient, make it seem more reasonable to attribute a facial palsy to the diabetes. Conversely, in the presence of well-controlled diabetes and in the absence of other diabetic neuropathies, the diagnosis of Bell's palsy seems not unreasonable.

The quoted incidence of facial paralysis in diabetics varies enormously. This is partly due to variations in the methods and criteria used to establish the diagnosis of diabetes. It is also partly due to the selection of patients in different series, since the type of medical practice and the age and race of the patients vary from series to series. Adour *et al.* (1974) quote that the incidence of diabetics in the U.S.A. is estimated to be 2–4 per cent of the population. In their large series of facial paralysis they found that 10 per cent had diabetes. Not only did they conclude that facial palsy was much more common in diabetics than in non-diabetics, but they found a greater degree of neural degeneration in diabetics and a correspondingly poorer degree of recovery of facial nerve function.

Autonomic visceral neuropathy The presence of vasomotor, trophic, and other autonomic disorders in diabetics is widely recognized. In the skin, sweating deficiencies, loss of vasomotor control, and neurogenic ulcers occur. Orthostatic hypotension, bladder and sphincter disturbances, and impotence are also well-established features of diabetic autonomic neuropathy. However, Watkins (1973) described facial sweating during eating (gustatory sweating) as a new sign of diabetic autonomic neuropathy. In his group of 6 patients the sweating was very severe and was provoked by many foodstuffs, cheese being the most powerful stimulus. Atropine inhibited the gustatory sweating and the unpleasant symptom was effectively controlled by oral anticholinergic drugs, e.g. propantheline. The area of skin involved in gustatory sweating extended from the scalp to the level of the third or fourth dermatome but was always restricted to the territory of the superior cervical ganglion. All 6 patients had other features of diabetic autonomic neuropathy, e.g. diarrhoea, postural hypotension, etc. Watkins suggested that the mechanism producing this gustatory sweating was degeneration of autonomic vagal fibres, followed by abnormal nerve regeneration between fibres of the vagus and sympathetic cholinergic sweat fibres at the level of the superior cervical ganglion.

Pathology of diabetic neuropathy The basic pathogenesis of diabetic neuropathy is unknown but there is general agreement that the major change which occurs in peripheral nerves is a patchy segmental demyelination. Whether the segmental demyelination is primary, i.e. due to a disturbance affecting the Schwann cells, or the myelin itself, or whether it is secondary to axonal (or neuronal) disease is not fully known. The majority of authorities hold that it is primary. Autopsy evidence of demyelination was found by Asbury *et al.* (1970). They recorded the findings in a diabetic lady who died one month after the onset of a left third nerve paralysis. She had had a right third nerve palsy three years previously which had recovered spontaneously. The autopsy showed demyelination of the left third nerve and a normal right third nerve. It was assumed that demyelination had been present in the right third nerve at the time of the original paralysis and recovery by remyelination had taken place.

De Jong (1976) states that most current investigators believe atherosclerosis and other vascular disease play little part in the development of symmetric peripheral neuropathy. However, they think that vascular disturbances may play a significant part in the development of the mononeuropathies, autonomic neuropathies, and the cranial neuropathies, all of which have an abrupt onset and may improve spontaneously.

Apart from diabetes mellitus, no other endocrine disorder regularly causes facial paralysis. Compression of the median nerve in the carpal tunnel syndrome is often seen in acromegaly and in hypothyroidism but entrapment neuropathy of the facial nerve does not occur in these conditions.

The interesting facial palsy due to hyperparathyroidism recorded by Page *et al.* (1975) must be an extraordinarily rare occurrence (Chap. 3, p. 103).

Amyloidosis

The occurrence of peripheral nerve disorders in amyloidosis is well known, both in the genetically determined variety and in the acquired types. The histological picture is one of massive endoneurial deposition of amyloid, which appears to cause impairment of nerve function by compression of the fibres. In a minority of cases, amyloid deposition may be almost completely restricted to blood-vessel walls, and narrowing of the vasa nervorum produces ischaemic nerve damage. Neuropathy from extrinsic compression also occurs and the carpal tunnel syndrome may be seen in this disease. Cranial nerve palsies are not common but paralysis of the facial, auditory, and hypoglossal nerves and ocular palsies have been noted.

Cranial neuropathy as the principal manifestation of the disease was described in a small group of patients with hereditary amyloidosis by Meretoja and Teppo (1971). Cranial nerve palsies appeared in the fifth decade of life in this small group and the facial nerve was the one most frequently involved.

Post-mortem examination in one case showed that a branch of the facial nerve was almost totally replaced by amyloid.

Porphyria

Neurological disturbances are found in the hepatic forms of porphyria, particularly in acute intermittent porphyria (Swedish type) and in variagate porphyria (South African type). Although the porphyrias are a group of genetically determined metabolic disorders, attacks of porphyric neuropathy are nearly always precipitated by certain drugs. The porphyria-inducing compounds include: barbiturates, oestrogens and progesterones, sulphonamides, chloramphenicol, griseofulvin, diazepam, meprobamate, hydantoins, succinamides, ergot, glutethemide, methyldopa, chlorpropamide, and tolbutamide.

The most prominent feature of porphyric neuropathy is a symmetrical polyneuropathy affecting the upper limbs more severely than the lower limbs. This may progress to involve the trunk and bulbar muscles and cause death from respiratory failure. Focal cranial and peripheral nerve involvement is also common. The tenth and seventh cranial nerves are the most frequently affected and bilateral facial paralysis may occur. Ocular disturbances are a well-recognized feature of porphyric neuropathy and the fifth, eleventh, and twelfth cranial nerves are also occasionally involved.

The primary neuropathologic lesion in porphyria is axonal degeneration together with some demyelination. It is not known whether the axonal and neuronal metabolic disorder is primary or whether it is secondary to disordered porphyrin metabolism in the liver.

Beriberi

This disease is said to be named from the Hindustani word meaning 'swelling of the legs' or 'unsteady gait'. It is a deficiency disorder due to lack of vitamin B_1 (thiamin). The oedema of the legs is often accompanied by pericardial, pleural, and peritoneal effusions.

In the subacute and chronic forms of the disease neurological defects are a prominent feature and take the form of a severe motor and sensory polyneuropathy in half of the cases.

The vagus is the commonest cranial nerve to be involved in this disease and this results in tachycardia, vocal cord paralysis, and dysphagia in severe cases.

Victor (1975) quotes an article by Pekelharing and Winkler (1887) who found facial weakness in 5 cases in a series of 80 patients, '. . . four times in the muscles around the angles of the mouth and once in the orbicularis palpebrum'.

Bilateral facial paresis has also been reported in association with severe beriberi by Denny-Brown (1947), and more recently Erbslöh and Abel (1970) state that electromyographic studies show that the facial nerve is far more often involved than was previously realized.

Other metabolic neuropathies

Lower motor facial paralysis or facial weakness is sometimes seen in other rare metabolic neuropathies, e.g. metachromatic leucodystrophy (sulphatide neuropathy) and Tangier disease. It is, however, only a minor and occasional feature of these uncommon conditions. In Refsum's disease the only two cranial nerves that appear to be involved occasionally are the first and eighth, causing anosmia and deafness.

References

Adams, G. L., Paparella, M. M., and El Fiky, F. M. (1971). Primary and metastatic tumors of the temporal bone. *Laryngoscope* **81**, 1273.

Adour, K. K., Bell, D. N., and Wingerd, J. (1974). Bell's palsy. Dilemma of diabetes mellitus. *Arch. Otolaryngol.* **99**, 104.

Aitken, R. S. and Brain, R. T. (1933). Facial palsy and infection with the zoster virus. *Lancet* **i**, 19.

Aleksic, S. N., Budzilovich, G. N., and Lieberman, A. N. (1973). Herpes zoster oticus and facial paralysis (Ramsay Hunt Syndrome). *J. neurol. Sci.* **20**, 149.

Alfrey, A. C., Mishell, J. M., Burks, J., Contiguglia, S. R., Rudolph, H., Lewin, E., and Holmes, J. H. (1972). Syndrome of dyspraxia and multifocal seizures associated with chronic haemodialysis. *Trans. Amer. Soc. Artificial inter. Organs* **18**, 257.

——, Le Gendre, G. R., and Kaehny, W. D. (1976). The dialysis encephalopathy syndrome. Possible aluminium intoxication. *New Eng. J. Med.* **294**, 184.

Amberg, S. (1929). Hypertension in the young. *Amer. J. Dis. Child.* **37**, 335.

Andermann, F., Cosgrove, J. B. R., Lloyd Smith, D. S., Gloor, P., and McNaughton, F. L. (1961). Facial myokymia in multiple sclerosis. *Brain* **84**, 31.

Asbury, A. K., Aldredge, H., Hershberg, R., and Fisher, C. M. (1970). Oculomotor palsy in diabetes mellitus: a clinico-pathological study. *Brain* **93**, 555.

Austin, J. H. (1958). Recurrent polyneuropathies and their corticosteroid treatment. *Brain* **81**, 157.

Ballantyne, J. W. (1904). *Manual of antenatal pathology and hygiene. The embryo.* London Green.

Beeson, P. B., and McDermott, W. (1975). *Textbook of medicine* (14th edn). Saunders, Philadelphia.

Bell, W. E., and McCormick, W. E. (1975). *Neurologic infections in children*, p. 196. Saunders, Philadelphia, London, and Toronto.

Blackley, B., Friedmann, I., and Wright, I. (1967). Herpes zoster auris associated with facial nerve palsy and auditory nerve symptoms. *Acta Otolaryngol. (Stockh.)* **63**, 533.

Boudouresques, J., Khalil, R., Vigouroux, R. A., Daniel, F., and Gosset, A. (1970). In *Handbook of clinical Neurology* (ed. E. J. Vinken and G. W. Bruyn), Vol. 7. North-Holland, Amsterdam.

Bradley, W. G. (1971) Nerve, muscle, and muscular dystrophy. *Develop. Med. Child Neurol.* **13**, 528.

Breadon, G. E., Cody, D. T. R., and Weiland, L. H. (1977). Facial palsy. Unusual etiology. *Laryngoscope* **87**, 26.

Buxton, P. H., and Hayward, M. (1967). Polyneuritis cranialis associated with industrial trichloroethylene poisoning. *J. Neurol. Neurosurg. Psychiat.* **30**, 511.

Cayler, G. C. (1967). An epidemic of congenital facial paresis and heart disease. *Paediatrics* **40**, 666.

Chandler, J. R. (1972). Pathogenesis and treatment of facial paralysis due to malignant external otitis. *Ann. Otol.* (*St. Louis*) **81**, 648.

Chisholm, J. J. (1882). Congenital paralysis of the sixth and seventh pairs of cranial nerves in an adult. *Arch. Ophthal.* **11**, 323.

Clarke, E., and Murphy, E. A. (1956). Neurological manifestations of malignant hypertension. *Brit. med. J.* **2**, 1319.

Cochrane, R. G. (1964). In *Leprosy in theory and practice* (ed. R. G. Cochrane and T. F. Davey), 2nd ed*n*, p. 4. John Wright, Bristol.

Conley, J. (1975). In *Salivary glands and the facial nerve*, p. 197. Georg Thieme, Stuttgart.

——, and Janecka, I. (1974). Schwann cell tumors of the facial nerve. *Laryngoscope* **84**, 958.

Danis, P. (1945). Les paralysies oculofaciales congenitales. *Ophthalmologica* (*Basel*) **110**, 113.

Dastur, F. D., Shahani, M. T., Dastoor, D. H., Kohiyar, F. N., Bharucha, E. P., Mondkar, V. P., Kashyap, G. H., and Nair, K. G. (1977). Cephalic tetanus: demonstration of a dual lesion. *J. Neurol. Neurosurg. Psychiat.* **40**, 782.

Debain, J. J., Siardet, J., Francois, J., and Rouberol (1966). Meningiome du nerf facial intra-tympanique. *Ann. Oto-laryng.* (*Paris*) **83**, 397.

De Jong, R. N. (1976). In *Handbook of neurology* (ed. P. J. Vinken and G. W. Bruyn), Vol. 27, p. 110. North-Holland, Amsterdam.

Denny-Brown, D. (1947). Neurological conditions resulting from prolonged and severe dietary restrictions. *Medicine* (*Baltimore*) **26**, 41.

——, Adams, R. D., and Fitzgerald, P. J. (1944). Pathologic features of herpes zoster. A note on "geniculate herpes". *Arch. Neurol. Psychiat.* (*Chic.*) **51**, 216.

Drachman, D. A. (1963). Neurological complications of Wegener's granulomatosis. *Arch. Neurol.* (*Chic.*) **8**, 145.

Edgerton, M. T. and Williams, G. S. (1972). In *Davis-Christopher Textbook of surgery.* (ed. D. C. Sabiston Jr), p. 1268. Saunders, Philadelphia, London, and Toronto.

Eneroth, C. M. (1972). Facial nerve paralysis. A criterion of malignancy in parotid tumours. *Arch. Otolaryngol.* **95**, 300.

Engler, C. W., and Missal, S. C. (1955). Involvement of the cranial nerves in poliomyelitis. *Trans. Amer. Acad. Ophthalmol. Otolaryngol.* **59**, 732.

Engström, H., and Wohlfart, G. (1949). Herpes zoster of the seventh, eighth, ninth and tenth cranial nerves. *Arch. Neurol. Psychiat.* (*Chic.*) **62**, 638.

d'Eramo, N., and Levi, M. (1972). In Neurological symptoms in blood diseases. Ch. 5, p. 95. Harvey Miller and Medcalf, London.

Erbslöh, F., and Abel, M. (1970). In *Handbook of clinical neurology* (ed. P. J. Vinken and G. W. Bruyn), Vol. 7, p. 561. North-Holland, Amsterdam.

Evans, P. R. (1955). Moebius syndrome: the congenital facial diplegia syndrome. *Arch. Dis. Child.* **30**, 237.

Farber, S. (1941). The nature of "solitary or eosinophilic granuloma" of bone. *Amer. J. Path.* **17**, 625.

Figi, F. A., and Hempstead, B. E. (1943). Malignant tumors of middle ear and mastoid process. *Arch. Otolaryngol.* **37**, 149.

Fondu, P., and De Meuter, F. (1969). Facial palsy, a manifestation of acquired toxoplasmosis. *Helv. Paediat. Acta* **24**, 208.

Ford, F. R. (1973). *Diseases of the nervous system in infancy, childhood, and adolescence*, 6th Edn, p. 66. Charles C. Thomas, Springfield, Illinois.

Francois, J. (1963). *La toxoplasmose et ses manifestations oculaires*, p. 144. Masson et Cie, Paris.

Gordon, G. (1966). The mechanism of thalidomide deformities correlated with the pathologic effects of prolonged dosage in adults. *Develop. Med. Child. Neurol.* **8**, 761.

Guttmann, M. R., and Simon, M. U. (1951). Neurofibrosarcoma of the facial nerve involving the tympanomastoid. *Arch. Otolaryngol.* **54**, 162.

Hanson, P. A., and Rowland, L. P. (1971). Moebius syndrome and facioscapulo-humeral muscular dystrophy. *Arch. Neurol.* (*Chic.*) **24**, 31.

Harlan, G. C. (1881). *Trans. Amer. ophthal. Soc.* **3**, 216.

Head, H., and Campbell, A. W. (1900). The pathology of herpes zoster and its bearing on sensory localization. *Brain* **23**, 353.

Henderson, J. L. (1939). The congenital facial diplegia syndrome; clinical features, pathology, and aetiology. *Brain* **62**, 381.

Hoefnagel, D., and Penry, J. K. (1960). Partial facial paralysis in young children. *New Eng. J. Med.* **262**, 1126.

Huebner, O. (1900). Uber angeborenen Kernmangel (infantiler Kernschwund, Moebius). *Charite-Ann.* **25**, 211.

Hunt, J. R. (1907). On herpetic inflammation of the geniculate ganglion; a new syndrome and its complications. *J. nerv. ment. Dis.* **34**, 73.

——. (1915). The sensory field of the facial nerve; a further contribution to the symptomatology of the geniculate ganglion. *Brain* **38**, 418.

Hussain, K. K., and Koilpillai, H. (1960) Toxic effects of furaltadone. *Lancet* **ii**, 490.

Illis, L. S. (1975). In *Viral diseases of the central nervous system*, p. 8. Ballière and Tindall, London.

Joachims, H. Z. (1976). Malignant external otitis in children. *Arch. Otolaryngol.* **102**, 236.

Keith, M. N., Wagener, H. P., and Kernohan, J. W. (1928). The syndrome of malignant hypertension. *Arch. intern. Med.* **41**, 141.

Kettle, K. (1950). Intratemporal sarcoma of the facial nerve. *Arch. Otolaryngol.* **52**, 778.

——. (1959). In *Peripheral facial palsy; pathology and surgery*. Thomas, Springfield, Illinois.

Lambert, V., and Richards, S. H. (1964). Facial palsy in Heerfordt's syndrome. *J. Laryngol. Otol.* **78**, 684.

Larson, D. L., and Auchincloss, J. H. (1950). Multiple symmetric bilateral cranial nerve palsies in patients with unregulated diabetes mellitus. *Arch. intern. Med.* **85**, 265.

Lee, M. L. H. (1960). Toxic effects of prolonged treatment with furaltadone. *Lancet* **ii**, 374.

Lichtenstein, L. (1953). Histiocytosis X. *Arch. Path.* **56**, 84.

Lieberman, P. H. (1975). In *Textbook of medicine* (ed. P. B. Beeson and W. McDermott), p. 1529. Saunders, Philadelphia, London, and Toronto.

Livingstone, G. (1965). Congenital ear anomalies due to thalidomide. *Proc. roy. Soc. Med.* **58**, 493.

Lloyd, A. V. C., Jewitt, D. E., and Still, J. D. L. (1966). Facial paralysis in children with hypertension. *Arch. Dis. Child.* **41**, 292.

Mann, W. N. (1975) (ed.) *Coneybeare's Textbook of medicine*, 16th edn, p. 770. Churchill Livingstone, Edinburgh, London, and New York.

Marino, H. (1953). Paralysis of muscles of chin: surgical treatment. *Surg. Gynec. Obst.* **96**, 433.

Mathews, W. B. (1975). *Peripheral Neuropathy* (ed. P. J. Dyck, P. K. Thomas, and E. H. Lambert), Vol. 2, p. 1203. Saunders, Philadelphia, London, and Toronto.

McComas, A. J., Sica, R. E. P., and Currie, S. (1970). Muscular dystrophy: evidence for a neural factor. *Nature* **226**, 1263.

McLaughlin, A. I. G., Kazantzis, G., King, E., Teare, D., Porter, R. J., and Owen, R. (1962). Pulmonary fibrosis and encephalopathy associated with the inhalation of aluminium dust. *Brit. J. industr. Med.* **19**, 253.

Menkes, J. H. (1974). In *Textbook of Child Neurology*, p. 245. Lea and Febiger, Philadelphia.

Meretoja, J., and Teppo, L. (1971). Histopathological findings of familial amyloidosis with cranial neuropathy as principal manifestation *Acta. path. microbiol. scand.* Section A, **79**, 432.

Merwarth, H. R. (1942). The occurrence of peripheral facial paralysis in hypertensive vascular disease. *Ann. intern. Med.* **17**, 298.

Miehlke, A. (1965). Anatomy and clinical aspects of the facial nerve. *Arch. Otolaryngol.* **81**, 444.

Moebius, P. J. (1888). Ueber angeborenen doppelseitige Abducens-Facialis-Lähmung. *Munch. med. Wschr.* **35**, 91.

——. (1892). Ueber infantilen Kernschwund. *Much. med. Wschr.*

Monier-Vinard, and Puech, P. (1930). Nephrite chronique et paralysie faciale. *Bull. Soc. med. Hôp Paris* **54**, 977.

Moxon, W. (1869). Apoplexy into canal of Fallopius in a case of Bright's disease causing facial paralysis. *Trans. path. Soc. Lond.* **20**, 420.

Muller, R. (1949). Studies in disseminated sclerosis. *Acta. med. scand.*, Suppl. 222.

Nager, G. T. (1975). Paget's disease of the temporal bone. *Ann. Otol.* (*St. Louis*) **84**, Suppl. 22.

Naufal, P. M. (1973). Primary sarcomas of the temporal bone. *Arch. Otolaryngol.* **98**, 44.

Neely, J. G., and Alford, B. R. (1974). Facial nerve neuromas. *Arch. Otolaryngol.* **100**, 298.

Nelson, K. B., and Eng, G. D. (1972). Congenital hypoplasia of the depressor anguli oris muscle. Differentiation from congenital facial palsy. *J. Pediat.* **81**, 16.

Nicholas, D. D., Kratzer, J. H., Ofosu-Amaah, S., and Belcher, D. W. (1977). Is poliomyelitis a serious problem in developing countries? *Brit. med. J.* **i**, 1009.

Oberman, H. A. (1961). Idiopathic histiocytosis. *Paediatrics* **28**, 307.

Oppenheim, H. (1911). In *Textbook of nervous diseases.* Translated by Bruce. T. N. Foulis, London.

Page, J. R., Jash, D. K., and Patel, J. B. (1975). Seventh and eighth cranial nerve palsies due to parathyroid adenoma with associated osteitis fibrosa cystica. *J. Laryngol. Otol.* **89**, 761.

Paley, R. G., and Truelove, S. C. (1948). Diphtheria in the Army in the United Kingdom. *J. roy. Army med. Cps* **90**, 109.

Paparella, M. M., and El Fiky, F. M. (1972). Ear involvement in malignant lymphoma. *Ann. Otol.* (*St. Louis*) **81**, 352.

Pape, K. E., and Pickering D. (1972). Asymmetric crying facies. An index of other congenital anomalies. *J. Pediat.* **81**, 21.

Park, D. M. (1970). Cephalic tetanus. *J. Neurol. Neurosurg. Psychiat.* **33**, 212.

Parker, N. (1963). Dystrophia myotonica presenting as congenital facial diplegia. *Med. J. Aust.* **2**, 939.

Pekelharing, C. A., and Winkler, C. (1887). Mittheilung uber die Beriberi. *Dtsch med. Wschr.* **13**, 845. Translation by J. Cantlie (1893). John Bale and Sons, London.

Pitner, S. E., Edwards, J. E., and McCormick, W. F. (1965). Observations on the pathology of Möbius syndrome. *J. Neurol. Neurosurg. Psychiat.* **28**, 362.

Pulec, J. L. (1969). Facial nerve tumors. *Ann. Otol.* **78**, 962.

——. (1972). Facial nerve neuroma. *Laryngoscope* **82**, 1160.

Rainy, H., and Fowler, J. S. (1903). Congenital facial diplegia, due to nuclear lesion. *Rev. Neurol. Psychiat.* **1**, 149.

Remillard, G. M., Andermann, F., Rhi-Sausi, A., and Robbins, N. M. (1977). Facial asymmetry in patients with temporal lobe epilepsy. *Neurology* **27**, 109.

Revilla, G. A. (1948). Differential diagnosis of tumors at the cerebellopontile recess. *Bull. Johns Hopk. Hosp.* **83**, 187.

Reichart, P. (1976). Facial and oral manifestations in leprosy. *Oral Surg.* **41**, 385.

Richter, R. B. (1958). Congenital hypoplasia of the facial nucleus. *J. Neuropath. exp. Neurol.* **17**, 520.

Rubinstein, A. E., Lovelace, R. E., Behrens, M. M., and Weisberg, L. A. (1975). Moebius syndrome in association with peripheral neuropathy and Kallman syndrome. *Arch. Neurol.* **32**, 480.

Sabin, T. D., and Swift, T. R. (1975). In *Peripheral Neuropathy* (ed. P. J. Dyck, P. K. Thomas and E. H. Lambert), Vol. 2, p. 1181. Saunders, Philadelphia, London, and Toronto.

Saito, H., and Baxter, A. (1972). Undiagnosed intratemporal facial nerve neurilemomas. *Arch. Otolaryngol.* **95**, 415.

Sand, G. (1953). In *Lélia: The life of George Sand*, by André Maurois, p. 372. Translated by Hopkins. Cape, London.

Schuknecht, H. F., Allam, A. F., and Murakami, Y. (1968). Pathology of secondary malignant tumors of the temporal bone. *Ann. Otol. Rhinol. Laryngol.* **77**, 5.

——, ——, and ——. (1977). Discussion. Case record of Massachusetts General Hospital. *New Eng. J. Med.* **296**, 271–6.

Spillane, J. D. (1973). *Tropical neurology.* Oxford University Press.

Starzecka, B. (1960). Tetanic paralysis (Polish) *Przegl. epidem.* **14**, 153. Quoted in *Handbook of clinical neurology* (ed. P. J. Vinken and G. W. Bruyn), Vol. 7, p. 476. North-Holland, Amsterdam.

Takemori, S., Tanaka, Y., and Suzuki, J-I. (1976). Thalidomide anomalies of the ear. *Arch. Otolaryngol.* **102**, 425.

Thomas, H. M. (1898). Congenital facial paralysis. *J. nerv. ment. Dis.* **25**, 571.

Thomas, P. K., Lascelles, R. G., Hallpike, J. F., and Hewer, R. L. (1969). Recurrent and chronic relapsing Guillain–Barré polyneuritis. *Brain* **92**, 589.

Toothill, R. J., Kidder, T. M., and Eby, L. G. (1973). Eosinophilic granuloma of the temporal bone. *Laryngoscope* **83**, 877.

Tos, M. (1969). Facial palsy in Hand–Schüller–Christian disease. *Arch. Otolaryngol.* **90**, 563.

Vakil, B. J., Singhal, B. S., Pandya, S. S., and Irani, P. F. (1973). Cephalic tetanus. *Neurology (Minneapolis)* **23**, 1091.

Van Allen, M. W., and Blodi, F. C. (1960). Neurologic aspects of the Möbius syndrome. *Neurology* **10**, 249.

Victor, M. (1975). In *Peripheral neuropathy* (ed. P. J. Dyck, P. K. Thomas and E. H. Lambert), p. 1034. Saunders, Philadelphia, London, and Toronto.

Von Graefe, A. (1880). *Graefe–Saemisch's Hanbuch der Augenheilkinde*, Vol. 6, p. 60. Engelmann, Leipzig.

Wallis, P. G. (1960). Creatinuria in Möbius' Syndrome. *Arch. Dis. Child.* **35**, 393

Watkins, A. L. (1939). Facial paralysis in cephalic tetanus. *Arch. Neurol. Psychiat.* **41**, 788.

Watkins, P. J. (1973). Facial sweating after food: A new sign of diabetic autonomic neuropathy. *Brit. med. J.* **i**, 583.

Ziter, F. A. Wiser, W. C., and Robinson, A. (1977). Three-generation pedigree of a Möbius syndrome variant with chromosome translocation. *Arch. Neurol.* **34**, 437.

4 Facial nerve disorders of unknown aetiology

4 Facial nerve disorders of unknown aetiology

Abnormal facial movements

A GREAT deal of confusion surrounds the subject of abnormal facial movements. This confusion springs from well-meaning, and indeed ingenious, attempts to classify in an area where our ignorance exceeds our knowledge. Attempts have been made to separate involuntary movements into those due to organic disease and those due to emotional disorder. Movements which are precipitated or aggravated by emotional stress and movements which can be voluntarily inhibited were held to be psychogenic. Such a classification is not constructive, because it runs contrary to the basic principles of facial nerve anatomy and physiology. Organic disease can involve the supranuclear pathways for emotional and associated movements of the face. Since both organic disease and psychic disorder can affect the emotional control of facial muscles, in the absence of other signs of disease there is no way of apportioning responsibility. No attempt will be made, therefore, to separate semivoluntary and involuntary facial movements into rigid compartments.

Other efforts have been made to define the abnormal facial movements according to their visual appearance. Separate disorders have been classified according to whether they produce tics, twitches, or tremors, flickering, quivering, or grimacing, myokymia, fasciculation, or spasm. Such a system of classification is based more upon the clinician's powers of observation and description than on disease processes.

Perhaps the most logical attempt at classification is based on anatomical location. The fibrillation of bulbar motor neurone disease and the myokymia of brain-stem disorders are two examples. Unfortunately our knowledge is insufficient at present to permit such a classification to include all abnormal facial movements. We are ignorant of the locations of the lesions responsible for hemifacial spasm, drug-induced facial dyskinesia, and the facial grimacing of hepatic encephalopathy, for example. It is not proposed, therefore, to adopt any of these three types of classification. Our lack of knowledge prompts a pragmatic approach and we will deal first with those abnormal movements which are harmless and then go on to discuss those of a more serious nature. To be able to recognize and identify those abnormal facial movements which belong to the harmless variety or group is a very worthwhile objective. It enables one confidently to reassure the patient that the abnormal movement is more of a nuisance than a disease, that no dire consequences need be feared, and best of all perhaps, that no treatment is necessary—*primum non nocere*. Since the majority of these abnormal facial movements are of unknown aetiology they are discussed together in this chapter.

Hereditary quivering of the chin

This is a fascinating medical curiosity in which involuntary movement of the muscles of the chin is inherited as a dominant characteristic. The movement is confined to the mentalis muscle with only occasional spread to other muscles. It begins at birth and exists throughout life, becoming progressively less severe with increasing age. The flickering or quivering movement is not present continuously but disappears and reappears in a very random manner. It is precipitated by a great variety of mechanical stimuli and is aggravated by emotional stress. Laurance *et al.* (1968) were able to obtain an EMG recording of the mentalis muscle in an affected patient and found that it was quite unlike the EMG pattern in myokymia. Diagnosis depends primarily on an awareness of the existence of the disorder and on a positive family history. Since the condition is harmless treatment is seldom warranted. Occasional cases have been treated by division of the marginal mandibular nerve or by excision of the mentalis muscle.

Facial tics

(Synonyms: habit spasms, mimic spasms, winking tics)

Facial tics consist of sudden brief and recurrent movements of the facial muscles, e.g. winking, grimacing, wrinkling the nose, etc. The movement often extends beyond the facial muscles and involves tongue, glottic, and neck muscles. For each patient the tic is stereotyped and is a repetitive, purposeless, semi-automatic movement. It can be actively reproduced at will, and can be voluntarily suppressed at least for a brief period. Tics are aggravated by emotion and fatigue and disappear during sleep. They usually begin in children of 5–12 years old and are thought to start as purposeful movements which continue after their original purpose has ceased to exist. They then develop into a complex compulsive movement or series of movements. Frequently, tics which appear in childhood are transient and tend to diminish spontaneously and finally disappear. For those tics which persist, there is no effective drug treatment. Various forms of psychotherapy have been tried, with some success. It is important, however, to recognize these tics for the harmless habits that they are (Fig. 4.1).

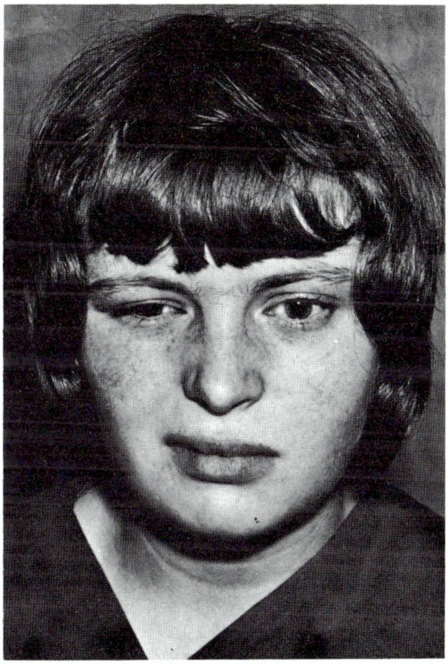

Fig. 4.1. Facial tic (habit spasm). Sudden, brief, recurrent movements of the right side of the face, ceasing when the patient's attention was diverted and increasing when she was embarrassed. Periodic sniffing, shrugging movements of the shoulder, and moodiness. (Spillane 1975)

Blepharospasm

(Bilateral facial spasm; facial paraspasm; Meige's median spasm)

It is not claimed that these terms are synonymous but they would appear to represent different degrees of the same condition rather than separate disorders. In many ways they resemble tics but they are distinguished by the bilateral symmetrical nature of their movements. The condition always affects the orbicularis oculi muscles of both sides. Initially the twitching and spasms are limited to these muscles. Later on there is an increased tendency to involve other facial muscles. The syndrome described by Meige (1910) occurs in elderly people and consists of forced blinking of both eyes, wrinkling of the nose, and twitching of both sides of the upper lip. Understandably, blepharospasm is aggravated by any stimulus which triggers the blink reflex (Chapter 1) including bright light. Many sufferers find that dark sunglasses offer the double advantage of reducing the severity of the blepharospasm and of concealing it. In mild forms of the condition the bilateral blinking movements can be inhibited by distraction techniques deliberately invoked by the patient, such as whistling, etc. However, the movements are more automatic than tics and have fewer semivoluntary features. Occasionally patients are so incapacitated by the extreme frequency of their spasmodic eye closure that they are rendered, in effect, blind for several seconds at a time (Fisch and Esslen 1972).

The EMG pattern is highly characteristic (Fig. 4.2). It reveals that the twitching is produced by bilateral synchronous group discharges of motor units in the orbicularis oculi muscles. The group discharges on each side begin and end at the same time, but there is usually an uneven distribution of motor units involved in the contractions. This demonstrates that although the eyelids on both sides close and open at the same time, one side may be closed more forcibly than the other. Because both eyes are involved simultaneously the lesion is deemed to be supranuclear. The multi-synaptic pathway is generally thought to be a more likely location of the lesion than the direct cortico-nuclear tract. The condition occurs principally in middle-aged and elderly people. Since the majority of patients have no preceding history of neurological disorder a localized ischaemic or degenerative lesion is often invoked. Medical treatment with benzhexol (Artane) is seldom helpful. Surgical treatment by division of several of the terminal nerve fibres supplying the orbicularis oculi is temporarily beneficial. The muscles tend to become reinnervated after a while with a recurrence of the blepharospasm. Apart from the small number of cases with impaired vision, the majority of patients with blepharospasm can be regarded as suffering from a harmless form of abnormal facial movement requiring nothing more in the way of treatment than provision of dark spectacles in appropriate cases. Blepharospasm is not a feature of some serious neurological disease and, while acknowledging that it is a serious nuisance, one can reassure the patient that it is not the herald of some more sinister disorder.

Synkinesis

This has already been discussed in Chapter 2 and only brief mention need be made of it here. Synkinetic movements are a sequel of lower motor neurone facial paralysis and are seen in patients who have an incomplete recovery. The movements occur only during voluntary contraction of the facial muscles. They consist of involuntary movements of one part of the face which occur when a separate region of the face is moved voluntarily. In this way an involuntary winking movement of the peri-orbital muscles may accompany voluntary movement of the peri-oral muscles during speech. The synkinetic movement is always confined to the side of the preceding paralysis and residual facial weakness can usually be detected. Synkinesis is thought to be due to either faulty regeneration of nerve fibres or a 'short circuit' in the nerve trunk due to an artificial synapse.

Dyskinesis

Dyskinetic movements are attributed to upper motor neurone lesions and are not associated with paralysis or weakness of the facial muscles. The move-

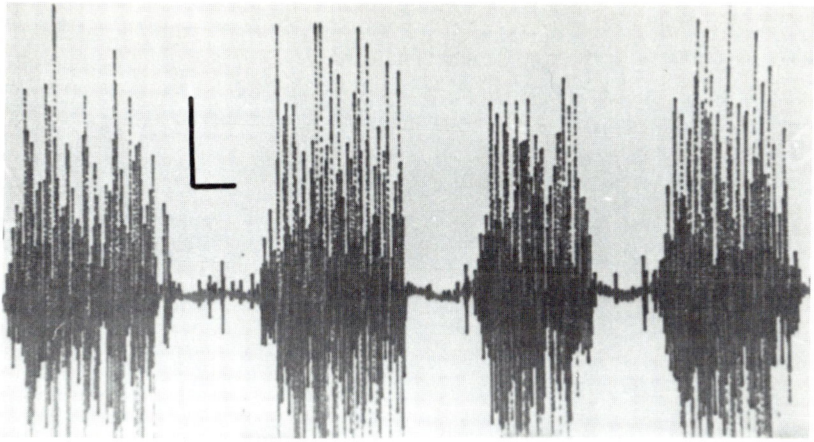

Fig. 4.2. Blepharospasm. A concentric needle electrode in the orbicularis oculi. There is excessive, abrupt recruitment of motor units in a series of contractions in blepharospasm. (Calibration 50 μV:10 ms)

ments affect both sides of the face and extend beyond the facial muscles to involve the tongue and neck and more distant parts of the body as well. They consist of writhing, twisting, grimacing, facial movements which are involuntary and often unnoticed by the patient. The features may be distorted into grotesque gargoyle shapes as though the patient was trying to make a series of extremely unpleasant and rude faces (Fig. 4.3). The dyskinesia may be produced by either drugs or disease.

The phenothiazine group of drugs and levodopa are two well-recognized causes. The tardive dyskinesia seen with phenothiazine therapy may begin early in treatment in patients with a personal idiosyncrasy. In these cases the dyskinesia usually disappears when the drug is withdrawn. More often the dyskinesia occurs after prolonged therapy with high dosage of phenothiazines and may persist indefinitely after medication has ceased. With levodopa, symptoms may develop during the early progression of dosage or they may appear after several months therapy on a fixed dosage. In either event, the involuntary movements usually cease when the blood level of the drug falls. It may be possible in some cases to return to the previous dose levels without the reappearance of dyskinesia, but often one has to sacrifice some symptomatic control of the Parkinson's disease by maintaining a lower dosage of the drug. Bromocriptine and piribedil, which also affect dopamine receptors, can produce similar dyskinesia.

A number of neurological disorders also produce these involuntary movements. It is often seen in 'spastic' patients born with brain damage and in Huntingdon's chorea. On clinical grounds the lesion would appear to be located in the cortical motor centres for emotional and associated movement or in their multisynaptic pathways. The facial grimacing which is sometimes seen in patients with hepatic encephalopathy is thought to be similarly produced.

Hemifacial spasm

(Synonyms: clonic facial spasm; tic convulsif)

Hemifacial spasm is the term used to describe repeated and involuntary twitches of the muscles supplied by one facial nerve (Fig. 4.4). There is seldom an associated weakness of the affected muscles. The peri-orbital, perinasal, and peri-oral muscles are principally involved in the twitching but the frontalis and platysma muscles sometimes participate also. The spasm is essentially unilateral. In a few cases both sides of the face have been involved but the spasms are never synchronous on each side. The resultant clinical picture is of right and left unilateral spasms occurring independently of each other. Hemifacial spasm can neither be voluntarily reproduced or suppressed and persists during sleep. It is aggravated by physical fatigue and psychic stress. It does not occur in children and is more frequently seen in middle-aged and elderly patients than in young adults. The ratio of female to male sufferers is said to be 3:2 (Ehni and Woltman 1945). The spasm is made up of

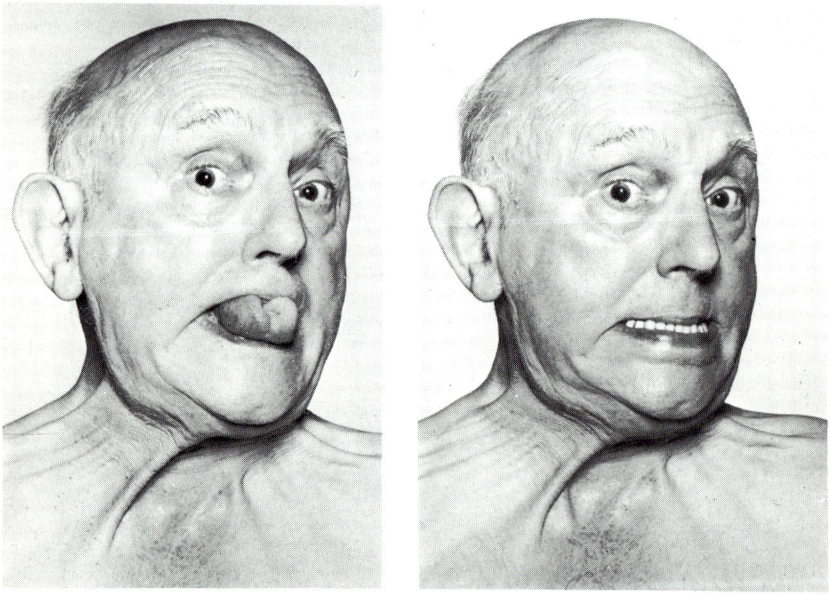

Fig. 4.3. Facial dyskinesia in a patient taking L-dopa 4 g-daily for one year. There was an almost complete disappearance of the facial movements and grimacing on reducing the dose of L-dopa by 1 g daily. (Spillane 1975).

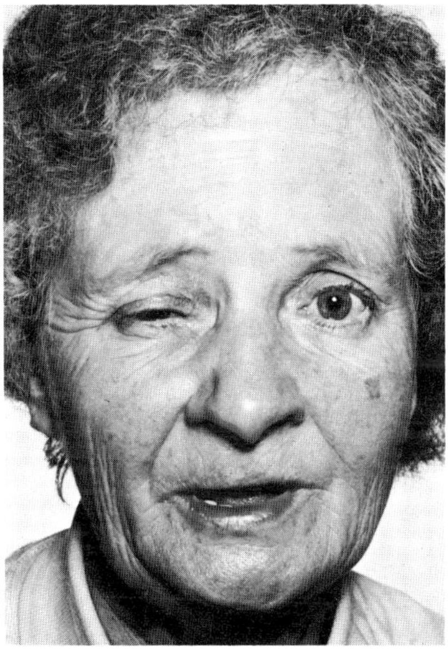

Fig. 4.4. Hemifacial spasm. Recurring clonic spasm of right facial muscles. (Spillane 1975)

rapidly recurring clonic twitches and can last for up to five minutes at a time. The prolonged or tonic contraction of muscle which results in a facial contracture is probably a separate entity.

The twitching movements of hemifacial spasm are usually painless but obviously can be the source of considerable emotional distress. Occasional cases have been recorded in which the twitches have been accompanied by pain in the trigeminal region but fortunately this is rare.

The diagnosis of hemifacial spasm can be confirmed if necessary by electromyography (Fig. 4.5, p. 132). By simultaneous recording of groups of muscles, completely synchronous bursts of motor activity are revealed. The bursts consist of very rapid firing of motor units at a rate of 200–400 impulses per second. Between 5 and 20 of these bursts per second are often recorded.

In the majority of patients no cause for the condition can be identified and prolonged follow-up fails to reveal evidence of progressive disease. Because of this the hemifacial spasm has been held to be due to a central rather than an axonal lesion. Toremalm *et al.* (1977) expressed the view that the simultaneous action of muscles supplied by different branches of the facial nerve suggests a central action rather than cross-firing in the nerve. Nonetheless, a lesion involving the peripheral nerve is responsible for hemifacial spasm in a number of cases. A cerebellopontine angle tumour, aneurysm of the basilar artery, and arachnoiditis of the posterior fossa have been known to be responsible on rare occasions (*British Medical Journal* 1972). The acoustic neuroma shown in Fig. 5.4 (p. 169) produced hemifacial spasm as the initial clinical sign. Nussbaum (1977) has recorded hemifacial spasm due to a benign parotid tumour. The spasm ceased completely within a few months of the surgical removal of the tumour. The case is probably unique and is especially interesting as it shows hemifacial spasm from a lesion involving the terminal branches rather than the trunk of the facial nerve. Although the majority of cases will turn out to be due to no identifiable disease, a very thorough investigation must be carried out in every case to ensure that no organic disease is overlooked.

This investigation should include angiography in suitable patients for there is now increasing evidence that abnormalities of the vertebrobasilar circulatory tree are responsible for a significant proportion of cases. Nappi *et al.* (1977) found an increase in length and diameter in one or more segments of the vertebrobasilar tree in three patients with hemifacial spasm. They considered the lesion to be a manifestation of arteriosclerotic disease with the characteristics of dilating arteriosclerosis. Such an aetiology would help to explain why hemifacial spasm occurs principally in middle-aged and elderly people. In a much larger series of 47 patients Jannetta *et al.* (1977) found that 46 had vascular compression of the facial nerve root exit zone by an arterial loop. In 38 (84 per cent) of these patients they obtained relief of hemifacial spasm by surgically manipulating the vessel away from the nerve.

No medical treatment abolishes the twitches but psychotropic drugs can relieve the emotional stress and thereby reduce the severity of the spasm. The details of surgical treatment will be dealt with in Chapter 7, but the basic principle can be stated here that in idiopathic hemifacial spasm surgery offers a naked choice between spasm and paralysis. Complete section of the facial nerve will completely eliminate the spasm and produce a complete facial paralysis. Partial section of either the nerve trunk or its terminal branches will result in partial relief of the spasm and partial facial paralysis. If reinnervation takes place the facial paralysis recovers and the spasm returns. An alternative surgical compromise has been recommended by Harrison (1976). He divides either the whole facial nerve or, in less severe cases, the temporofacial trunk. He then anastomoses the hypoglossal nerve to the distal cut end of the facial nerve. He finds that this successfully abolishes the spasm and achieves a satisfactory degree of voluntary facial movement. In his view, the inevitable permanent loss of emotional movement on the affected side of the face and the neurogenic hemiatrophy of the tongue are lesser evils.

Facial myokymia

Facial myokymia is an interesting and intriguing disorder of facial nerve function. A few decades ago it would have been classified as a disorder of known aetiology, for it was then thought to be a condition associated exclusively with multiple sclerosis. Many authorities believed that not only was it a specific sign of multiple sclerosis but that it was also an early sign of the disease. Indeed the presence of facial myokymia in the absence of any other symptoms and signs of neurological disorder was thought to be diagnostic of multiple sclerosis, since myokymia was known to be the first sign of the disease in some cases. Myokymia was also thought to be a very rare condition and in their excellent review Andermann *et al.* (1961) were able to cull only seven cases besides their own from the world literature. Increased awareness of the existence of the condition together with the use of EMG studies brought many more cases to light. Lambert *et al.* (1961) demonstrated that facial myokymia occurred in patients with brain-stem tumours and Radu *et al.* (1975) showed that it was present in many other diseases as well. Knowledge of the condition was further expanded when it was shown that myokymia was not confined exclusively to the muscles supplied by the facial nerve. Susac *et al.* (1973) described myokymia in the superior oblique muscle, Radu *et al.* (1975) described it in the masseter, and Kaeser and Skorpil (1976) have recorded the only case to date of myokymia involving the muscles supplied by six cranial nerves.

Although knowledge of the condition is expanding, the pathophysiology of myokymia remains obscure. Paradoxically this expansion of knowledge compels us to remove myokymia from the list of disorders of known aetiology, and place it among those of unknown aetiology, where we hope its stay will be brief.

Clinical features Facial myokymia is a condition with distinct clinical and electromyographical features. It usually begins abruptly and patients may complain that their face feels screwed up or swollen, and that certain movements are difficult to perform because of facial 'stiffness'. Surprisingly, patients may be unaware of the condition and Radu *et al.* (1975) recorded that this was the case in about half of their series of 43 patients.

In affected patients the muscles on one side of the face appear to be in slight contraction so that the palpebral fissure is narrowed, the angle of the mouth is drawn up, and the lips are slightly pursed. A continuous flickering movement is seen in all the muscles from the frontalis to the platysma in a fully developed case. Contractions of small bands or strips of muscle transmit a ripple, like a 'bag of worms', to the overlying skin. The lay term 'live flesh' is very apt.

Initially myokymia begins in a group of muscles, commonly the peri-orbital or peri-oral, and may remain confined to one group or spread to other muscles. It remains unilateral, however, and is an involuntary continuous activity which is not significantly altered by sleep or by voluntary or reflex facial movements. The rapid undulating waves of movement are too

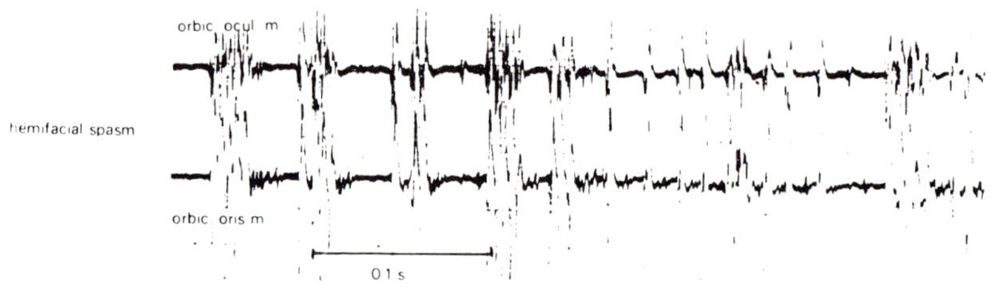

Fig. 4.5. Hemifacial spasm EMG recording of synchronous bursts of motor units from ipsilateral facial muscles. (Fisch and Esslen 1972). Copyright 1972, American Medical Association.

fast and too complex for visual analysis. The EMG pattern shows motor units of normal shape and duration appearing as single, double, or group discharges with a definite rhythmic pattern. On voluntary contraction a normal interference pattern is obtained (Fig. 4.6). The frequency of the bursts is relatively stable in each case. Two types of discharge have been described, a 'continuous' and a 'discontinuous'. The continuous type is particularly associated with multiple sclerosis and the discontinuous type with brain-stem tumours, but this is only a general rule to which there are an increasing number of exceptions. In multiple sclerosis myokymia tends to disappear spontaneously after a period of a few weeks or months. In keeping with the nature of the underlying disease, however, relapse or recurrence of the myokymia can occur on the same and on the opposite side of the face. In brain-stem and posterior fossa tumours the myokymia usually persists and is accompanied by a slowly progressive peripheral facial palsy. Myokymia ceases when facial palsy becomes complete. Radu *et al.* (1975) reported a series of 43 patients with myokymia in 3 of whom the condition was not detectable clinically but was demonstrated by EMG studies. Six patients (14 per cent) had a brain-stem or posterior fossa tumour, 18 patients (42 per

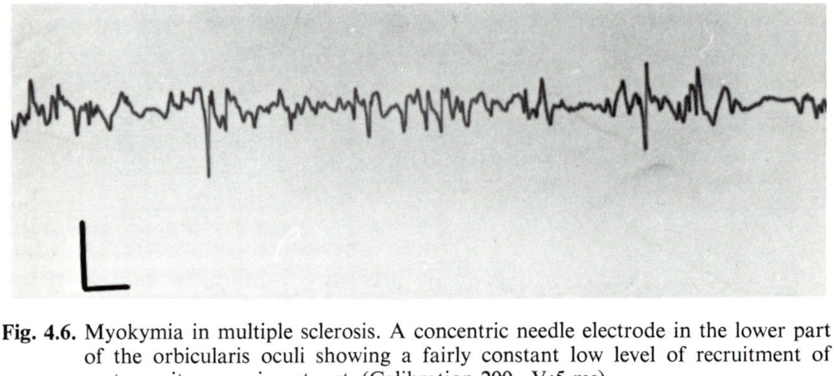

Fig. 4.6. Myokymia in multiple sclerosis. A concentric needle electrode in the lower part of the orbicularis oculi showing a fairly constant low level of recruitment of motor units occurring at rest. (Calibration 200 μV:5 ms)

cent) had multiple sclerosis, and 19 patients (44 per cent) formed a miscellaneous group with a great variety of neurological disorders, but without evidence of tumour or multiple sclerosis during a prolonged period of follow-up. The diseases encountered in this last group included 3 patients with vertebrobasilar insufficiency, 1 with probable syringo-bulbia, 1 with cerebral palsy and continuous myokymia since birth, and a case of phosgene poisoning.

Pathophysiology Facial myokymia is a clear-cut sign of organic disease involving principally the brain-stem or posterior fossa, but the precise location and the mode of action of the responsible lesion is not known. In tumour cases most autopsies have shown fairly extensive damage to the pons. Sethi *et al.* (1974) were able to localize very precisely the metastatic deposits which were responsible for their case of myokymia. The deposits were rostral to the nucleus and interrupted the corticonuclear fibres. They suggested that myokymia was due to a supranuclear lesion which released the neurones from the inhibitory influences of higher centres. Radu *et al.* (1975) favour the idea of a perinuclear lesion which affects the neurones by oedema or pressure and thereby presumably heightens their excitability. However, one of their tumour cases was a cholesteatoma in the region of the middle ear, labyrinth and fundus of the internal auditory meatus where it would be adjacent to the facial nerve but not the brain-stem. In another case the autopsy showed no contact between the posterior fossa tumour and the brain stem. These authors do not attempt to explain the mechanism whereby their miscellaneous group of disorders produce myokymia. Perhaps as our knowledge of the variety of conditions which produce myokymia grows, we may come to the conclusion that there is no one single mechanism of production and that supranuclear, nuclear, infranuclear, and even axonal mechanisms can evoke myokymia.

The facial myokymia we have discussed is referred to as 'true myokymia' by some authors. This is to distinguish it from so-called 'benign myokymia'. This latter term has unfortunately been applied to the momentary quivering of the eyelids that occurs in healthy people during fatigue.

Melkersson–Rosenthal syndrome

In 1928 Melkersson reported the case of a 35-year-old woman who had recurring facial paralyses and recurring swelling of her lips. Rosenthal (1931) described two families in which three individuals had lingua plicata, facial paralysis, and facial oedema. The tongue anomaly is not in itself pathological. It is thought to be a congenital variant and Rosenthal regarded it as evidence of a constitutional stigma. The terms lingua plicata, fissured tongue, furrowed tongue, and scrotal tongue are synonymous. Lüscher (1949) suggested that the syndrome be named after both Melkersson and Rosenthal and this practice will be followed here. It is also referred to more briefly throughout the literature as Melkersson's syndrome.

Clinical features

The classical triad consists of recurring episodes of facial oedema and of recurring facial palsy, frequently associated with the anomaly of a congenital fissured tongue. The facial oedema is usually maximal in the lips and has a characteristically abrupt onset. Since the eyelids are also frequently affected, the clinical appearances resemble angioneurotic or Quincke's oedema. The swelling lasts for more than a week and then disappears almost as quickly as it came. The oedema recurs in the same site at highly irregular intervals of weeks, months, or years, and instead of clearing up completely between attacks, it eventually begins to persist. The affected part then remains chronically swollen with exacerbations of even greater swelling. The oedema most commonly begins in the upper lip and after several recurrences it gradually extends to involve the lower lip, cheek, face and tongue. If the swelling invades the tongue, the patient may develop macroglossia. The tongue is then sometimes too bulky and stiff to allow comfortable speaking and swallowing.

Peripheral facial paralysis is the commonest neurological sign in this disorder and is estimated to occur in a third of all cases (Hornstein 1970). It affects all branches of the nerve as a rule but occasionally the paralysis is limited to a few branches only. The onset is very similar to that seen in Bell's palsy or the Ramsay Hunt syndrome. It may be accompanied by pain around the ear or, less frequently, by tinnitus, deafness, or vertigo. The facial paralysis may occur before any swelling is evident or there may be several recurrences of facial oedema before the paralysis becomes manifest. The natural history of each episode of facial paralysis is the same as that seen in Bell's palsy. After each episode of paralysis, signs of incomplete recovery such as synkinesis and residual muscle weakness may become more obvious.

The paralysis is characteristically unilateral and bilateral involvement appears to be rare. The paralysis more often recurs on the side of the original facial palsy. The history in most cases is therefore one of recurring ipsilateral paralysis rather than alternating facial paralysis. Other cranial nerves may be involved whether facial paralysis is present or absent. Trigeminal pain or paraesthesia, diplopia, and symptoms of eighth nerve dysfunction occur. Secretory disturbances of the salivary glands (facial and glossopharyngeal nerves) and neurogenic hemi-atrophy of the tongue can also occur. Sometimes involvement of the central nervous system produces a clinical picture resembling multiple sclerosis, with disseminated and remitting lesions.

In addition to the major dermal and neural features mentioned, several less common disorders have been described as marginal features of the disease. These are generally attributed to abnormal function of the autonomic nervous system. Hyperhidrosis, vasomotor rhinorrhoea, and disturbed lacrimal secretion are reported fairly consistently. A number of patients have also been found to suffer from megacolon.

Pathology

A post-mortem study by Schwarz and Elsässer (1961) showed angiopathy of the small arteries of the brain and many other visceral organs. The angiopathy resulted in arterial narrowing and obstruction similar to endarteritis obliterans. A granular atrophy of the cerebral cortex was found. More autopsy reports are required before the significance of these findings can be properly evaluated.

Kettel (1959) described the appearance of the facial nerve seen during decompression operations on patients with the Melkersson–Rosenthal syndrome. The nerve showed degenerative changes without signs of inflammation. These were identical to his findings in Bell's palsy patients. In both disorders Kettel occasionally found signs of aseptic bone necrosis in the mastoid bone adjacent to the Fallopian canal. He was uncertain of what significance to attach to this; the majority of other surgeons engaged in decompression operations have not encountered any bone pathology.

The histological appearances of the skin have been widely studied. There is a diffuse oedema of the interstitial connective tissue with some atrophy of facial muscle fibres. Occasional blood-vessels are found to have thickened walls which narrow the lumen. Other small blood vessels and the lymphatics are often dilated. Miescher (1945) drew attention to the presence of small granulomas scattered throughout the oedematous subepithelial tissue. These granulomas vary in their histological appearance and three varieties have been described, lymphonodular plasmocytic, tuberculoid, and sarcoid. The erythrocyte sedimentation rate is either normal or slightly elevated and a differential white count often shows a moderate lymphocytosis of around 50 per cent.

Pathogenesis

The cause of the disease is unknown but many authorities believe that constitutional factors play a large part. Lingua plicata is regarded as an irregularly inherited, dominant anomaly. The frequent association of this anomaly, together with reports of a familial incidence of the disease, lend support to the importance of constitutional factors. Further support is given by the recognition that a number of people with the syndrome also have congenital megacolon. The facial swelling is attributed to an angioneurotic oedema although subepithelial granulomas are not a feature of angioneurotic oedema associated with other disorders. In addition, Quincke's oedema affects other parts of the body as well as the face and always clears up completely between each attack. The facial paralysis is attributed by most writers to vasomotor injury to the nerve in the same way that Bell's palsy is held to be due to a vasomotor disturbance. The aetiology of Bell's palsy will be discussed later but it is worthwhile pointing out here that the vasomotor or ischaemic theory of causation of facial paralysis in Bell's palsy and in the Melkersson–Rosenthal syndrome is unproved.

Treatment

In the absence of a known aetiology, it is difficult to devise treatment. However, it is generally agreed that antibiotic therapy is without benefit. Corticosteroids are the agents most frequently employed. They are used systemically and also topically by intralesional injection. They are believed to reduce both the frequency and the duration of the recurring attacks or relapses.

Occurrence

The disease either occurs more often or is recognized more often in Scandinavian countries. Reported cases in Great Britain and the United States of America are relatively few in number. However, the disease is not confined to the continent of Europe and it has been reported among the Japanese, the Arab races, and in African negroes.

Bell's palsy

Definition During the last century and the early part of this century the term 'Bell's palsy' was used as a synonym for peripheral facial paralysis. Older textbooks refer to 'traumatic Bell's palsy' and 'Bell's palsy due to otitis media' and so on. The practice today is to exclude all known causes of facial paralysis and to restrict the term to isolated peripheral facial paralysis of unknown aetiology. The recurring facial paralysis of unknown aetiology associated with recurring facial oedema and lingua plicata, named the Melkersson–Rosenthal syndrome, is a different nosological entity. We may define Bell's palsy as a unilateral lower motor neurone facial paralysis of sudden onset, unrelated to disease elsewhere in the body. The term, therefore, excludes all those facial paralyses discussed in the previous chapter.

Incidence and epidemiology

It is often stated that the face is more frequently paralysed than any other part of the body, and Hauser *et al.* (1971) calculated the annual incidence of Bell's palsy in Minnesota to be 22·8 per 100 000 population. Adour *et al.* (1972) express the incidence somewhat more dramatically by stating that

Bell's palsy occurs once every 13 minutes in the United States of America. Verjaal (1955) estimated the annual incidence of Bell's palsy in Holland was 20 per 100 000 for adults; and 5 per 100 000 for children. Many series contain a higher proportion of females than males but other series show the opposite finding, and it is difficult to draw any valid conclusions on this point. Similarly there is no agreement on whether the condition is commoner in pregnancy. Hauser *et al.* (1971) and Adour (1970) found no increased incidence but later Adour, writing with Hislinger *et al.* (1975), found that pregnant women had 3·3 times greater incidence of Bell's palsy than non-pregnant women of the same age group. Interestingly enough, 36 (85 per cent) of the 42 pregnant women in this series developed facial palsy either in the third trimester or in the first two weeks of the puerperium. This corresponds with reports by Korczyn (1971) and Furakawa *et al.* (1975) of a greater incidence of Bell's palsy in pregnant women, especially around the time of parturition.

The age incidence is also subject to debate but the results of many series may be summarized by saying that the disease occurs in all age groups and that it seems to be more prevalent in the third, fourth, and fifth decades of life. The seasonal incidence of Bell's palsy has been recorded in a number of investigations into the epidemiology of the disease. Once again, conflicting results have been obtained. Adour *et al.* (1972) and Hauser *et al.* (1971) found a random distribution throughout the year. El Ebiary (1971) and many others have reported seasonal clustering. Allowance has to be made for the fact that the seasons of the year occur during different months in different parts of the world. Even when this is done, however, the various studies report conflicting seasonal clusterings. This suggests that while clusters of cases may well occur, the clustering is related to factors other than the season of the year.

Familial incidence There have been few reports of a familial incidence of Bell's palsy in the literature and as a result one gets the impression that either it is rare or it is overlooked. In a controlled series Alter (1963) found a 3 per cent incidence of facial paralysis reported in first degree relatives of patients with Bell's palsy. De Santo and Schubert (1969) reported the occurrence of 10 cases of Bell's palsy in a family spread over a period of 83 years. The highest recorded incidence of Bell's palsy in a family was 29 cases over three generations during a 40-year period. (Willbrand *et al.* 1974). This record seems in little danger of being broken because there were two consanguinous marriages in the first generation, four in the second generation, and eight consanguinous marriages in the third. The same authors report a 6 per cent positive family history in a series of 230 consecutive patients with Bell's palsy. A positive family history was defined as the occurrence of Bell's palsy in parent, grandparent, child, or grandchild, sibling or first cousin, aunt or uncle, nephew or niece. To account for this they suggest an autosomal dominant inheritance with incomplete penetration. It will be very interesting to see if future reports support this finding.

As knowledge increases it is to be expected that the percentage of facial paralysis labelled as idiopathic will decrease. Certainly the percentage today is very different from that in the past, partly due to more sophisticated diagnostic methods and partly due to the decreased incidence of facial paralysis from bacterial infection today. Every series will be subject to a certain amount of selection bias based on the nature of their authors medical or surgical speciality.

In Table 4.1 the results of three children's series and four adult series are listed.

Table 4.1
The percentage of cases attributable to Bell's palsy in seven series of facial paralysis

Children's series		Adult series	
Lloyd *et al.* (1966)	47	Swan (1952)	66
Manning and Adour (1972)	60	Cawthorne and Haynes (1956)	63
Alberti and Biagioni (1972)	28	Zülch (1970)	80
		Tomita *et al.* (1972)	66

Symptoms

Pain Pain around the ear and tenderness often accompany Bell's palsy and may even precede the paralysis by a few days. The pain may be felt in the ear, the occiput, the jaw, or the neck. Sometimes the whole side of the head and face feels painful. The pain has been attributed to both vascular and nervous mechanisms but no entirely satisfactory explanation has been found. Similar pain often accompanies the facial paralysis of diabetic neuropathy, sarcoidosis, and the Ramsay Hunt syndrome. Many writers hold the view that the severity of the pain is directly proportional to the severity of the paralysis, and that the presence of pain, therefore, worsens the prognosis. This view is supported by Taverner (1959), Dalton (1960), Alford *et al.* (1966), and by McGovern (1966). However, the presence of pain was found to be of no prognostic value by Park and Watkins (1949) and Jongkees (1973). About half of the patients with Bell's palsy complain of some pain.

Taste disturbance and hyperacusis Approximately one-third of patients have a disturbance of taste sensation. The symptom is not often volunteered by patients, perhaps because they are unaware of any relationship between taste loss and facial paralysis. However, if asked directly, about one-third of patients will admit to the symptom. Hyperacusis or phonophobia seems to be slightly less common than taste disturbance. In a series of 1080 patients with Bell's palsy reported by Byl and Adour (1977) 29 per cent had auditory symptoms but none showed any deafness on audiometric testing. Their auditory symptoms were attributed to stapedius paralysis. We have been struck by the number of patients who have a proven stapedius paralysis and who insist that they have noticed no change in their tolerance to loud sounds. It may well be that the percentage of patients who complain of phonophobia seriously understates the true incidence of stapedius paralysis. Crocodile tears and gustatory sweating are fortunately rare complications of Bell's palsy which occur in less than 10 per cent of cases.

The clinical features of facial paralysis have been dealt with in Chapter 2, and the prognostic significance of taste loss, and reduced lacrimal and salivary secretion will be dealt with in Chapter 6.

Natural history

The paralysis has a characteristically sudden onset, and usually reaches its maximum development within 48 hours. Occasionally it continues to increase after the first week. The taste loss may precede the motor paralysis and recovery of taste sensation can herald the return of muscle movement.

Some degree of spontaneous recovery is to be expected in every case of Bell's palsy and it is universally agreed that over 60 per cent of patients have a good recovery. Most writers agree that approximately 80 per cent get such good recovery that facial symmetry at rest is restored and patients are satisfied with the result. Recovery usually begins within eight weeks and has generally reached its maximum in nine months or a year. It is widely believed that those who show signs of recovery within the first two weeks will go on to achieve a higher degree of recovery in a shorter course of time. There are many exceptions to this, however. The degree of paralysis seems to be a more reliable indicator of the recovery to be expected than the latent time before recovery commences. The milder the paralysis in the first two weeks, the more complete the recovery is likely to be. It is often said that patients over 50 years of age tend to have a poorer degree of recovery.

The most common sequel of incomplete recovery in Bell's palsy is synkinesis, and minor degrees of this can be detected in approximately half the patients if a careful examination is made. Some degree of residual muscular weakness persists in 25–50 per cent of cases. Contracture, due in part to tonic facial spasm, occurs in roughly a quarter of patients with Bell's palsy. Hemifacial spasm is a dubious complication of Bell's palsy, however. It was reported by earlier writers but the term was used more loosely in the past and included tonic spasm as well as clonic spasm. Thus what was described in previous years as hemifacial spasm might be termed a contracture today.

Hemifacial spasm as defined in this chapter has never been seen following a Bell's palsy by the authors.

Recurrent Bell's palsy A small number of patients have more than one attack of Bell's palsy on the same or the opposite side of the face. Recurring attacks always prompt renewed investigation to exclude a neurinoma, diabetes mellitus, sarcoidosis, cholesteatoma, or the Melkersson–Rosenthal syndrome. After all the known causes of recurring facial paralysis have been excluded there remains a hard core of patients with truly idiopathic recurring facial palsy. By the third or fourth attack most recurring cases have generally involved each side of the face. The patient seen in Fig. 6.7 (p. 209) had a Bell's palsy on the opposite side two years previously. This interesting variant form of Bell's palsy has not been the subject of much discussion, perhaps because no one worker has gathered a large series, although most practitioners have seen a few cases. The authors have had two patients who suffered five attacks of alternating facial paralysis each during an eight-year period. Both patients were young women under 30 years of age.

Unfortunately the signs of imperfect recovery tend to become more apparent after each attack of facial paralysis. Despite having repeated attacks the residual facial deformity is often not severe; this is partly because if both sides of the face have been affected the asymmetry is less obvious. Synkinesis tends to be a greater problem than deformity. It was previously believed that decompression of the facial nerve would prevent recurrence of paralysis. It is now known that despite expert decompression the facial paralysis does recur in a number of cases (Miehlke 1973). The cause of recurring facial paralysis is unknown. However, the failure of decompression to prevent it adds to our difficulty in accepting that compression of the nerve in the bony canal is responsible for Bell's palsy.

De Vriese and Pelz (1969) classified recurrences of Bell's palsy into those that recurred on the same (ipsilateral) side and those that recurred on the opposite (contralateral) side. They labelled them recurrent and alternating Bell's palsy respectively. Boddie (1972) felt there was no essential difference in the nature of these repeated attacks and recommended that the term alternating Bell's palsy be discarded and that all repeated attacks should be called recurrent Bell's palsy.

Boddie estimates the total incidence of recurrent Bell's palsy to be less than 5 per cent of all cases. The quoted incidence varies between 7–15 per cent but he suggests that all the reported series represent a highly selected group of patients.

Bilateral Bell's palsy This might be regarded as a contradiction in terms since we have defined Bell's palsy as a unilateral facial paralysis. However, there are occasional reports in the literature of Bell's palsy occurring in one side of the face and being followed a few days later by Bell's palsy on the other side (McGovern 1965). Unlike recurrent Bell's palsy where the episodes of paralysis are separated in time, in bilateral Bell's palsy they are present at the same time. Bilateral Bell's palsy appears to be a much more rare variant than recurrent Bell's palsy. No specific factor is known which accounts for these variant forms and their explanation must await the elucidation of the aetiology of Bell's palsy.

Involvement of other nerves in Bell's palsy There is growing evidence that Bell's palsy is not always the simple mononeuropathy it appears to be on routine clinical examination. Subclinical involvement of other nerves has been detected by electromyography and nerve conduction studies. Hopf (1963) reported abnormal ulnar nerve conductivity in patients with clinically evident mononeuropathies. His series included three cases of Bell's palsy and implied the existence of a polyneuropathy. A number of studies have been carried out on the electrical changes in the facial nerve of the uninvolved side in Bell's palsy. Waylonis and Johnson (1964) reported evidence of bilateral facial nerve pathology in 5 out of 9 patients. Delayed latencies in nerve conduction tests were found. Similar results were obtained by Safman (1971) who demonstrated a subclinical neuropathy on the clinically uninvolved side in 14 out of 18 cases of Bell's palsy. In the majority of these 14 cases a neuropraxic lesion was found by electromyography and nerve conduction latency studies. The electrical tests in the non-paralysed side returned to normal within six months.

A very thorough electrophysiological study was carried out by Olsen (1975) and he found no evidence of subclinical involvement of the non-paralysed side. He examined 45 patients with Bell's palsy without a history of previous facial paralysis, and 17 patients with traumatic facial palsy. Comparison of the involved and uninvolved sides in both groups showed normal electromyograms and nerve conduction latencies in the non-paralysed side. Adour (1976) points out that there is often clinical evidence of slight involvement of other cranial nerves in Bell's palsy. He quotes that in 40 per cent of cases there is evidence of an abnormal response in the vestibular system, in 35 per cent sensation in the afferent arc of the gag reflex (glossopharyngeal nerve) is absent or decreased, and in 25 per cent the trigeminal nerve is involved.

Pathology

There has been a surprisingly small number of autopsy reports in this disease. Although the disease is not fatal it is a common enough condition and many autopsy subjects must have had an unrelated Bell's palsy in their medical history. It would be helpful to know what changes are present in the nerve and the nucleus some years after the paralysis. If one excludes cases of facial paralysis due to hypertensive haemorrhage in the Fallopian canal, then there have been fewer than a dozen autopsy reports in the literature. In essence they all showed degeneration in the myelin sheaths and axons with no inflammatory changes. Some autopsies before 1910 did show inflammatory changes, but it has been argued that these may have been undiagnosed herpes zoster facial palsies in the days before the syndrome was defined by Ramsay Hunt. Similarly, the autopsy reported by Proctor *et al.* (1976), on a man who died 10 days after the onset of a presumed Bell's palsy, revealed the histological picture of a viral neuritis.

The other source of histological material comes from biopsies performed during an episode of paralysis. Biopsies have been taken from the chorda tympani and facial nerves, usually in association with decompression surgery and nerve grafting procedures. Most of the biopsies of the facial nerve have also shown degenerative changes without inflammatory features (Hall 1951; Kettel 1959). Similar changes have been found in the chorda tympani nerve. McGovern (1970) and Miehlke (1973) biopsied the chorda tympani nerve and found oedema without inflammatory changes. Blatt and Freeman (1966) claimed to show evidence of inflammation in the chorda tympani but their interpretation of the histology has been disputed by Sanchez Fernandez *et al.* (1977) and other writers. Most of the reports from operations in Bell's palsy patients are confined to the naked eye changes in the facial nerve. There have been a great number of reports of swelling of part of the nerve or 'herniation' of the nerve when the sheath is incised (Cawthorne 1946; Kettel 1959; Jongkees 1965). These authors regard this as proof of an abnormal oedematous nerve. Herniation or bulging of the nerve after incision of the sheath has been regarded as a normal finding by Sunderland (1946) and Sadé (1972). Sadé supported his opinion by taking a biopsy of the sheath and showing that although the nerve bulged through the incision there was no oedema of the sheath. Decompression surgery involves the removal of bone from the mastoid process and Fallopian canal by the use of a drill. It seems inevitable that this must disturb some of the anastomoses between the blood-supply of the middle ear cleft and the facial nerve. In addition the drilling may on occasion cause some direct trauma to the nerve. When Crabtree (1972) re-explored four facial nerves which had been decompressed elsewhere he found two cases in which the previous surgery had produced a traumatic neuroma of the facial nerve. Even if one were to accept that the reported macroscopic swelling of the nerve is due to abnormal oedema, a lingering doubt remains that in some cases the oedema could be due to the surgical exposure rather than to the paralytic lesion. This problem does not exist with chorda tympani nerve biopsies which are easily obtainable with the minimum of surgical trauma and a number of recent electronmicroscopic studies of this branch of the nerve have been most instructive. Karatay *et al.* (1976) demonstrated the co-existence of degenerative and regenerative changes in the nerve in Bell's palsy with no inflammatory changes. This has been confirmed by Sanchez Fernandez *et al.* (1977). These authors showed that a similar pattern of degenerative changes in the chorda tympani was present in other facial nerve paralyses. Similar degenerative changes were found in ascending order of severity in (a) Bell's palsy, (b) traumatic facial paralysis, (c) congenital facial paralysis, and (d) the Melkersson–Rosenthal syndrome.

Aetiology

In the previous chapter the different mechanisms which produce facial paralysis were examined. The causal mechanism of Bell's palsy must be one which can produce sudden facial paralysis with a high degree of spontaneous recovery. It must also be capable of producing a monophasic illness in the majority of patients while causing recurrent paralyses in a small minority. Five main hypotheses have been put forward to explain the mystery of Bell's palsy and these will be discussed in turn. The hypotheses should not, however, be regarded as mutually exclusive and many believe in a combination or synthesis of several of them.

The rheumatic hypothesis Berard (1836) put forward the view that a rheumatic swelling pressed the nerve against the walls of the Fallopian canal. The meaning of the term rheumatic has changed over the years and the theory is now obsolete.

The cold hypothesis (paralysis a frigore or ex frigore) Sir Charles Bell believed that peripheral facial palsy could have a variety of causes, including exposure to draughts and chills. Almost a century and a half later the debate continues, and Zülch (1970) lays great stress on rapid cooling or chilling as a factor in the production of Bell's palsy. The evidence in favour of the hypothesis is mainly anecdotal and is based on the unreliable principle *post hoc ergo propter hoc*. Many writers have identified a history of exposure to cold preceding the onset of paralysis in a large number of their patients. Since exposure to draughts or cold is an everyday occurrence one might not be too surprised to find such a history in any group of people. Other writers have gone to great lengths to show that people with occupational exposure to draughts and cold, such as train drivers, frozen-food packers, soldiers guarding high mountain passes, etc., suffer no increased incidence of Bell's palsy. The enclosure of the nerve in the Fallopian canal should be a protective advantage as far as cold injury is concerned and the adjacent cranial and cervical nerves would appear to be immune from this proposed lesion. It is probably true to say that many modern doctors pay only lip service to the hypothesis of exposure to cold. However, patients certainly find it reassuring to be told that their alarming facial paralysis is due to nothing more serious than sitting in a draught or a chill and that the paralysis will soon start to improve.

The ischaemic hypothesis The essence of this hypothesis is that ischaemia from disturbed circulation in the vasa nervorum causes facial nerve paralysis. Originally it was believed that primary ischaemia was sufficient to account for the paralysis and this formed the theoretical basis of treatment with vasodilator drugs. Later the hypothesis of combined primary and secondary ischaemia was advocated by a number of writers (Hilger 1949; Blunt 1956; Sullivan and Smith 1956). According to this theory primary vascular spasm does not of itself produce sufficient ischaemia to cause paralysis. However, the initial ischaemia does produce a swelling or oedema of the nerve. This swelling of the nerve in the confined space of the Fallopian canal produces a secondary compressive ischaemia which results in facial nerve paralysis. A great number and variety of factors are thought to be capable of producing the vasospasm which initiates the primary ischaemia. These include cold injury, anoxia, carbon dioxide excess, constitutional vasomotor instability, and toxic, allergic, infective, hormonal, and emotional factors. The ischaemic hypothesis represents the current orthodox view and is supported by the majority of eminent authorities in the field (Cawthorne and Haynes 1956; Bosatra 1956; Fowler 1958; Korkis 1959; Williams 1959; Kettel 1959; Jongkees 1972). In addition, Zülch (1970) and Miehlke (1973) now regard the ischaemic hypothesis as so firmly established that they substitute the term 'ischaemic facial paralysis' for Bell's palsy. The concepts of ischaemia and oedema have formed the theoretical basis of treatment by vasodilators, stellate ganglion block, and surgical decompression of the nerve and are at least tacitly accepted by the large number of specialists who employ these modes of therapy. The ischaemic hypothesis is supported almost entirely by the eloquence of its distinguished advocates: there is a dearth of scientific evidence. A great medley of animal experiments has been carried out in which various fluids have been injected into the Fallopian canal, and in which ligatures and spring clips have been applied to the facial nerve distal to the stylomastoid foramen. The majority of these interesting experiments prove only what is already widely known, that compression damages the nerve. What they do not prove is that ischaemia, compression, or oedema occur in Bell's palsy. Evidence that these do occur is based principally on the appearance of the nerve during decompression surgery which has already been discussed.

That gross vascular lesions can cause facial palsy is proven by the occurrence of the paralysis due to haemorrhage seen in patients with malignant hypertension (Chapter 3). Recently Calcaterra *et al.* (1976) have shown that embolism involving the petrosal branch of the middle meningeal artery can also cause facial palsy. Three of their patients who had pre-operative ferrosilicone embolization of the middle meningeal artery quickly developed an ipsilateral peripheral facial paralysis, and recovery took place over a period of some months. One of the difficulties in accepting that vasospasm can cause similar ischaemic paralysis is that vasospasm is essentially a recurring phenomenon, as seen in Raynaud's disease and migraine for example. All the factors held to be responsible for producing vasomotor disturbance in the facial nerve are recurring factors. Bell's palsy, on the other hand, is generally a once-in-a-lifetime event. Furthermore, no other nerve paralysis is attributed to such vasospastic ischaemia. Supporters of the hypothesis blame the Fallopian canal and claim that instead of being a protective factor it predisposes the nerve to compression injury. They explain the uniqueness of the facial nerve lesion by claiming that no other nerve has a prolonged course through a bony tunnel. This is incorrect. The inferior alveolar nerve has a similar, although admittedly less tortuous, course through the mandibular canal. It is even more exposed than the interosseous facial nerve to cold and focal (dental) sepsis. The bony canal is highly protective, and paralysis of this sensory nerve is a rarity.

The viral hypothesis Many clinicians, troubled by the lack of evidence for an ischaemic cause of Bell's palsy, have turned to a viral hypothesis secure in the knowledge that viruses do cause some types of facial paralysis. Some speculate that many cases of Bell's palsy are cases of herpes zoster infection without a rash. Others believe that herpes simplex virus is the likeliest culprit or that the viruses of mumps, measles, and influenza are responsible in some instances.

Aitken and Brain (1933) demonstrated complement-fixing antibodies to varicella zoster virus in 4 (18 per cent) of 22 cases of facial palsy without a zoster rash. Mair *et al.* (1976) carried out viral studies on 133 consecutive cases of peripheral facial palsy. Nine patients (6·8 per cent) had virological evidence of simultaneous infection with herpes zoster virus. Seven of these were clinically obvious cases of the Ramsay Hunt syndrome but 2 patients (1·8 per cent) had neither rash nor auditory symptoms and would have been classified clinically as Bell's palsy cases. Berg *et al.* (1976) in a series of 44 patients with peripheral facial paralysis found that the herpes zoster antigen was raised only in those patients with clinically obvious herpes zoster oticus. Laboratory evidence of recent viral infection in 16 (31·3 per cent) of 51 consecutive cases of acute non-traumatic peripheral facial palsy was found by Djupesland *et al.* (1976). The viruses implicated were herpes zoster (9 cases), herpes simplex (3 cases), influenza B (2 cases), and cytomegalovirus and mumps virus (1 case each). In other virological studies essentially negative serological findings were reported (Dodge and Poskanzer 1962; McCormick 1972; Korczyn *et al.* 1973).

From these and other highly instructive papers it would appear that viruses are in some way associated with a number of apparently idiopathic facial palsies. It would also appear that in over two-thirds of cases no such association exists. Even if greatly improved methods of viral detection are developed in future, viral neuritis as a cause of Bell's palsy seems an unlikely possibility on histological grounds. Viral infections are characterized by an inflammatory response and lymphocytic infiltration of the facial nerve would be the expected finding. In Bell's palsy no inflammatory response is seen and the histological picture is one of degeneration without inflammation.

The immunological hypothesis This is by no means a new theory but it has recently received considerable experimental support. The occasional cases of bilateral Bell's palsy have often prompted comparison with the Guillain–Barré syndrome. In 1916 Patrick wrote: 'Clinically there seems to be no dividing-line between facial diplegia of polyneuritis and facial diplegia ex frigore. To go one step further, one might ask what is the essential difference between rheumatic facial diplegia and ordinary unilateral facial palsy ex frigore?' One very important difference between the Guillain–Barré syndrome and Bell's palsy is that the cerebrospinal fluid protein is increased in the former and is normal in the latter. However, Charous and Saxe (1962) pointed out the following similarities between the two conditions:

(a) both have a rapid onset and spontaneous recovery;
(b) oedema of the nerve and myelin degeneration have been reported in both; and
(c) aetiology is unknown but an allergic response has been postulated in both.

To these we might add:

(d) steroids are used to treat both conditions;
(e) recurrent forms of both conditions occur in a small number of patients;
(f) in a number of patients a preceding viral infection is associated with both diseases;
(g) unilateral facial paralysis sometimes occurs in the Guillain–Barré syndrome;
(h) there is sometimes evidence of a polyneuropathy in Bell's palsy patients.

It is suggested that Bell's palsy mononeuropathy with normal cerebrospinal fluid protein, and Guillain–Barré polyneuropathy with raised cerebrospinal fluid protein, may represent the opposite ends of a single spectrum of disease.

Recent experimental work on the production of facial palsy in animals by immunological methods has given strong support to the hypothesis. Coassolo (1953) induced facial paralysis by placing ice over the mastoid process of rabbits sensitized to horse serum. No paralysis was produced by ice in non-sensitized animals acting as controls. McGovern and Hansel (1961) were not able to reproduce Coassola's findings in rabbits. However, in 1972 McGovern *et al.* used non-sensitized dogs as controls and showed that sensitized dogs suffered a more severe facial paralysis with more intense histological nerve damage when the facial canal was injected with saline or horse serum. Later

McGovern *et al.* (1977) showed that, in immunized dogs, the severity of facial nerve damage was directly proportional to the degree of mast cell degranulation which occurred. Mast cell degranulation is a characteristic feature of immunological reactions. The infusion of cromolyn sodium—a mast cell degranulation inhibitor—lessened both the degree of experimental paralysis and the severity of the histological nerve injury.

A very much closer link between Bell's palsy and the Guillain–Barré syndrome in humans has been demonstrated by Abramsky *et al.* (1975). They found a striking immunological similarity in both conditions. The *in vitro* lymphocyte response to peripheral nerve basic protein P_1L was strongly positive in both. There was no lymphocyte response in either condition to the three other neural antigens (P_2, BE, and AChR) commonly used in experimental auto-immune neurological disease. The basic protein P_1L produces experimental allergic neuritis in animals, which is thought to be an appropriate animal model of the human Guillain–Barré syndrome. The lymphocyte response to neural antigen P_1L was found exclusively in patients with Bell's palsy or the Guillain–Barré syndrome. In 26 control subjects with other types of facial weakness or with chronic neuropathy no such response occurred. It is postulated that an *in vivo* sensitization of lymphocytes to peripheral nerve myelin gives rise to a cell-mediated auto-immune response in Bell's palsy and the Guillain–Barré syndrome. Abramsky and his colleagues suggested that the immunological theory of causation justified the use of steroid therapy on account of its immunosuppressive action.

Conclusion None of the aetiological hypotheses of Bell's palsy can be regarded as proven. However, we are strongly attracted by the immunological hypothesis. At present, therefore, we regard Bell's palsy as a mononeuritic variant or '*forme fruste*' of the Guillain–Barré syndrome. It must be admitted that the immunological hypothesis attempts to explain the mechanism of Bell's palsy rather than the cause. Indeed the reason why the facial nerve is so frequently involved in the Guillain–Barré syndrome may remain obscure after the basic cause of this syndrome has been found. It seems possible that some local facial nerve factors may account for the increased susceptibility of the nerve. The correctness of a theory is of course less important than its fruitfulness. Despite its limitations, the immunological theory would appear to provide a fertile path of enquiry.

Geniculate neuralgia

This condition is also called Hunt's neuralgia, facial nerve neuralgia, nervus intermedius neuralgia, and *tic douloureux* of the chorda tympani. In spite of this variety of titles some authors (Reichert 1933) deny that the condition exists and all who believe it does exist agree that it is rare. The concept of geniculate neuralgia is based on the theory of the cutaneous nerve supply of the facial nerve proposed by Hunt (see the section on the Ramsay Hunt syndrome, p. 70). The cell bodies of the sensory fibres of the facial nerve are located in the geniculate ganglion. Geniculate neuralgia can be defined as neuralgic pain occurring in the area of distribution of the cutaneous fibres of the facial nerve. It consists of paroxysms of severe pain in the deep part of the external auditory canal. Initially, at least, the pain is highly localized and only occasionally radiates for a distance of a few centimetres around the ear. Later the pain may be continuous for prolonged periods, and may spread beyond the ear. Trigger points, which when stimulated will precipitate neuralgic pain, are found less frequently in geniculate neuralgia than in trigeminal and glossopharyngeal neuralgia. Because the fifth, ninth, and tenth cranial nerves contribute to the cutaneous innervation of the ear, it can be difficult to be certain to which nerve the neuralgia should be attributed. The otalgia may be indistinguishable from that of glossopharyngeal neuralgia, and Reichert (1933) held that all cases of geniculate neuralgia were simply misdiagnosed cases of glossopharyngeal neuralgia. The differential diagnosis of otalgia is made more difficult by the number of sites in which disease causes referred earache. The tongue, tonsils, teeth, temporomandibular joints, pharynx, and the larynx are all well-recognized sources of otalgia. The diagnosis of geniculate neuralgia is based on the character and history of the pain and the exclusion of other local or referred causes. Medical treatment has not been accompanied by much success. Fortunately, spontaneous cures and prolonged remissions do occur.

Several surgical procedures have been reported to abolish the pain. Intracranial section of the nervus intermedius (Clark and Taylor 1909), glossopharyngeal neurectomy (Reichert 1933), and chorda tympani neurectomy (Rosen 1953) have all been reported to give at least temporary, if not permanent, relief. Kunc (1965) recommended selective tractotomy. More recently, Pulec (1976) has used a middle cranial fossa approach and excised the geniculate ganglion and the nervus intermedius. In his successful series of 15 cases he also carried out selective section of the trigeminal and glossopharyngeal nerves in some patients, and in others he removed 10 per cent of the motor trunk of the facial nerve. These series illustrate the difficulty in attributing the neuralgia to a single nerve because of the overlapping of the sensory nerve supply around the ear, and the numerous anastomoses between the facial nerve and adjacent nerves.

References

Abramsky, O., Webb, C., Teitelbaum, D., and Arnon, R. (1975). Cellular immune response to peripheral nerve basic protein in idiopathic facial paralysis (Bell's palsy). *J. neurol. Sci.* **26**, 13.

Adour, K. K. (1970). Bell's palsy (letter to editor). *Arch. Otolaryngol.* **91**, 310.

——. (1976). Cranial polyneuritis and Bell's palsy. *Arch. Otolaryngol.* **102**, 262.

Adour, K. K., Wingerd, J., Bell, D. N., Manning, J. J., and Hurley, J. P. (1972). Prednisone treatment for idiopathic facial paralysis (Bell's palsy). *New Engl. J. Med.* **287**, 1268.

Aitkén, R. S., and Brain R. T. (1933). Facial palsy and infection with zoster virus. *Lancet* **i**, 19.

Alberti, P. W., and Biagioni, E. (1972). Facial paralysis in children. A review of 150 cases. *Laryngoscope* **82**, 1013.

Alford, B. R., Dickey, J. R., and Pratt, F. E. (1966). Management of facial paralysis. *Tex. St. J. Med.* **62**, 56.

Alter, M. (1963). Familial aggregation of Bell's palsy. *Arch. Neurol.* (*Chic.*) **8**, 557.

Andermann, F., Cosgrove, J. B. R., Lloyd-Smith, D. L., Gloor, P., and McNaughton, F. L. (1961). Facial myokymia in multiple sclerosis. *Brain* **84**, 31.

Berard, A. (1836). Névralgies rebelles: section des nerfs malades. *J. Connais. med. chir.* **3**, 441.

Berg, R., Fosgren, M., and Schiratzki, H. (1976). Acute facial palsy. Some clinical and virological observations. *Acta Otolaryngol.* **81**, 462.

Blatt, I. M. and Freeman, J. A. (1966). Bell's palsy. Pathogenetic mechanism of idiopathic peripheral facial paralysis. *Trans. Amer. Acad. Ophthalmol. Otolaryngol.* **70**, 381.

Blunt, M. J. (1956). The possible role of vascular changes in the aetiology of Bell's palsy. *J. Laryngol. Otol.* **70**, 701.

Boddie, H. G. (1972). Recurrent Bell's palsy. *J. Laryngol. Otol.* **86**, 1117.

Bosatra, A. (1956). Some observations on the vascularisation of the seventh nerve. *J. Laryngol. Otol.* **70**, 605.

British Medical Journal (1972). Leading article. **iv**, 624.

Byl, F. M., and Adour, K. K. (1977). Auditory symptoms associated with Herpes Zoster or idiopathic facial paralysis. *Laryngoscope* **87**, 372.

Calcaterra, T. C., Rand, R. U., and Bentson, J. R. (1976). Ischaemic paralysis of the facial nerve—a possible aetiologic factor in Bell's palsy. *Laryngoscope* **86**, 92.

Cawthorne, T. (1946). Peripheral facial paralyses: some aspects of its pathology. *Laryngoscope* **56**, 653.

——, and Haynes, D. R. (1956). Facial palsy. *Brit. med. J.* **ii**, 1197.

Charous, D. I., and Saxe, B. I. (1962). The Landry–Guillain–Barré syndrome. Report of an unusual case with a comment on Bell's palsy. *New Engl. J. med.* **267**, 1334.

Clark, L. P., and Taylor, A. S. (1909). True tic douloureux of the sensory filaments of the facial nerve. *J. Amer. med. Ass.* **53**, 2144.

Coassolo, M. (1953). Studio della eccitabilita elettrica del nervo faciale nella paralise 'a frigore' sperimentale. *Minerva otorinolaring.* **3**, 31.

Crabtree, J. A. (1972). Facial nerve decompression. *Arch. Otolaryngol.* **95**, 395.

Dalton, G. A. (1960). Bell's palsy: some problems of prognosis and treatment. *Brit. med. J.* **ii**, 1765.

Djupesland, G., Berdal, P., Johanessen, T. A., Degre, M., Stien, R., and Skrede, S. (1976). Viral infection as a cause of acute peripheral facial palsy. *Arch. Otolaryngol.* **102**, 403.

De Santo, L. W., and Schubert, H. A. (1969). Bell's palsy, ten cases in a family. *Arch. Otolaryngol.* **89**, 700.

De Vriese, P. P., and Pelz, P. G. (1969). Recurrent and alternating Bell's palsy. *Ann. Otol.* (*St. Louis*) **78**, 1091.

Dodge, P. R., and Poskanzer, D. C. (1962). Varicella-zoster and herpes simplex antibody responses in patients with Bell's palsy. *Neurology* (*Minneap.*) **12**, 34.

Ehni, G., and Woltman, H. W. (1945). Hemifacial spasm: review of one hundred and six cases. *Arch. Neurol. Psychiat.* **53**, 205.

El Ebiary, H. M. (1971). Facial paralysis: a clinical study of 580 cases. *Rheumatol. phys. Med.* **11**, 100.

Fisch, U., and Esslen, E. (1972). The surgical treatment of facial hyperkinesia. *Arch. Otolaryngol.* **95**, 400.

Fowler, E. P. (1958). Medical and surgical treatment of Bell's palsy. *Laryngoscope* **68**, 1655.

Furakawa, Y., Tamaoki, H., and Nomura, A. (1975). Facial paralysis in pregnancy. *Practica Otologica* (*Kyoto*) **68**, 1115.

Hall, A. (1951). Pathology of Bell's palsy. *Arch. Otolaryngol.* **54**, 475.

Harrison, M. S. (1976). The facial tics. *J. Laryngol. Otol.* **90**, 561.

Hauser, W. A., Karnes, W. E., Annis, J., and Kurland, L. T. (1971). Incidence and prognosis of Bell's palsy in the population of Rochester, Minnesota. *Mayo Clin. Proc.* **46**, 258.

Hilger, J. A. (1949). The nature of Bell's palsy. *Laryngoscope* **59**, 228.

Hislinger, R. L., Adour, K. K., and Doty, H. E. (1975). Idiopathic facial paralysis, pregnancy, and the menstrual cycle. *Ann. Otol.* (*St. Louis*) **84**, 433.

Hjorth, R. J., and Willison, R. G. (1973). The electromyogram in facial myokymia and hemifacial spasm. *J. neurol. Sci.* **20**, 117.

Hopf, H. C. (1963). Electromyographic study on so-called mononeuritis. *Arch. Neurol.* **9**, 307.

Horstein, O. P. (1970). *Handbook of clinical neurology* (ed. P. J. Vinken and G. W. Bruyn), Vol. 8, p. 215. North-Holland, Amsterdam.

Jannetta, P. J., Abassy, M., Maroon, J. C., Ramos, F. M., and Albin, M. S. (1977). Etiology and definitive treatment of hemifacial spasm. *J. Neurosurg.* **47**, 321.

Jongkees, L. B. J. (1965). Bell's palsy: a surgical emergency? *Arch. Otolaryngol.* **81**, 497.

——. (1972). On peripheral facial nerve paralysis. *Arch. Otolaryngol.* **95**, 317.

——. (1973). Practical application of clinical tests for facial paralysis. *Arch. Otolaryngol.* **97**, 220.

Kaeser, H. E., and Skorpil, V. (1976). Myokymia involving the muscles innervated by the Vth, VIth, VIIth, IXth, Xth and XIIth cranial nerves with brain stem tumor. *Europ. Neurol.* **14**, 408.

Karatay, S., Katircioglu, S., and Erbengi, T. (1976). Ultrastructural investigations on the degenerative and regenerative processes in chorda tympani in Bell's paralysis. *Acta Otolaryngol.* **81**, 304.

Kettle, K. (1959). *Peripheral facial palsy: pathology and surgery*. Charles C. Thomas, Springfield, Illinois.

Korczyn, A. D. (1971). Bell's palsy and pregnancy. *Acta neurol. scand.* **47**, 603.

——, Swirski, R., and Henig, E. (1973), Bell's palsy and viral infections. *Europ. Neurol.* **10**, 191.

Korkis, F. B. (1959). The treatment of recent Bell's palsy on a rational etiological basis. *Arch. Otolaryngol.* **70**, 562.

Kunc, Z. (1965). Treatment of essential neuralgia of the ninth nerve by selective tractotomy. *J. Neurosurg.* **23**, 494.

Lambert, E. H., Love, J. G., and Mulder, D. W. (1961). Facial myokymia and brain tumor: electromyographic studies. *Amer. Ass. Electromyogr. Electrodiag. News Letter* **8**, 8.

Laurance, B. M., Mathews, W. B., and Diggle, J. H. (1968). Hereditary quivering of the chin. *Arch. Dis. Childh.* **43**, 249.

Lloyd, A. V. C., Jewitt, D. E., and Still, J. D. LL. (1966). Facial paralysis in children with hypertension. *Arch. Dis. Childh.* **41**, 292.

Lüscher, E. (1949) Syndom von Melkersson–Rosenthal. *Schweiz. med. Wschr.* **79**, 1.

Manning, J. J., and Adour, K. K. (1972). Facial paralysis in children. *Pediatrics* **49**, 102.

McCormick, D. (1972). Herpes simplex virus as cause of Bell's palsy. *Lancet* **i**, 937.

McGovern, F. H. (1965). Bilateral Bell's palsy. *Laryngoscope* **75**, 1070.

——. (1966). The use of the nerve excitability tests in paralysis of the facial nerve. *Laryngoscope* **76**, 955.

——. (1970). Chorda tympani neurectomy for Bell's palsy. *Arch. Otolaryngol.* **92**, 189.

——., and Hansel, J. S. (1961). Decompression of the facial nerve in experimental Bell's palsy. *Laryngoscope* **71**, 1090.

——., Konigsmark, B. W., and Sydnor, J. B. (1972). An immunological concept for Bell's palsy. *Laryngoscope* **82**, 1594.

——., Estevez, J., and Jackson, R. (1977). Immunological concept for Bell's palsy. Further experimental study. *Ann. Otol. (St. Louis)* **86**, 300.

Mair, I. W. S., Flugsrud, L. B., and Emmanuel, I. A. (1976). Peripheral facial palsy and herpes zoster infection. *J. Laryngol. Otol.* **40**, 373.

Meige, H. (1910). Les convulsions de la face. Une forme clinique de convulsion faciale bilaterale et médiane. *Rev. neurol.* **20**, 437.

Melkersson, E. (1928). Ett fall av recidiverande facialispares i samband med angioneurotiskt ödem. *Hygiea (Stockh.)* **90**, 737.

Miehlke, A. (1973). *Surgery of the facial nerve*. Saunders, Philadelphia, London, and Toronto.

Miescher, G. (1945). Über essentielle granulomatöse Makrocheilie (*Cheilitis granulomatosa*). *Dermatologia (Basel)* **91**, 57.

Nappi, G., Moglia, A., Poloni, M., and Arrigo, A. (1977). Hemifacial spasm associated with dolichomegavertebrobasilar anomaly. *Europ. Neurol.* **15**, 94.

Nussbaum, M. (1977). Hemifacial spasm associated with a benign parotid tumour. *Ann. Otol. (St. Louis)* **86**, 75.

Olsen, P. Z. (1975). Prediction of recovery in Bell's palsy. *Acta neurol. scand.* **52**, (Suppl. 61).

Park, W. P., and Watkins, A. L. (1949). Facial paralysis. Analysis of 500 cases. *Arch. phys. Med.* **30**, 749.

Patrick, H. T. (1916). Facial diplegia in multiple neuritis. *J. nerv. ment. Dis.* **44**, 322.

Proctor, B., Corgill, D. A., and Proud, G. (1976). The pathology of Bell's palsy. *Trans. Am. Acad. Ophthalmol., Otolaryngol.* **82**, ORL 70.

Pulec, J. L. (1976). Geniculate neuralgia: diagnosis and surgical management. *Laryngoscope* **86**, 955.

Radu, E. W., Skorpil, V., and Kaeser, H. E. (1975). Facial myokymia. *Europ. Neurol.* **13**, 499.

Reichert, F. L. (1933). Tympanic plexus neuralgia. *J. Amer. med. Ass.* **100**, 1744.

Rosen, S. (1953). Tic douloureux of the chorda tympani; report of cases. *Arch. Neurol. Psychiat.* **69**, 375.

Rosenthal, C. (1931). Klinisch-erbbiologischer Beitrag zur Konstitutionspathologie. Gemeinsames Auftreten von (rezidivierender familiärer) Facialislähmung, angioneurotischem Gesichitsödem und Lingua plicata in Arthritismus-Familien. *Z. ges Neurol. Psychiat.* **131**, 475.

Sadé, J. (1972). Pathology of Bell's palsy. *Arch. Otolaryngol.* **95**, 406.

Safman, B. L. (1971). Bilateral pathology in Bell's palsy. *Arch. Otolaryngol.* **93**, 55.

Sanchez Fernandez, J. M., Rivera Pomar, J. M., Marco, J., and Lopez Campos, J. L. (1977). Macroscopic and ultrastructural findings in some diseases of the facial nerve. *Acta Otolaryngol.* **83**, 211.

Schwarz, K., and Elsässer, K. H. (1961). Klinischer und neuropathologischer Beitrag zur cerebralen Symptomatik beim Melkersson–Rosenthal Syndrom. *Arch. Psychiat. Nervenkr.* **202**, 281.

Spillane, J. D. (1975). *An atlas of clinical neurology*, second ed. Oxford University Press, Oxford.

Sullivan, J. A., and Smith, J. B. (1950). The otological concept of Bell's palsy and its treatment. *Ann. Otol. (St. Louis)* **37**, 233.

Sunderland, S. (1946). The effect of rupture of the perineurium on the contained nerve fibres. *Brain* **69**, 149.

Susac, J. O., Smith, J. E., and Schatz, N. J. (1973). Superior oblique myokymia. *Arch. Neurol. (Chic.)* **29**, 432.

Swan, D. M. (1952). Stellate block in Bell's palsy. *J. Amer. med. Ass.* **150**, 32.

Taverner, D. (1959). The prognosis and treatment of spontaneous facial palsy. *Proc. roy. Soc. Med.* **52**, 1077.

Tomita, H., Hayakawa, W., and Hondo, R. (1972). Varicella-zoster virus in idiopathic facial palsy. *Arch. Otolaryngol.* **95**, 364.

Toremalm, N. G., Elmqvist, D., Elner, A., and Mercke, U. (1977). Hemifacial spasm. *Acta Otolaryngol.* **83**, 341.

Verjaal, A. (1955). Acute Periphere Facialisparalyse. *Ned. T. Geneesk.* **99**, 3767.

Waylonis, G. W., and Johnson, E. W. (1964). Facial nerve conduction delay. *Arch. phys. Med.* **45**, 539.

Willbrand, J. W., Blumhagen, J. D., and May, M. (1974). Inherited Bell's palsy. *Ann. Otol. (St. Louis)* **83**, 343.

Williams, H. (1959). Bell's palsy. *Arch. Otolaryngol.* **70**, 436.

Zülch, K. Z. (1970). In *Handbook of clinical neurology* (ed. P. J. Vinken and G. W. Bruyn), Vol. 8. North-Holland, Amsterdam.

5 Trauma involving the facial nerve

5 Trauma involving the facial nerve

WE HAVE chosen to describe trauma to the facial nerve and its effects, together with the subject of regeneration. When one sees a patient with recognizable clinical signs of facial nerve trauma, one immediately sizes up the chances of his or her return to normality. Therefore, in this chapter we start with a short introduction to the subject of regeneration, and follow this with a detailed assessment of aetiological factors in trauma.

Introduction

One of the sources of much research into regeneration up to the present day is the classic study on the regeneration of animal tissues by Lazzaro Spallanzani (1729–99). Since regeneration is a physiological process, restoration of function must be considered along with restoration of structure. Comparative animal studies are also instructive. To keep within the limitations of this book we shall confine our attention mainly to the restoration of function, for which neurological regeneration is of course necessary. Detailed information on all aspects of regeneration is available in the book by Goss (1969).

Regeneration is a normal continuing function of cells in the body, blood cells for example have a life-span of only 100 days. If regeneration perpetually balanced degeneration, there would be no death. We maintain, all being well, an equilibrium between one and the other, and in man this should last, so we are told, about three score years and ten. Conditions such as disease and trauma will, of course, affect the equilibrium. The most important form of regeneration is the reproduction of our species. Other regenerative processes have changed little in man over the time of evolution (Flickinger 1967; Barr 1964).

Protozoa can synthesize molecules, and thus adapt to the changing biochemical surroundings in which they must survive. Metazoa can synthesize cells, and in man this process is more efficient in some tissues than in others. There are, of course, varying degrees of regeneration. Often it is not sufficient merely to reproduce cells. Organs must be built up, appendages grown, and function, for example, neurological function, restored. It is generally true to say that as evolution proceeded regenerative capabilities were reduced. The more specialized or complex the tissue, the less its reparative ability. Perhaps some definitive selection of the regenerative powers to be retained took place. The complexity of this study is enormous. Have human beings in the course of evolution had to discard the greatest powers of regeneration in order to retain higher intellectual capabilities? Could it be that we can better adapt to the loss of a limb, eye, or ear, or survive degrees of cerebral damage because of our better brain?

Considerable work has been carried out to try and determine in more detail the importance of neural stimulus in the process of regeneration. Readers are referred to the work by Singer (1959). Perhaps in our own species the repair of injury is better described as healing, rather than regeneration, which is more appropriate in other vertebrates. Carlson (1970) has written an interesting account of muscle regeneration as opposed to simple muscle healing. Our skin usually heals if not too severely injured, but if we lose a finger it will never re-grow. If a nerve is torn, its function is lost, but may be restored by inserting a graft between the torn ends, or by anastomosing the distal end to another nerve. If a cutaneous nerve is transferred in order to repair the peripheral seventh cranial nerve, it does not remain as a nerve, but becomes only a guide to the repair process from the regenerating cut end of the damaged seventh nerve (Berrill and Karp 1976).

While studying lower vertebrates during the first half of this century, it was discovered that irradiation appeared to make cells lose their regenerative competence. We now know that cytotoxic drugs will also in certain cases inhibit regeneration which is becoming harmful to the patient. We have also learned that such drugs can damage the patient because they lack selectivity and interfere with normal regeneration.

Peripheral nerve axons can regenerate after injury, although with varying degrees of success and return of function. Lieberman (1971) remarks that the regeneration is prevented when the affected neurone or neurones 'die'. This can happen not only when the neurone itself is damaged, but also if the axon is severed close to the parent cell. Should the neurone survive, then the axon can extend and spread over a considerable area (Cajal 1928; Sunderland 1968). Great differences exist between the regenerative capacities of axons in the central nervous system and those of peripheral nerves. In mammals attempts at rejoining and restoring function in the upper motor neurone are in vain. Little is known of the metabolic responses to neurone damage in the central nervous system. Cole (1968) provided some limited histochemical evidence suggesting differences between central and peripheral neurones in the reaction of axons to damage. Work progresses in this extremely difficult area of investigation. Myelin is a membrane-like structure surrounding most of the large axons in higher animals, and serves as an extremely efficient electric insulator. In man the myelin membranes originate from the Schwann cells in the peripheral nervous system. The homologous cells in the central nervous system are called oligodendroglial cells. There are, however, proportionately less of the latter. At present there is no absolute evidence that local injury stimulates any proliferation of neurones or oligodendrocytes in the central nervous system. This means that if upper motor neurones are extensively damaged, then, as elsewhere in the nervous system, they will not recover. Even after relatively minor injury there is apparently no stimulus to restore function.

Upper motor neurone trauma

This chapter is devoted to trauma of the seventh cranial nerve, and the major part necessarily relates to lower motor lesions. However, much of the morbidity associated with neurological damage arises in the course of, and because of, the upper motor neurones being damaged. Significantly, an article in *The Lancet* (1976) was entitled 'What hope is there in the realms of investigation and experiment for the upper motor axon?'. Many basic problems remain unresolved in humans. Consider, for example, the following idea. Do the regenerating central nervous system axons start off in the right direction? Work by Adams *et al.* (1969) suggests that this is possible in the axons of the hypothalamo–hypophyseal tract. However, in humans, unlike some of the lower vertebrates, they do not arrive at their destination. Distance in man must surely play some part in the intricate task of investigation. It is difficult to ascertain what happens between the injured site and the peripheral muscle or sense organ. All this refers in degree to the upper motor neurone connections of the seventh cranial nerve.

The upper motor neurone area of the facial nerve includes the motor cortex, cortico-bulbar tracts, and the brain-stem. Trauma to these vital sections of the nerve may produce an upper motor paralysis, or, after healing, result in focal epilepsy, involving the face. Road accidents and missile injuries can account for much of this trauma. Brain injury can result in facial weakness of upper motor neurone type. In skull injuries, fractures may also tear the dura, and allow cerebrospinal fluid to leak into cavities which have direct access to the outside. Examples are tympanic membrane and middle ear damage. Leakage of cerebrospinal fluid along the eustachian tube into the post-nasal space will occur if the drum remains intact. Fractures of the anterior cranial fossa may also result in communication with the nasal cavity. In this way infection can develop, and further influence the prognosis of upper motor neurone damage. Sometimes an intracranial haematoma develops only slowly, and so the effects of increasing pressure may take several days to become evident. This perhaps accounts for those cases of late onset upper motor neurone lesions that may affect the face. Lateral blows tend to produce middle meningeal vessel damage, with all its associated hazards. Readers are invited to study Sutherland (1974) and Hooper (1969) for detailed reading on the patterns of skull trauma. The subsequent degree of recovery after trauma to the upper motor neurone of the facial nerve depends entirely on the amount of tissue left potentially intact, and this is apparent only after the initial shock phase has worn off.

There are conditions which are reversible, an obvious one being the presence of an extra, or sub-dural haematoma. Continued pressure would gradually destroy more and more cells, and unless decompression is carried out, restoration of function is unlikely. There is no method of grafting the upper motor neurone, and permanent damage to the face can result from injury in this area.

Lower motor neurone trauma

Historical introduction

One of the best-known names in the study of peripheral nerves, and their disorders, must be that of Schwann (1839). Virchow (1858) was also initially associated with the new science of cellular biology. Further discoveries were made by Louis Antoine Ranvier (1871, 1872, 1875, 1876) who was then Professor of Histology in Paris. He described the interruptions which are seen in the myelin sheath—now known as the nodes of Ranvier. Gombault in 1881 described demyelination, and Waller (1850, 1852) showed that since the neurone was a trophic centre, then damage to, or section of, the process or axon, could lead to degeneration in the distal portion. It has always been fortunate that peripheral nerves were readily available for macroscopic and microscopic study. This section of the book is devoted to a discussion of damage occurring to the nucleus and the ongoing peripheral nerve.

Certain basic terms must be mentioned before we continue to the aetiology of trauma. Chronologically: Nissl (1892) described the retrograde cell change and, in 1893, Stroebe wrote of chromatolysis, both effects occurring in the cell body after sectioning of the axon. The latter also demonstrated the primary changes of the nerve fibres which occur after crush injuries or pressure, resulting in swelling of the interrupted nerve fibre proximal and distal to the site of injury. Nissl's discoveries were immediately accepted. The later findings of Stroebe, however, met with less credence, despite the earlier descriptions of Ranvier (1875). Ranvier and Stroebe had demonstrated actual sprouting of new axons from the stump of axis cylinders in a regenerating nerve. Much important work has been carried out since and is still continuing.

Effects of injury

In higher animals contraction has become the specialized function of muscle cells and the transmission of nerve impulses has become the function of the neurones. The seventh nerve is insulated very effectively by a myelin sheath, which is interrupted at roughly millimetre intervals by the nodes of

Ranvier. However long the axon processes, it is the cell body which maintains their function and anatomical integrity. Protein material necessary for axon maintenance is produced in the neurone, and transported down the axon by so-called axoplasmic transport. Ganong (1975) discusses this physiological process in detail. The neurone, or central trophic centre, as it is sometimes described, contains the organelles and nucleus that control the metabolic processes of the entire neurone. Apparently there is no significant protein synthesis along the course of the axon (Droz 1969). Hence, the entire nerve is dependent on the proper functioning of the parent cell, in which there is a relatively high level of protein synthesis. The exact origin of the driving force for axoplasmic transport is not entirely clear. Original work on this form of transport was done by Weiss and Hiscoe (1948), who noticed that if a ligature was placed around a regenerating nerve, then a distension would occur above the point of constriction. Axoplasmic flow can be affected by factors other than trauma. Colchicine, barbiturates, and immunosuppressive agents have been implicated, as we shall see later; see also Weiss (1969) and Pollard *et al.* (1971). Damage to the axon close to the neurone can result in a reduction in the number of brain stem neurones. Torvik and Skjösten (1971) showed that, in the mouse, a considerable number of cells in the seventh nerve nucleus disappeared after extracranial nerve section. Crushing of the nerve, however, produced only minimal neurone loss. Diphtheria neurotoxin is toxic to the peripheral nerve, causing segmental demyelination at the nodes of Ranvier.

Cortico-steroids have been advocated as a means of reducing scarring and diminishing tissue overactivity in cases of lower motor neurone trauma. These drugs can also have adverse catabolic and growth-retarding effects. Some workers have shown that cortisone can inhibit myelin deposition by the Schwann cells (Lytton and Murray 1954). It is important to distinguish several terms. 'Axonal degeneration' need not be associated with transection of nerve fibres. 'Segmental demyelination' indicates that the myelin sheath is absent for various segments of the length of the fibre, but that the axon has remained basically intact.

Parent cell or neurone If a neurone survives injury, the cell body enlarges progressively, beginning to enlarge on around the third day subsequent to injury and persisting in enlargement as long as active regeneration is required. For many years, it was thought that such enlargement, and the changes which took place within the cell, were part of a degenerative process. It is now recognized as an integral part of the regeneration process.

The total amount of cell RNA increases, but no longer remains in the Nissl particles. These migrate to the outer edges of the cell, and break up into smaller particles, a process known as chromatolysis (Cragg 1970). There is also an increase in enzyme activity, and protein synthesis. Animal experiments using the seventh nerve were carried out by Cammermeyer (1963), who demonstrated various aspects of chromatolysis occurring after the division of the facial nerve in the mouse.

Once the regeneration process is complete, the neurone returns to its normal size and activity. Hydén (1960) showed that the neurone produces great volumes of organic protein material during the regeneration process. The nearer the injury is to the neurone cell body, the greater is the metabolic effort for survival.

Proximal nerve stump Within about an hour of the section of a peripheral nerve, there is a marked swelling extending about a centimetre towards the parent cell. Work on the facial nerve by Campbell and Luzio (1964) has suggested this swelling contains fluid, consisting of muco-polysaccharides. Demyelination occurs over a few adjacent segments. Providing all goes well, after about seven days, there is evidence of new axons sprouting from the damaged end of the nerve stump. The concentration of enzymes, including acetylcholinesterase, and succine hydrogenase is increased. This is essential to the process of regeneration.

Distal nerve stump It is in this portion of the damaged nerve that the process known as Wallerian degeneration takes place after injury. When the neuronal elements are separated from their trophic centre, they die and disintegrate within about seven days. During this time, the surrounding myelin sheath disintegrates and is digested by the Schwann cells. Macrophages eventually remove all the debris. Weiss (1944) suggested that the Schwann cells themselves could act as macrophages, but this is now doubtful.

It is interesting to enquire as to why and how the Schwann cells change from protective sheath cells to active removers of broken-down myelin. According to Singer (1959) the stimulus may come from a decrease in, or actual cessation of axoplasmic flow. The cells may have such a positive stimulus, or else their transformation may be due to some loss of this inhibitory effect of the axon on the Schwann cells and their function (Nathaniel and Pease 1963). Various authorities have quoted the appearance of mast cells during Wallerian degeneration, and have suggested that these are connected with the break-down of myelin (Enerbäck *et al.* 1965; Olsson 1968, 1971). The basement membranes surrounding the Schwann cells persist, and form Schwann tubes. Inside the latter, cells proliferate, and give rise to the longitudinal bands of Büngner. These bands provide the optimal pathways along which regenerating axons can reach their destination. Most of the original layer of myelin will have been removed after about eighteen days. Regeneration, however, is evident by the fifth day, and some of the Schwann cells proliferate to produce remyelination.

Schwann cells The Schwann cells appear to play an important role in the complex mechanism of trauma and repair. Therefore nerves, such as the optic nerves, or the central nervous system tracts do not appear capable of much regeneration. There is, however, a considerable chemical difference between peripheral and central nervous system myelin. Reference to biochemistry text books is necessary for a review of this complex subject.

When a damaged nerve starts regeneration, axon outgrowth starts from both ends of the injured part. This plays an essential part in the mechanisms by which any gap may eventually be bridged. If the nerve is crushed or cut it will continue to conduct impulses for about three days, and, if the damage was severe, will then degenerate and die. In amphibia function may continue for two or three weeks (Barker and Ip 1966).

Supportive glial cells It is essential to remember that the four areas of nervous tissue which we have been discussing could not function without the supportive glial cells. These glial cells provide the surroundings in which the neurones exist within the central nervous system. They facilitate the passage of amino acids, sugars, and other nutrient materials to the neurones. Trauma to their blood supply, or tearing injury will damage not only the neurone, but also this highly important cellular background. There appears to be no doubt that the glial cells play an active part in regenerative processes (Pinner and Campbell 1965; Sjöstrand 1965).

Summary Injuries that destroy axonal continuity will lead to the following:

(a) Retrograde changes in the system central to the injury, i.e. in the stump of the nerve, and up to the parent body, provided that the axon damage is not close enough to the parent body. These changes include degeneration in one or two nodes, the axon diameter eventually decreases, and occasionally areas of demyelination and remyelination appear. Central chromatolysis takes place in the parent cell.

(b) Wallerian degeneration, with axolysis and myelinolysis, takes place in the nerve fibre at, and below the site of injury.

(c) The Schwann cell–fibroblast reaction.

(d) Chemical changes which are a direct result of the Wallerian degeneration, and are necessary for the immediate stimulus of regeneration.

(e) Increased activity in the supporting glial cells.

All these processes are described in great detail by Sunderland (1968), and Ducker (1972).

Degrees of damage

Neuropraxia This is a blockage of nerve conduction without any loss of continuity in the axon. The effect of such damage is entirely transitory once the aetiological factor has been removed, and recovery is complete.

Axonotmesis This is a term denoting damage to the axon, following which Wallerian degeneration has occurred. Eventual regeneration takes place at the rate of 1–4 mm per day. The regenerating axons will rapidly enter the empty endoneural tubes. Following axonotmesis, scar tissue does not obstruct regeneration, and recovery will be very satisfactory. Examples of lesions which can produce axonotmesis are listed below.

1. Compression, of a mild degree.
2. Crushing, as long as the nerve is not actually severed.
3. Cooling below 5 °C for over 30 minutes.
4. Transient ischaemia.

Neurotmesis This is the total physiological severance of a nerve. The axon and the connective tissue are damaged, but in some cases the fascicular architecture is retained. Such cases will show regeneration which will be less complete than that following axonotmesis. However, recovery of function may still be acceptable.

Maximum nerve damage If the injury is much more extensive, and involves damage to the axon, connective tissue, and the perineurium, regeneration will be poorly orientated, and much less effective than with any of the previously described degrees of nerve damage. The nerve will still appear macroscopically intact after this degree of injury.

Nerve division The nerve may not only be severed, but there may be a gap if a portion of the nerve has been torn out by injury. For recovery from this type of trauma a graft will be required to close the gap.

We can now consider the Schwann cell fibroblast reaction which takes place at the ends of the severed nerve. After rupture of the neural tube, the proliferating Schwann cells and the regenerating axons are no longer confined to a tube during their growth; Schwann and fibroblast elements proliferate in all directions at the ends of the cut tube, forming outgrowths which, depending on the distance to be covered, may or may not bridge the gap formed by the tear in the axon. The end result of this reaction could be merely the production of scar tissue, containing mainly Schwann cells and fibroblasts. The capacity of Schwann cells to sprout is apparently retained for long periods after injury. Clinically there is good reason for believing that this ability may be retained up to several years after the injury. If repair is to be made by surgery, the resultant scar tissue must first be removed from the cut ends of the nerve.

Classification of traumatic agents

Many peripheral nerves are exposed to possible injury, either in surgical proceedings, or in other forms of trauma such as accidents on the roads, at home, or in heavy industry. The spread of urban guerilla warfare has increased the incidence of missile trauma to all peripheral nerves. We suggest the following as a reasonably comprehensive method of classification of traumatic agents (Sunderland 1970).

1. *Missile injuries* These can produce trauma in the following ways;
   (a) As they enter, traverse, or leave the body they can tear away portions of the nerve.
   (b) They can produce traction on nerves which have some degree of elasticity. The magnitude of the effects will depend on the actual physical forces on the nerve and its blood-supply.
   (c) Damage may occur in nerves which are adjacent to the wound, and are unable to withstand the stresses and strains produced by the missile. In World War II, severe injuries of this 'stretch variety' were caused to the facial nerve by high velocity missiles. The facial nerve is protected by its long bony course, but this also means that injuries which involve it may be more severe than those affecting more vulnerable nerves. As the seventh nerve is more sheltered, greater degrees of force are necessary to reach and injure what may be extensive sections of the nerve. Animal experiments have shown that up to 60 per cent elongation can take place in peripheral nerves before the epineurium tears. Once this happens the nerve remains both elongated and perhaps damaged. Even a lesser degree of tension can leave the nerve up to one-fifth longer (Hapter 1970).

2. *Surgical section* The facial nerve can be damaged either accidentally or intentionally during surgery. The latter may be necessary in petrosectomy or in parotid gland surgery.

New techniques have lessened the risk of facial nerve damage in surgery. Use of the microscope during operations was first described in the 1920s but it was truly popularized only by the introduction of the Zeiss instrument in 1950 (Fig. 5.1). Advances in anaesthesia and in positioning techniques have allowed the development of more intricate procedures in the middle ear and temporal bone. Improved drills and other small instruments have aided in the speed and precision of ear surgery, and allowed new materials to be used as protheses in the restoration of hearing function. The use of temporal bone laboratories have provided means of training new surgeons in simulating theatre conditions (Fig. 5.2). Better training means less surgical trauma to the facial nerve.

All these new techniques have had two main effects. First, a higher proportion of patients are now submitted to surgery for the treatment of disease and the restoration or possible improvement of hearing; the most common operations are stapedectomy and tympanoplasty. Ear disease is fairly well controlled in Western countries. Secondly, operations in the region of the ear are now much safer in terms of all degrees of morbidity, including damage to

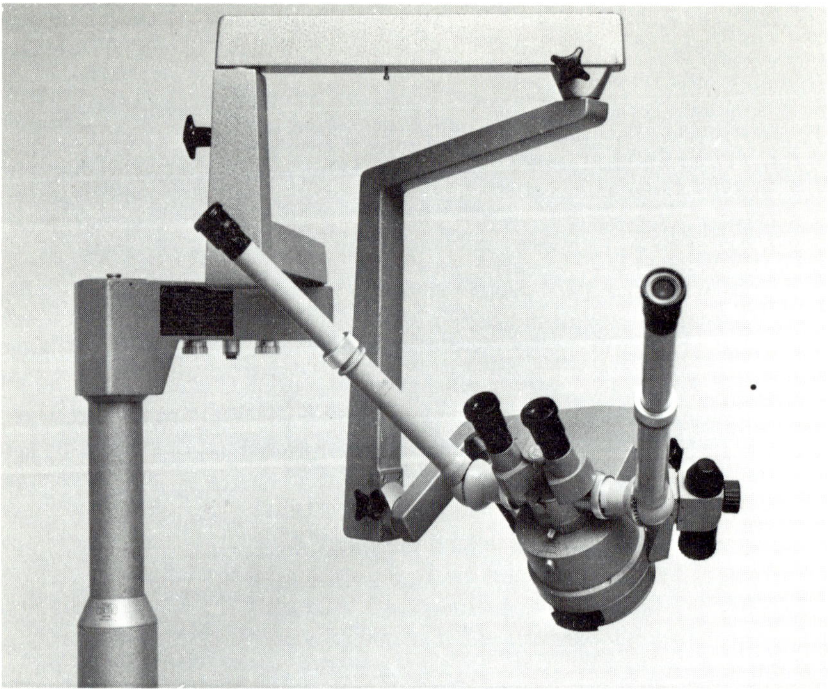

Fig. 5.1. Operating microscope.

the facial nerve. The question we would like to answer in this section is how much safer is the facial nerve from damage as a result of improved surgical techniques? The reply must be slightly evasive, for two reasons. Improved training of surgeons and the wider use of advanced techniques should in theory safeguard the seventh nerve. However, the nerve is still occasionally damaged, although usually only temporarily. Greater magnification means greater safety only if the surgeon has an exact knowledge of the area in which he is working. High-speed drills remove bone quickly, but generate potentially harmful heat if not properly controlled. A neighbouring nerve can easily be damaged if the drill slips. For a modern review the reader is referred to Hammond (1975).

It is relatively easy to assess the small morbidity arising from facial nerve damage in the large number of articles published over the past twenty years. The great imponderable is—how many accidents to facial nerves are never reported? Only by continual insistence on adequate training, a sufficiency in practice, and above all, an awareness of the potential hazards along its entire course and to the structures it subserves, will the facial nerve be protected from accidental damage during surgery.

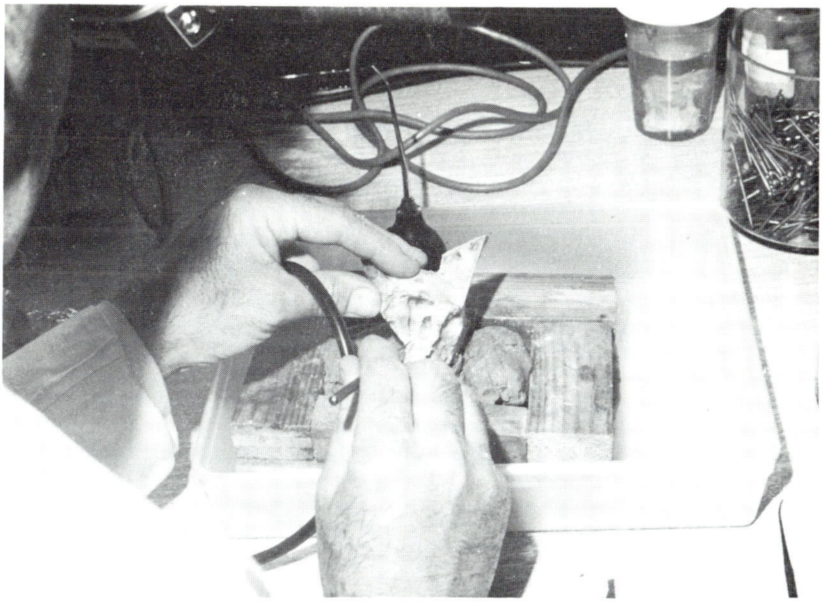

Fig. 5.2. Temporal bone laboratory. Dissection in progress.

3. *Compression* This type of injury may be permanent or temporary. All degrees of nerve damage can occur, from neuropraxia to more severe injury.

4. *Traction* This type of nerve injury has been discussed in association with missile injuries. Such injuries are also found following fractures of the skull and face which cause loss of soft tissue. These are commonly seen in industrial, road traffic accidents, or missile injuries.

5. *Ischaemia* Depending upon its severity, ischaemia can result in either permanent or temporary loss of function.

6. *Cold injury* The long-term effects of cold on the facial nerve depend on the type and duration of the cooling process. Cold exposure could produce neuropraxia, or, at the other extreme, complete nerve destruction. It is well known that nerve conduction velocity is reduced by cooling, and that transmission ceases altogether at a certain temperature; see Thomas *et al.* (1975). Frostbite may affect the nose and ears, but we cannot find any reference to seventh nerve damage. Perhaps the relatively unprotected part of the seventh nerve in the face is shielded by a good surrounding blood-supply, and a tendency towards better external protection by clothing. Injury by cryosurgery is discussed by Holden (1976).

Cold damage may be produced if cryosurgery is used close to the facial nerve anywhere along its course. Probably the most common site of injury is in the middle ear, and will occur during cryosurgical treatment of glomus jugulare or other vascular tumours. Reported trauma varies from complete nerve damage to only a mild and temporary paralysis (Holden 1975). In general, motor function is the first to be affected by cooling, and vasomotor properties are the last to cease functioning.

7. *Heat injury* In the seventh nerve this injury can be produced from adjacent heat set up by drilling, especially if there is inadequate cooling around the actual drill head. How much nerve damage can be attributed to nearby drilling is not clearly understood. In surgery, the new high-speed instruments certainly raise the local temperature. Such an increase may be sufficient to injure the nearby facial nerve either directly or via the blood supply. Surgeons should use irrigation fluid at a known temperature, say 20 °C, to cool the area adjacent to the drill head, as well as to remove bone dust. Call (1978) discusses how to protect the nerve from such thermal injury. Diathermy injury is most commonly encountered during operations carried out in the internal auditory meatus, or posterior fossa.

8. *Radiation neuropathy* Much controversy has arisen over this subject. It is often difficult to determine whether or not facial nerve paralysis which develops during or after treatment for a tumour of the temporal bone is due primarily to the radiation (patients receive an average of 50–60 Gy rads over five weeks). It is seldom possible to exclude the ongoing tumour as the cause of the paralysis and, occasionally, infection set up by disintegrating and subsequently infected neoplasm or bone may involve the nerve. Post-irradiation damage by scarring and ischaemia are also possible. Any of the above processes may produce a facial paralysis, so it is not possible to show that any change has been inflicted on the nerve by the irradiation. Our previous experience (Frew and Finney 1963) and a further assessment of 40 cases of glomus jugulare and middle ear neoplasms would seem to suggest that the nerve is resistant—at least to the irradiation doses now being administered. Lea (1946) stated that nerves appear to be insensitive to irradiation only because we cannot detect changes in the DNA of the chromosomes. In general, doses of less than 100 Gy appear to have no effects detectable by conventional electrophysiological methods. This could be explained by the fact that normal nerve tissue is composed of non-mitotic material. Neurones do not divide once established, and are not therefore significantly altered by irradiation within the therapeutic dose range.

The discussion about post-irradiation necrosis of central nervous tissue, as opposed to effects on peripheral nerves, is well documented by Bailey (1962), Scholtz and Hsu (1938), Crane and Dutton (1963), and Holdorff (1975). McGuirt and McCabe (1977) discuss experimental effects of radiation therapy on seventh nerve grafts carried out on animals.

9. *Electrical injuries* Uncommonly, peripheral nerves may be injured when an electrical shock from lightning or generated electricity is received. Few references can be found concerning immediate facial nerve damage. However, effects delayed by some days have been documented (Richards 1973; Panse 1970; Dale 1954; Di Vincenti *et al.* 1969). Hann (1957) quoted a report of a patient who was struck by lightning on the mastoid process. This produced a rupture of the tympanic membrane, some cochlear loss, and a lower motor neurone facial paralysis. Vestibular function was also decreased (Silverside 1964).

10. *Ultrasound* Irradiation of a peripheral nerve with ultrasonic irradiation may produce a reversible block, or account for axonal degeneration (Young and Henneman 1961; Lele 1963). Lele considered that the effects were due to heat. Further studies are relevant for otologists, with the increasing use of ultrasonic therapy both for Ménières disease, and the post-traumatic positional vertigo of the peripheral labyrinthine type. No ill-effects have been documented by the use of diagnostic ultrasound, from obstetricians, neurologists, physio-therapists, or neurosurgeons. However, for diagnostic purposes, ultrasound at 3 MHz is used, the intensity being about 1 mW/cm^2. In otology the required destructive effects of ultrasound necessitate a frequency of 3·5 MHz, at an intensity level of 10 W/cm^2. However, Boyle (1972) showed that extensive ultrasonic irradiation of the seventh nerve in animal experiments did not produce axonal degeneration, although it did produce lesser degrees of damage. He also showed that dexamethasone did not hasten recovery from the damage to the nerve.

Since the labyrinthine destruction in the treatment of Ménières disease is apparently produced by a combination of heat and fluid vibration, it is very easy to imagine the most disastrous effect this could have should it involve the neighbouring facial nerve (Fig. 1.7). The ultrasonic transducer is placed on the thinned-down posterior end of the lateral semi-circular canal (Fig. 5.3). Exactly the same structures are involved in a cryosurgical labyrinthine destruction for relief of vertigo in Ménières disease. Baxter (1971) showed that about 50 per cent of the temporal bones which he investigated had dehiscences in the facial canal in the middle ear, and this provides an explanation for facial nerve damage by ultrasound. The fluid through which the ultrasound is transmitted flows over the mastoid and middle ear area. Should this fluid enter any facial canal dehiscence, then the ultrasound will follow, generate heat, and damage the seventh nerve. It is fortunate that no permanent damage to the nerve has occurred in any recent large series of cases (Angell-James 1976; Stahle 1976, personal communications).

11. *Chemical* Application of silver nitrate or chromic acid to the middle ear or to a mastoid cavity may damage an exposed nerve. Alcohol injected into the lateral semicircular canal, in the technique of Mollison, could

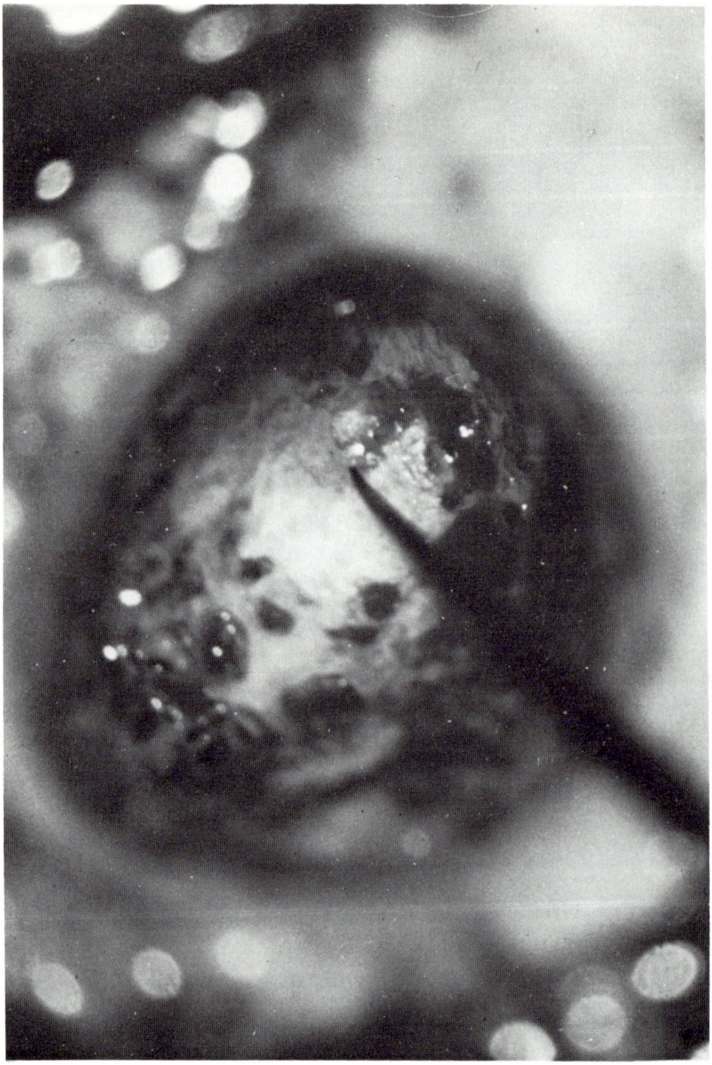

Fig. 5.3. Mastoid cavity. Position of ultrasonic transducer on the lateral semi-circular canal.

overflow and damage the nerve via a canal dehiscence. This method of labyrinthectomy is no longer used; many better techniques are available.

12. *Laser* Light amplification by stimulated emission of radiation is now an accepted surgical instrument in various fields, especially ophthalmology.

Laryngeal application has been described, and it is possible that accidental damage to the facial nerve could occur. We cannot trace any injury to the seventh nerve as yet. However, the extremely high temperatures generated by the utilization of 0·5–10 kJ/cm^2 makes nerve damage probable if inaccuracy were to occur in the use of a laser beam anywhere near the course of the facial nerve.

Sites of facial nerve damage

The following is suggested as a reasonable method of subdividing the areas in which seventh nerve trauma may occur.

Cerebellopontine angle Operations in this area (e.g. to remove an acoustic neuroma; Fig. 5.4) are potentially dangerous to the collective bundle of the seventh and eighth nerves. Accidental touching with diathermy may produce complete or partial damage, either from interference with the blood supply to a nerve, or by actual nerve involvement.

Complete tearing of the facial nerve in removal of an acoustic neuroma, or a meningioma, will produce a complete paralysis. Often the site of damage to the nerve occurs as it is emerging from the pons, and in this case no immediate repair is possible. Operations for the division of the vestibular nerve in Ménières disease, may result in damage to the seventh nerve, especially if anatomical landmarks become confused.

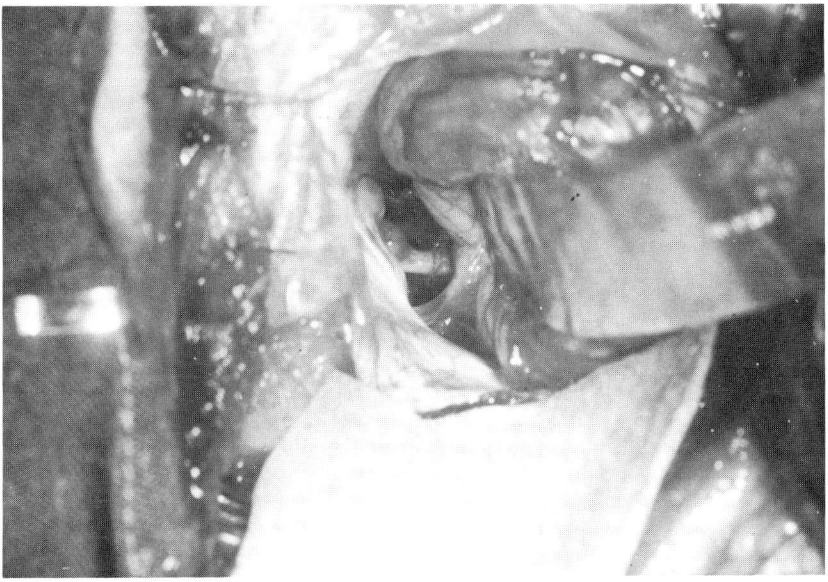

Fig. 5.4. Left acoustic neuroma filling internal auditory canal. Cerebellar retractor in position.

Internal auditory meatus Injury to the facial nerve in this area can be sustained during surgical approaches such as the accepted posterior craniotomy. The nerve can also be at risk during translabyrinthine operations to reach the internal auditory canal. Damage can occur by stretching the nerve, actual transection, or thermal injury. Translabyrinthine operations to remove small acoustic neuromas are safe only in very experienced hands. The limitations of the working area, possible bleeding, and the difficulty of distinguishing the various nerves, can often lead to permanent seventh nerve damage. Fisch (1970) believes the lesion in Bell's paralysis lies just within the internal canal, and an attempt to reach and decompress such areas—said to be oedematous parts of the nerve—could produce accidental injury.

House and Hitselburger (1976) report on four patients in whom a new approach to the base of the skull is described. He calls it the transcochlear approach to the skull base. The facial nerve has to be dissected out most carefully in order to avoid damage. Occasionally, if it is found to be involved in a tumour, the nerve cannot be preserved. Portman *et al.* (1975) give great detail on all aspects of surgery in the region of the internal auditory meatus.

The middle fossa Facial nerve damage in this area is nearly always caused by head injury. The skull may be fractured, even though this may not be demonstrable radiologically. Injury to the nerve can vary from a mild oedema to complete section of the nerve in severe injuries. Occasionally small spicules of bone can penetrate the nerve (Kettel 1959a, b).

Some authors have described facial paralysis associated with subtemporal decompression of the Gasserian ganglion carried out for relief of trigeminal neuralgia. Love and Svien (1954) remarked on the fact that 16 patients out of a consecutive 100 suffered lower motor neurone facial paralysis as a result of surgery to decompress the Gasserian ganglion. This may be explained by the finding of Hall *et al.* (1969) that in 15 per cent of the temporal bones they dissected, there was a gap in the bony cover of the geniculate ganglion. Good exposure and adequate illumination help to safeguard the facial nerve in this operation.

Foerster (1973) reported the incidence of facial nerve injury in a group of 3907 head injury casualties in World War I as being about 3 per cent. A comparable incidence was reported from World War II by Russell (1973). A remarkably similar proportion of facial nerve damage has occurred among civilian head injuries admitted to the Regional Neurological Centre at Newcastle General Hospital (Table 5.1), where the average incidence of facial nerve damage has been about 4 per cent. A lower rate in civilian injury of 1·6 per cent was reported by Friedmann and Merritt (1944). However, this was in a smaller group of 430 cases. Lathrop (1946) reports on his war injury cases.

Table 5.1
Newcastle General Hospital head injury admissions

1964	965
1965	703
1966	686
1967	578
1968	582

We have recently devised a method whereby the anaesthetists can monitor facial movements while the otologist is working in the posterior fossa, in which it is not always easy to determine with accuracy the exact location of the seventh nerve. Once the nerve has been located, dissection of a neuroma is much facilitated. By such advances, preservation of the facial nerve becomes feasible in the removal of large tumours, as well as small ones. Work is currently in progress on the insertion of small electrodes or one large electrode into the face, with monitoring on an oscilloscope. A facial nerve stimulator must be used, as moving the seventh nerve with instruments does not produce enough stimulation for recording purposes. We are hopeful that advances in this field will reduce morbidity from trauma in the near future. Such a method could be used in all operations involving the internal auditory meatus, or any location near the facial nerve. Mastoidectomy, stapedectomy, and facial nerve decompression are obvious examples.

General features of skull base fractures Considerable force is required to fracture the reinforced bone of the skull base. The lines of fracture may themselves produce complications, in particular by opening up spaces to the exterior, for example a fracture into the para-nasal sinuses, nasal cavity, middle ear, or external auditory meatus. Infection can easily be introduced into the cranial cavity. In addition, should the fracture lines involve foramina, nerves can be badly crushed at the time of impact, when maximum distortion occurs to the skull (Hooper 1969). A study of the fracture lines involving the middle ear will often show how very extensive this initial widening was at the time of impact. The series by Hough (1973) showed that the ossicular injuries, and actual displacements following skull injury could have occurred only if a considerable bone distortion had been momentarily present, i.e. at the time of impact. This is also shown by the frequency with which the tough dura mater is torn, resulting in cerebrospinal fluid otorrhoea or rhinorrhoea.

In considering a cranial fracture at least three factors are of importance.

1. The point of impact or injury to the skull.
2. The actual speed with which the lesion is inflicted. Obvious examples being high velocity missiles, or falling, as in a vasovagal attack.
3. The direction in which the force is exerted is also important. With a few

rare exceptions, fractures of the middle cranial fossa always involve the petrous portion of the temporal bone. Indeed fractures of the petrous bone are said to occur in approximately 75 per cent of all basal skull fractures. Although most authorities quote three main types of fractures, combinations can obviously occur, depending on the injury.

(a) *Transverse fractures* In these the line runs vertically through the squamous petrous bone, sometimes rupturing the lambdoid suture, into the labyrinth (Fig. 5.5).
(b) *Longitudinal fractures* The line now usually runs obliquely from above, through the squamous part of the temporal bone, then longitudinally along the posterior surface of the pyramid. The middle ear will be involved in this type of injury, and C.S.F. otorrhoea is often found either in the external auditory meatus, lateral to an intact drum, or leaking from the middle ear through a torn tympanic membrane (Leonard and Belafskey 1973).
(c) *Combined transverse and longitudinal fractures* Bilateral injuries are usually of the transverse type, and may produce bilateral facial paralysis.

Obviously, variations of the exact angle of these fracture lines will determine in each patient the structures involved, any possible damage caused, and which symptoms may be produced. Each patient could present a variety of clinical signs and symptoms. The seventh cranial nerve may be involved in any of these fracture cases. Combat injuries, which are discussed by Krekorian (1971) can damage bone, nerve, and soft tissue quite extensively.

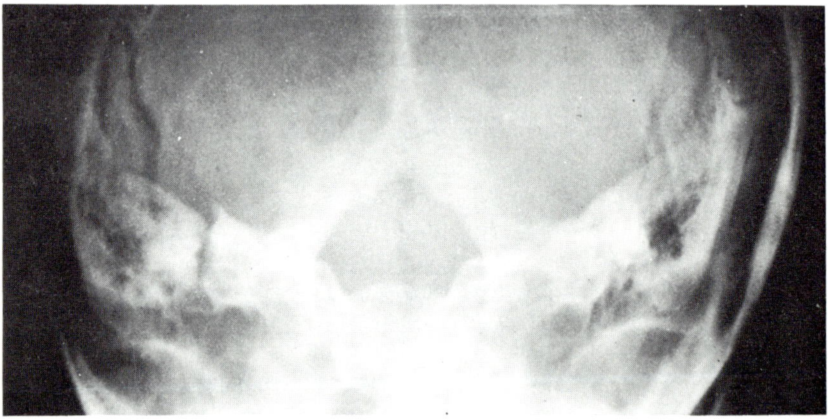

Fig. 5.5. Transverse fracture of the petrous temporal bone.

Skull base fractures in children Because of its greater flexibility, the immature skull can sustain a greater deformation before a fracture occurs. Unfortunately, this same flexibility can lead to greater deformation of the brain on impact, with shearing forces in the brain producing secondary neuronal damage to the facial nerve. Ramadier and Chaussé (1937) described occasional fractures of the mastoid process in children involving the descending segment of the seventh nerve. Longitudinal fractures extending into this area can produce ecchymoses behind the ear (Battle's sign). Such injuries are not, of course, limited to children.

A recent review by Craft (1975) discusses, in detail, a series of accidental and intentional head injuries occurring in children. Skull fractures at birth have been quoted as a possible cause of facial paralysis, but often radiological confirmation is lacking. McHugh (1963) said that the incidence was unknown, but considers it to be very low, and this is also our own experience. Fortunately, most cases recover spontaneously (Paine 1957). Manning and Adour (1972) review the subject of facial paralysis due to birth trauma in general.

The damage to the facial nerve Following injury to the temporal bone in the middle fossa, the facial nerve damage is most frequently to the lower motor neurone area. However, it is important to remember that upper motor neurone damage can also occur. Careful examination of the entire nervous system is necessary in order to arrive at the correct diagnosis.

Facial nerve paralysis of lower motor neurone type following head injury can be divided into three groups.

(a) *Immediate paralysis.* This is by far the most common presentation in patients who have sustained head injuries, and in whom accurate examination is possible. Facial paralysis will be apparent as soon as the patient is seen in hospital.

(b) *Delayed onset.* These are patients in whom no paralysis is detected on admission. A considerable interval may pass before the seventh nerve damage is apparent. A precise pathological cause may not be easily ascertained. Probably an infection, haemorrhage, oedema, or movement of a bone spicule occurring some interval after the original injury is the cause. It is generally agreed that if a facial paralysis after trauma is gradual in onset, the nerve is still in continuity. However, it does not follow that subsequent nerve recovery will be good. In general we have found delayed onset to occur within an average of 4–5 days, or sometimes longer, after skull injury. In the latter case, it is likely that the nerve is becoming involved in some healing fibrosis, and the prognosis for spontaneous recovery is, in our experience, not as good in these particular cases. However, it is now generally agreed that delayed onset of facial paralysis has a good prognosis, and thus operative intervention should be delayed.

(c) *Delayed diagnosis.* This classification can be used for upper or lower neurone damage. In our opinion a number of unconscious patients with multiple injuries have undiagnosed seventh nerve damage on admission. The facial paralysis is not apparent until there has been some improvement in the general and local condition of the patient. Unless very careful examination is carried out on all patients with head injuries facial paralysis may be missed for a considerable time. Then, when observed, it may be incorrectly labelled as delayed in onset. Occasionally, bilateral nerve damage makes diagnosis difficult at any stage.

Facial nerve damage following fractures Fractures to the base of the skull can involve the facial nerve (McGovern 1968). The transverse fracture accounts for about 10 per cent of all temporal bone fractures, according to Tos (1971). Approximately 40 per cent of patients sustaining such a fracture show a lower motor neurone paralysis. This is likely to be immediate in onset, and probably complete, with a relatively poor prognosis. The more common longitudinal fracture comprises about 90 per cent of all temporal bone fractures. Generally it involves the facial nerve close to the geniculate ganglion, but this depends on the precise angle. There is general agreement that facial paralysis appears in about 10–20 per cent of patients with this fracture. Recovery is usually complete without any operative intervention. There is not yet agreement on the incidence of delayed damage in this group of patients. Some authors quote rather lower figures for seventh nerve involvement. As an example Grove (1939) in a study of 211 cases found seventh nerve damage occurred in 19 per cent of the longitudinal, and in 31 per cent of the transverse injuries. Such figures are also supported by the studies of Hough (1973), Proctor (1956), McHugh (1959), and Harker (1974).

Table 5.1 on page 171 shows the total number of recorded head injuries admitted to the Newcastle General Hospital between 1964 and 1968. The distribution of fractures was as follows:

(1) Longitudinal—75 per cent, with 20 per cent showing facial paralysis.
(2) Transverse—25 per cent, with 40 per cent showing facial paralysis.

Over this period 141 patients, approximately 4 per cent of head injury admissions showed some evidence of seventh nerve damage. All these patients had a lower motor neurone lesion. Only one patient showed a bilateral facial paralysis, and he had no evidence of skull damage. These figures were obtained by reviewing case sheets prepared during a survey to obtain the number of patients suffering conductive hearing loss; fortunately seventh nerve paralysis was also noted. Since 1969 statistical information has been much easier to obtain, and will in future allow studies to be carried out more efficiently. The distribution of fractures remains approximately the same as in previous years, but the number of patients with seventh nerve damage is now only about 3 per cent (Table 5.2).

Table 5.2
Newcastle General Hospital—head injuries

Code	*Description*	1969	1970	1971	1972	1973	1974	1975
N.800	Fracture of vault of skull	98	43	94	93	68	54	40
N.801	Fracture of base of skull	39	13	69	35	35	43	47
N.802	Fracture of face bones	—	—	—	—	—	—	—
N.803	Other and unqualified skull fractures	5	9	19	33	5	11	12
N.804	Multiple fractures involving skull or face with other bones	34	31	77	56	30	55	41
N.850	Concussion	127	56	127	130	155	137	101
N.851	Cerebral laceration or contusion	14	7	19	31	20	26	18
N.852	Subarachnoid, subdural, and extradural haemorrhage following injury (without mention of cerebral laceration or contusion)	19	29	16	39	24	19	23
N.872	Open wound of ear	7	1	5	5	2	7	3

Patients who have a lower motor neurone facial nerve injury may also suffer otological damage. Guerrier (1967), in a review of a series of 2000 head injuries, found that 290, or about 15 per cent, had suffered acute otological disorders as a direct result of the trauma. This figure agrees with our own experience. Briggs and Potter (1971) and Potter and Braakman (1976), in their valuable work on the prophylaxis of delayed f acialparalysis, used middle ear damage as one of the indications for treatment. They found that if the fracture extended into the middle ear, a delayed facial paralysis might occur in up to 38·5 per cent of cases. This is a higher incidence than we have noted at Newcastle General Hospital.

The mastoid region In all surgery to the mastoid area, the seventh nerve is at risk. Statistics of damage at the time of operation are difficult to collate. It is generally agreed that the risk is greater during the course of a second operation, because of the presence of fibrous tissue masking the nerve from view. Bleeding may also be troublesome and occasionally, a detailed history of the previous operation may not be available to the surgeon. We are of the opinion that if technical difficulties occur in primary or secondary mastoid surgery, either further advice should be sought, or the operation should be abandoned before any damage to the seventh nerve occurs.

Jongkees (1965) quotes 139 patients in whom facial paralysis was produced by operative intervention. The same author writing in 1972 discusses 172 post-operative cases of peripheral seventh nerve damage of intra-temporal origin. Pollman (1937) reported an incidence of facial nerve damage in 0·6 per cent of a total of 1817 mastoid operations. Zuhlke (1956) reported that the danger is greater, as we remarked, in second operations. He had collected material concerning 1243 operations. In primary surgery, after 1171 operations 19 patients were shown to have facial nerve damage, an incidence of 1·6 per cent. For second operations, numbering 72, there were 8 cases of nerve trauma, an incidence of 11 per cent (Zuhlke 1956). In his book, Mawson (1974), writing on facial nerve damage, states that in his opinion 50 per cent of facial nerve injuries still occur during mastoid operations, in spite of improved facilities for temporal bone surgery. This appears to us a very high figure, and we have not found any series to confirm it. Cawthorne (1953, 1956), discussing 557 cases of lower motor neurone facial paralysis, found that 90 per cent were due to intra-temporal lesions, of which almost 60 per cent were due to Bell's paralysis. He quotes only 15 per cent as being due to surgical trauma, and of these only half were due to mastoid surgery complications. Although fenestration for otosclerosis is largely out-dated, it is of interest to note the figures of Shambaugh (1967). He noted damage to the facial nerve in 2 cases only out of 5000 patients, an incidence of only 0·04 per cent.

In labyrinthectomy performed by ultrasound the incidence of facial nerve damage at Newcastle General Hospital is only 0·5 per cent. No permanent injury has been recorded in any patient. In mastoid surgery carried out in our own department, a consecutive 1000 patients showed an incidence of 0·3 per cent with seventh nerve injury. Only one patient showed permanent damage. He had a congenital cholesteatoma (Fig. 3.12). These figures include first and second operations. In one early series Riskaer (1946) followed up 47 cases of facial nerve damage secondary to ear surgery. In 18 patients the paralysis was apparent immediately following the operation. Fairly predictably, there was no spontaneous recovery in 16 of these cases. A delayed paralysis occurred with 29 patients, and the majority made a good recovery. This would agree with modern views on the proportion of cases in which there is operative damage, compared with the number in which oedema or pressure occur later on. Riskaer (1946) noted an incidence of seventh nerve damage of about 2 per cent in otological surgery at that time. His article is interesting because it deals with cases collected between 1911 and 1943. Apart from the operative damage quoted above, some of the remaining patients also had a peripheral facial paralysis. The aetiology was otological disease or a tumour. His classification of aetiology is worthy of study, even many years after it was written. Kettel (1946) makes some criticism of this paper, and remarks on the difficulties of assessing patients from case sheets only.

Miehlke (1969), in an article which is predominantly concerned with the site of facial nerve lesions, quotes an incidence for post-operative paralysis of 1 per cent in Germany at that time. Palva *et al.* (1977) have written about their experiences with 2192 mastoid operations. They discussed the complications which arose from such surgery, and quote 10 patients who had a lower motor neurone facial paralysis. One patient required a graft during primary surgery. These figures include all types of ear operations, both first and repeated, and in 'clean' or infected temporal bones. Iodine is neurotoxic, and a bismuth and iodoform pack can occasionally produce a paralysis of toxic origin in a mastoid cavity. Actual pressure on an exposed nerve by any type of pack may result in a delayed paralysis. This will subside quite rapidly once the pressure has been removed. In general, the more complicated the operation, such as combined approach tympanoplasty, the greater the amount of experience required by the surgeon to avoid nerve injury. This is because the facial nerve is extremely close to the area of operation, more so than in other types of temporal bone surgery.

The middle ear *Congenital abnormalities* In patients with a conductive hearing loss of congenital origin, due to a malformation of the ossicles, the facial nerve can also pursue an erratic course. Very careful assessment of radiological studies is necessary to try and plot the course of an abnormal nerve. If a hearing aid will improve hearing, this may be preferable to the possibility of damaging the facial nerve by surgery. Rohrt and Lorentzen (1976) described 3 patients with congenital deafness and abnormal routing of the facial nerve in the middle ear. Surgery produced a temporary paralysis in one case, and some degree of permanent damage in another. The various anatomical abnormalities encountered in the facial nerve are discussed in Chapter 1. Most textbooks of otology deal with operative procedures in detail.

Stapedectomy for otosclerosis Injury to the facial nerve can occur during this operation. The damage may be produced by direct injury to the nerve in the facial canal, caused by, for example, careless instrumentation, touching with a drill, overheating of the drill, or, rarely, by encountering a misplaced nerve. A prosthesis may not retain its position, but move and damage the nerve in its canal. Plester (quoted by Miehlke (1975)) in his series, quotes an incidence for facial nerve injury during stapedectomy of only 0·3 per cent, all with a reversible paralysis. No patient had any permanent damage. Morrison (1971) gives his experience with 630 stapedectomies. Only one had a transient facial paralysis: an incidence of 0·15 per cent. At Newcastle General Hospital, no patient has suffered permanent damage since the operation was first carried out. Two patients have had transient seventh nerve paralysis. Leek (1974) discusses the difficulties encountered during a stapedectomy in which an aberrant facial nerve was inadvertently injured.

Fortunately, the patient made a good recovery, but he reminds us of the anxieties which can follow such an operation, or indeed any operation on the middle ear.

Myringoplasty Unless the facial nerve is abnormally routed, or a complete ignorance of the anatomy is displayed by the surgeon, these operations should not damage a facial nerve. However, Greison (1975) described an aberrant type of facial nerve which could have been damaged by almost any type of permeatal surgery. This again produced a post-operative paralysis, from which a good recovery was made.

Removal of a foreign body Operations to remove foreign bodies from the middle ear have been described as producing a facial paralysis. Similar damage has been recorded by pieces of hot metal entering the ear during welding procedures. Fortunately recovery in the reported cases has been spontaneous (Laumans 1962).

Chorda tympani nerve damage During all operations on the middle ear, whether any mastoid surgery is involved, not only the motor branch of the seventh nerve will be at risk but also the chorda tympani. This nerve carries taste fibres from the anterior two-thirds of the tongue on the same side, and damage to it can produce obtrusive symptoms. Injury may be bilateral or unilateral. The former is not commonly seen in our country, where, apart from myringoplasties, not many patients are submitted to operations on both ears. There has been much disagreement over the possible effects which can occur to the patient by injury to the nerve. Excessive strain on the chorda tympani has been suggested as a possible cause of lower motor neurone paralysis after surgery (Miehlke 1975). The pulling is said to damage the main facial nerve. We have never seen this in any of our patients. In our opinion the chorda tympani nerve will snap before such undue stress is imposed on the main nerve.

Symptoms which may follow injury to the chorda tympani are: (a) temporary or permanent alterations in taste; and (b) temporary or permanent alterations in the dryness of the mouth. Bull (1965) gives a detailed paper on his experiences with patients who have chorda tympani damage. Of 126 cases in which the nerve was sectioned to allow of better exposure of the operative field during stapedectomy, 100 (80 per cent) had one or both of the symptoms just described. However, in only 40 (32 per cent) were such symptoms persistent. He gives the duration in weeks, months, and in some cases over a year. Next he records 32 patients who had bilateral chorda tympani section. As might be expected, symptoms were found in over three-quarters of patients. However, the most persistent symptom was dryness of the mouth, which is surprising in view of the area of tongue from which taste sensation had been lost. Bull's third group consisted of 100 patients in whom the nerve had only been stretched. Hinchcliffe (1958) had shown that traction could predispose to loss of taste. In the group described by Bull, only 7 per cent had any persistent symptoms. It has often been suggested that sectioning the nerve, with some resulting anaesthesia, is preferable to traction with possible paraesthesia. This paper indicates that such statements are not true. In general our experience with chorda tympani damage supports Bull's findings.

As noted in Chapter 1, should the nerve damage be complete, then the involved areas of the tongue will show a clear, somewhat atrophied appearance. This will return to normal should re-innervation occur. The chorda tympani nerve may also be damaged during mastoid surgery, or in other permeatal operations such as myringoplasty. This is discussed by Arnold (1974), and more recently by Griffith (1977). The vulnerability of the chorda tympani nerve to middle ear disease is well discussed in the anatomical review by Anson *et al.* (1972).

Prognosis Following operations on the middle fossa, mastoid, or middle ear, facial damage may be apparent as soon as the patient wakes up. Accidental infiltration with local anaesthetic during the operation produces paralysis which rapidly wears off, and a differentiation between these cases and cases of trauma to the facial nerve should not be difficult. Onset delayed by some hours usually indicates lesser damage, or pressure from a pack, or even iodine toxicity. In these patients, of course, the prognosis is good once the cause is removed.

The stylomastoid foramen Post-auricular incisions, if made too low, may cut the facial nerve at the foramen. This is especially so in children, in whom the nerve is much more superficial. Accidental infiltration with local anaesthesics has also been mentioned, but such effects are only temporary.

Trauma at birth can damage the facial nerve in the stylomastoid foramen area. Hepner (1951) reported an interesting series of cases. In following a number of normal deliveries he came across 40 children with apparently spontaneous unilateral lower motor neurone facial paralysis. No external mark was apparent, and he ascribed the cause to pressure by the maternal sacrum on the face, close to the parotid gland. We have not seen any such cases. Temporary damage by forceps delivery is seen more frequently, and is easily recognizable by the usual marks just below the stylomastoid foramen. Fortunately, the paralysis is unilateral, and clears up very rapidly. Manning and Adour (1972) quote 5 such cases, all of which were forceps deliveries. All recovered spontaneously, but mild contracture and synkinesis developed in 2 of the children. Paine (1957), in an excellent review article including a discussion of 18 cases of birth trauma, argues against surgical intervention. He states that most traumatic facial paralyses in the neonatal period are due to swelling in the stylomastoid and facial area. Apart from any cases in which there are lacerations, or deep cuts, surgery is not required. Fractures to the overlying squamous temporal bone have been quoted as possible aetiological factors. There is little radiological evidence to support this view.

The face Injuries to the face can injure the facial nerve in its main trunk or smaller branches. Fractures of the jaw can involve the nerve close to the stylomastoid foramen, and slash injuries to the face, from above, downwards, and backwards, are especially dangerous. Despite the frequency with which such injuries are seen, it is remarkable how often the facial nerve seems to escape damage. Sometimes a few branches are severed, but the damage is not sufficient to produce any noticeable paralysis. However, more severe damage can occur, and all patients must be examined carefully when they are first seen or oedema and bruising may mask any paralysis for a considerable time.

When such patients are seen months, or even longer after the accident, considerable scarring may have produced its own limitations of movement, and no paralysis is noted. In the plastic repair of such scars a most careful search should be made for the nerve branches, or more damage will result.

In an operation to the upper neck area, for example to remove swollen upper deep cervical glands (Fig. 5.6), it is essential to be aware of all the nerves that are nearby. Dissection using a finger can damage a nerve by tearing or stretching, just as easily as can cutting it with scissors or scalpel. The use of a facial nerve stimulator is mandatory during these operations. Relying on the anaesthetist to watch the face is not sufficient. He will not notice the face twitching until after the nerve or a large branch has been cut.

The parotid area It is said that surgery in this area now produces more cases of seventh nerve damage than otological operations in children (Alberti and Biagoni 1972). The facial nerve is certainly more vulnerable in parotid surgery and, just as in otology, a thorough knowledge of anatomy, the use of facial nerve stimulators, and the increased use of magnification will help to reduce morbidity. In a recent article, Ward (1975) discussed the possibilities of injury to the facial nerve during limited or extensive parotid operations, giving an up-to-date assessment of injury in a great variety of cases. Frazell (1954), Conley (1975), and Eneroth (1972) give figures for the incidence of facial nerve surgery following parotid surgery. Damage is found to be greater in operations for recurrent tumours, as one would expect.

Frazell (1954) reviewed a series of 388 cases of benign mixed tumours of the parotid, occurring between 1930–45. After primary surgery on 269 patients the incidence of facial nerve damage was 14·5 per cent. This total was made up of 11·9 per cent with temporary damage, and only 2·6 per cent who showed any permanent deficit. However, in the group of 119 patients who were submitted to further surgery, the incidence of nerve damage rose

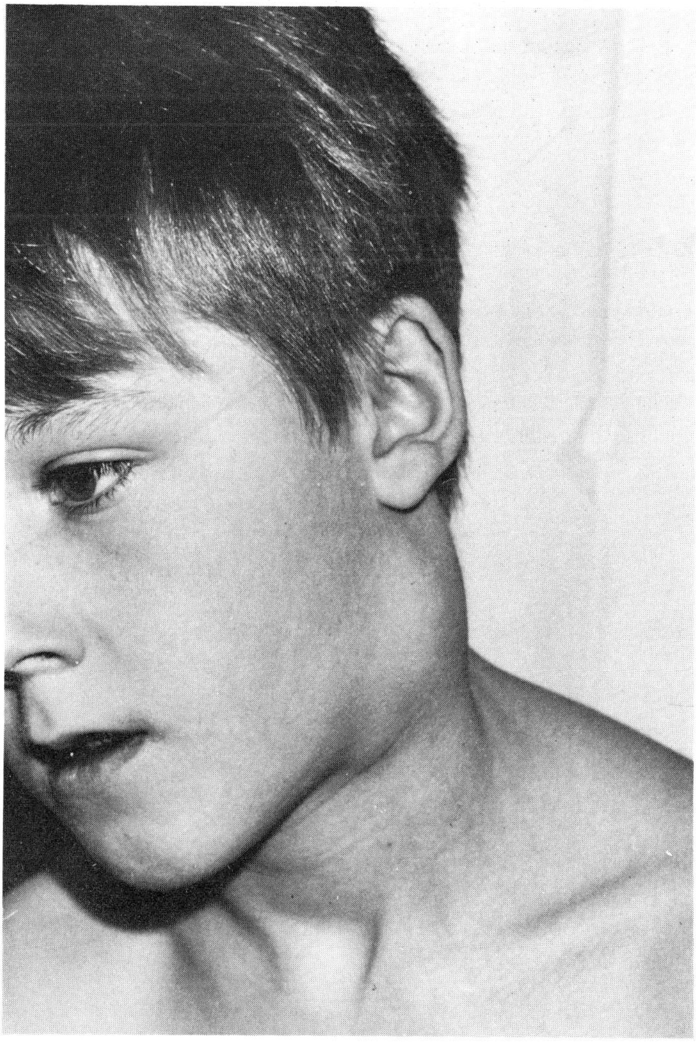

Fig. 5.6. Upper deep cervical glands.

to 29·4 per cent, of whom 13·4 per cent showed temporary injury, and 16 per cent suffered permanent effects, a significant increase.

Conley (1975) states that following surgery to benign tumours situated in what he calls the lateral lobe, and using a standardized technique, over 80 per cent of all patients should have no significant seventh nerve injury. He also discussed whole parotid gland surgery, and puts the incidence of facial nerve damage at 50 per cent, the majority with only a mild and temporary weakness. Eneroth (1972) discusses the results of a histological and clinical

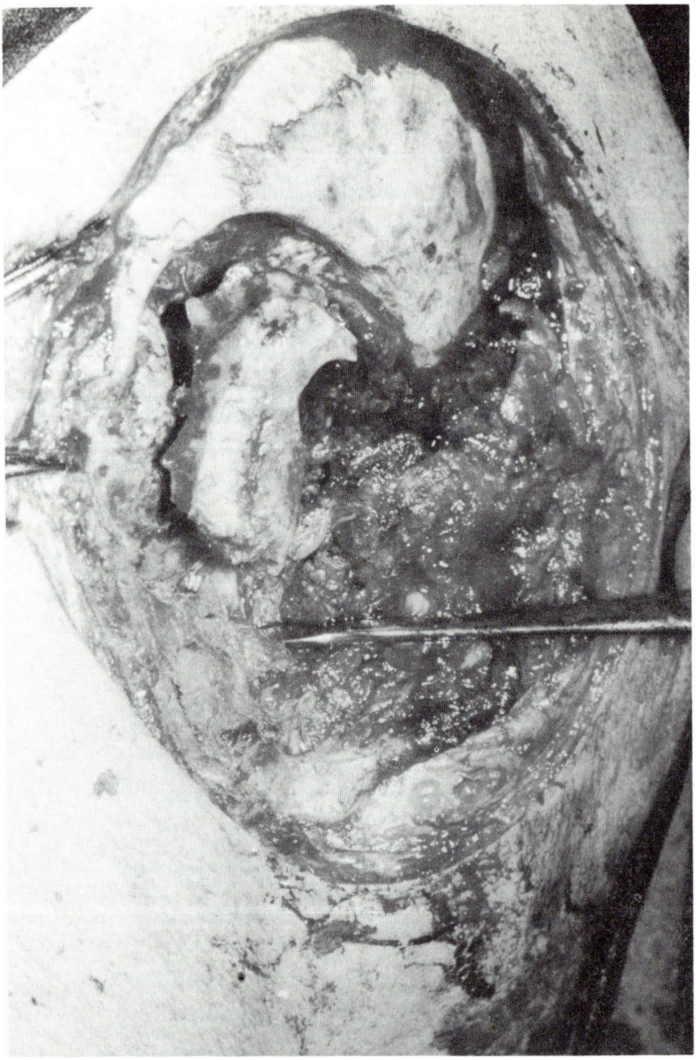

Fig. 5.7. Petrosectomy. The facial nerve has been sectioned.

survey of 2261 patients with parotid tumours. In the 1780 patients who had benign tumours, there was apparently no patient with a persistent facial paralysis before treatment was initiated. Only in the group of malignant tumours was pre-operative paralysis significant. Out of 378 patients, 46, that is 12 per cent, showed involvement of the nerve by tumour infiltration. This series demonstrates the order of pre-operative, or pre-radiotherapy, incidence to be expected in various types of parotid neoplasms. The chances of further injury to the nerve when operating on such patients is obviously very high.

Surgical section

Fortunately, there are now few patients who must be submitted to deliberate surgical section. In petrosectomy (Fig. 5.7) the nerve has to be cut in order to remove the bone. Most patients, however, already have a facial paralysis before operation. There was much confusion, even as late as the beginning of the nineteenth century, about distinction between the fifth and the seventh nerve. Sir Charles Bell (1821, 1829) finally established the differences, and showed the correct functional and anatomical distinctions between the nerves. This abolished the operation of cutting the seventh nerve in an attempt to relieve trigeminal neuralgia.

The few remaining therapeutic indications for partial or complete section of the facial nerve are discussed in Chapter 7 under facial spasm, and blepharospasm.

Medico-legal aspects of seventh nerve damage

The following questions should be clearly answered in any case of litigation.

1. Did the operation cause the facial paralysis?
2. Was this damage due to the negligence of the surgeon?
3. Could the facial paralysis have been prevented by an operation?

Litigation will usually be concerned with permanent facial damage. Temporary facial paralysis after an operation may cause a patient to consider legal action, but rapid improvement in his condition will, of course, reduce any chance of success in pursuing such a claim.

Operations in the region of the facial nerve can be divided into three groups.

1. Operations in which the facial nerve is bound to be damaged. This group includes petrosectomy, removal of extensive, probably malignant parotid tumours, or operations in which partial facial damage exists, and is likely to worsen, for example to remove a glomus tumour or middle-ear neoplasm, and whole or partial section for facial spasm. Before undertaking such an operation, the risks would have to be fully explained to the patient, and a form of consent signed.
2. Operations in which facial nerve may possibly be damaged. Examples would be during the exploration of ears which had congenital abnormalities, extensive cholesteatoma, and dissection of resectable parotid tumours. Retro-mandibular placing of forehead flaps comes into this group, as does surgery in the area of the mandible. Also included are operations in the internal auditory meatus, and posterior fossa areas.

3. Operations in which the surgeon does not expect any damage to occur. This group obviously includes the majority of operations on the ear or face, and raises a question discussed by surgeons all over the world. What should one tell a patient before operation? Should one mention every possible hazard, anaesthetic, surgical and post-operative, at the risk of alarming the patient unnecessarily? In Great Britain, every patient should be made fully aware of the reason, and expected end result of the proposed operation. In the case of children, parents must be given a similar explanation. Reasonable risks must be explained, and any special ones underlined. The Newcastle Area Health Authority consent form is reproduced in Fig. 5.8, as a guide line for use by responsible surgeons and anaesthetists, and others, such as radiologists who are using invasive techniques. It is also used as a basis for discussion with patients. Older forms have been described as being too vague; perhaps such a criticism is justified in some cases. Most medical practitioners, however, wish to make the patient fully aware of risks, without alarming them unduly, which might lead them to refuse to have a necessary operation. Litigation is probably more prevalent in the U.S.A. than in the U.K.; a full discussion of procedures in Europe and America can be found in Miehlke (1975) and Shambaugh (1975). In some countries poor results after the surgical treatment can be taken as possible evidence of negligence, an alarming thought for surgeons not presently exposed to such legal hazards.

Accidents do happen, even in the best of hands, and in cases of facial nerve damage it is sometimes very difficult dispassionately to distinguish between accidental or unavoidable damage, and negligence.

Summary

There is a great volume of literature about each area of nerve trauma, on the aetiological factors, and on related experiments on other cranial nerves. We have reported our own experiences, as well as authorities from whom more detailed information can be obtained.

The regenerative capacity of the nerve depends on the extent of damage. When neurone death occurs, only part of the nerve will be available for regeneration, and functional results will be poor. Complete separation of the nerve endings, and actual loss of an axonal segment are the worst forms of trauma. Unless surgical intervention takes place, no recovery will occur. It is apparent that only a slight force may cause the ends of the sectioned nerve to twist. Thus only a small number of neural elements are then available for onward transmission of function. The majority of endings would be opposed to the epineurium and perineurium which would effectively block any progress (Sunderland 1970). Even with a microscope it is not possible to

FORM OF CONSENT FOR OPERATION

CONSENT BY PATIENT

Record Number

I .... of ....

....

hereby consent to undergo the operation of ....

the nature and effect of which have been explained to me by Dr/Mr ....

I also consent to such further or alternative operative measures as may be found to be necessary during the course of the operation and to the administration of a general, local or other anaesthetic for any of these purposes.

No assurance has been given to me that the operation will be performed by any particular surgeon.

Date .... Signed .... (Patient).

I confirm that I have explained to the patient the nature and effect of this operation.

Date .... Signed ....

CONSENT BY PARENT OR GUARDIAN
*
CONSENT BY RELATIVE

I .... of.................................

....

hereby consent to the submission of ....

to the operation of...

the nature and effect of which have been explained to me by Dr/Mr...................

I also consent to such further or alternative operative measures as may be found to be necessary during the course of the operation and to the adminstration of a general, local or other anaesthetic for any of these purposes.

No assurance has been given to me that the operation will be performed by any particular surgeon.

Date .... Signed ....

Relationship to patient ....

I confirm that I have explained the nature and effect of this operation to the
child's parent / guardian
* patient's relative named above

Date ....Signed..............................

*Delete as necessary

Fig. 5.8. Consent form for operation as used in Newcastle General Hospital.

overcome these difficulties to any great extent. The capacity for nerve repair appears to be greatest in children, even taking into account the shorter distances. It is well known that axon regeneration rates are greater in the young patient.

Efficiency of regeneration declines with distance from the site of damage, and other unknown factors appear to influence the whole process. The motor area of the seventh nerve distribution, awaits reinnervation for renewed function, following nerve damage. It is fortunate that muscle fibres in the facial region appear to retain their capacity for re-starting activity for a long time—up to two or three years. Prognosis for function is much better than in muscles elsewhere. This difference has not yet been adequately explained, beyond the well known statement that muscles of the face have a better blood-supply than others in the body. Recovery therefore depends greatly on the integrity of the blood supply of the muscle.

Cragg and Thomas (1964) state that after crush injuries, nerve conduction velocity remains about 25 per cent below normal, and fibre diameter is also reduced. The axon diameter shrinks, by about 50 per cent, temporarily and probably never recovers to more than 80 per cent of its original size. All these factors play a part in the residual deficit produced by trauma to the seventh nerve.

It must be in the field of prevention that most reduction in nerve trauma will apply. Fewer road accidents and better protection in industry and the home in future years, will, we hope, lessen the amount of seventh nerve trauma that is seen. Further control of disease, especially infection, would mean fewer operations and would reduce possible nerve injury.

References

Adams, J. H., Daniel, P. M., and Prichard, M. M. (1969). Degeneration and regeneration of hypothalamic nerve fibres in the neurohypophysis after pituitary stalk section in the ferret. *J. Comp. Neurol.* **135**, 121.

Alberti, P. W., and Biagoni, E. (1972). Facial paralysis in children. A review of 180 cases. *Laryngoscope* **82**, 1013.

Angell-James. (1976). Personal communication.

Anson, B. J., Donaldson, J., and Shilling, B. (1972). Surgical anatomy of the chorda tympani nerve. *Ann. Otol.* **81**, 616.

Arnold, D. (1974). The vulnerability of the chorda tympani nerve to middle ear disease. *J. Laryng.* **88**, 457.

Bailey, O. T. (1962). Basic problems in the histopathological radiation of the central nervous system. In *Response of the nervous system to ionizing radiation*, (ed. T. J. Haley and A. S. Snider). Churchill, London.

Barker, D., and Ip, M. C. (1966). Sprouting and degeneration of mammalian motor axons in normal and deafferentated skeletal muscle. *Proc. roy. Soc. B* **163**, 538.

Barr, H. J. (1964). Regeneration and natural selection. *Amer. Naturalist* **98**, 183.

Baxter, A. (1971). Dehiscence of the Fallopian canal. An anatomical study. *J. Laryng.* **85**, 587.

Bell, C. (1821). On the nerves: giving an account of some experiments on their structure and function which lead to a new assessment of the system. *Phil. Trans. roy. Soc. Lond.* **111**, 398.

Bell, C. (1829). *The nervous system of the human body.* Longmans Green, London.

Berrill, N. J., and Karp, G. (1976). *Growth, development, and pattern.* Freeman, San Francisco.

Boyle, W. (1972). Experimental facial paralysis. *Arch. Otolaryng.* **95**, 313.

Briggs, M., and Potter, J. M. (1971). Prevention of delayed facial palsy. *Brit. med. J.* **3**, 458.

Bull, T. R. (1965). Taste and the chorda tympani. *J. Laryng.* **79**, 479.

Cajal, R. Y. (1928). *Degeneration and regeneration of the nervous system*, trans. R. M. May, Vol II, p. 510. Oxford University Press.

Call, W. H. (1978). Thermal injury from mastoid bone burrs. *Ann. Otol.* (*St. Louis*) **87**, 43.

Cammermayer, J. (1963). Peripheral chromatolysis after transection of mouse facial nerve. *Acta Neuropath.* **2**, 213.

Campbell, J. B., and Luzio, J. (1964). Symposium: facial nerve rehabilitation. *Trans. Amer. Acad. Ophthal. Otol.* **68**, 1068.

Carlson, A. M. (1970). Relationship between the time and epi-morphic regeneration of muscles. *Amer. Zool.* **10**, 175.

Cawthorne, T. (1953). The surgery of the temporal bone. *J. Laryng.* **67**, 377.
——. (1956). Facial palsy. *Brit. Med. J.* **2**, 1197.
Cole, M. (1968). Retrograde degeneration of axon and soma in the nervous system. In *The structure and function of nervous tisse* (ed. G. H. Bourne), Vol. 2, p. 269. Academic Press, London and New York.
Conley, J. (1975). *Salivary glands and the facial nerve.* Georg Thieme, Stuttgart.
Cooper, E. A. (1961). Tracheostomy and controlled respiration. *J. Laryng.* **75**, 142.
Craft, A. W. (1975). Head injuries in children. In: *Handbook of clinical neurology* (ed. P. J. Vinken and G. W. Bruyn), Vol. 23, Chap. 20. North-Holland, Amsterdam.
Cragg, B. G. (1970). What is the signal for chromatolysis? *Brain Res.* **23**, 1.
——, and Thomas, P. R. (1964). The conduction velocity of regenerated peripheral nerve fibres. *J. Physiol. Lond.* **171**, 164.
Crane, W., and Dutton, L. (1963). Experimental hypertension. *J. Path. Bact.* **86**, 83.
Dale, R. M. (1954). Electrical accidents. *Brit. J. Plast. Surg.* **7**, 44.
Di Vincenti, F. C., Moncrieff, F. J., and Pratt, B. (1969). Electrical injuries, a review of 65 cases. *J. Trauma.* **9**, 497.
Droz, B. (1969). Protein metabolism in nerve cells. *Int. Rev. Cytol.* **25**, 363.
Ducker, T. B. (1972). Metabolic factors in surgery of peripheral nerves. *Surg. Clin. N. Amer.* **52**, 1109.
Enerbäck, L., Olsson, Y., and Sourander, P. (1965). Mast cells in normal and sectioned peripheral nerve. *Z. Zellforsch.* **66**, 596.
Eneroth, C. M. (1972). Facial nerve paralysis. *Arch. Otolaryng.* **95**, 300.
Fisch, U. (1970). Transtemporal surgery of the internal auditory canal. *Fortschr. Hals–Nas–Ohrenheilk.* **17**, 203.
Flickinger, R. A. (1967). Biochemical aspects of regeneration. In: *The biochemistry of animal development* (ed. R. Weber), Vol. 2, p. 303. Academic Press, New York.
Foerster, (1973). In: *Textbook of neurology* (ed. H. H. Merritt), p. 369. Lea and Febiger, Philadelphia.
Frazell, E. L. (1954). Clinical aspects of major salivary gland tumours. *Cancer* **7**, 637.
Frew, I. (1961). Tracheostomy and controlled respiration. *J. Laryng.* **75**, 136.
——, and Finney, R. (1963). Neoplasms of the middle ear. *J. Laryng.* **77**, 415.
Friedmann, A. P., and Merritt, H. H. (1944). Damage to cranial nerves relating to head injury. *Bull. Los Angeles Neurol. Soc.* **9**, 135.
Ganong, W. F. (1975) *Review of medical physiology.* 7th ed. Lange Medical Publications, California.
Gombault, A. F. (1880, 1881). Nevrité segmentaire periaxils. Contribution a l'étude anatomique de la nevrité parenchymatous subaigue et chronique. *Arch. Neurol.* (*Paris*) **1**, 11–38, 177, 190.
Goss, R. (1969). *Principles of regeneration.* Academic Press, New York.
Greison, O. (1975). Aberrant course of the facial nerve. *Arch. Otolaryng.* **101**, 327.
Griffith, I. P. (1977). Observations on the pathology of the chorda tympani nerve. *J. Laryng.* **91**, 135.
Grove, W. (1939). Skull fractures involving the ear: a clinical study of 211 cases. *Laryngoscope* **49**, 678.
——. (1947). Hearing impairment due to cranio-cerebral trauma. *Ann. Otol.* **56**, 264.
Guerrier, Y. (1967). Le traitement chirurgical des traumatismes de l'oreille moyenne. *Montpellier Chir.* **4**, 483.

Guerrier, Y. and Dejean, Y. (1965). Les surdites de transmission dans les traumatismes fermes ducrâne cahiers. *Oto–rhino–laryng. Int.* **1**, 11.

Hall, G., Pulec, J., and Rhoton, A. (1969). Geniculate ganglion anatomy for the otologist. *Arch. Otolaryng.* **90**, 568.

Hammond, V. (1975). The indications for stapedectomy. Proc. 4th Brit. Academic Congress on Oto-laryngology. *J. Laryng.* **1**, 23.

Hann, J. (1957). In: *Handbook of clinical neurology* (ed. P. J. Vinken and G. W. Bruyn), p. 975. North-Holland, Amsterdam.

Hapter, J. (1970). Stretch injury of peripheral nerves. Acute effects on stretching on rabbit nerve. *J. Bone, J. Surg.* **52**, 354.

Harker, L. (1974). Temporal bone fractures and facial nerve injury. *Otolaryng. Clinics N. Amer.* **7**, 425.

Hepner, W. R. (1951). Some observations on facial paralysis in the new-born infant. Etiology and incidence. *Pediatrics* **8**, 494.

Hinchcliffe, R. (1958). Clinical quantitative gustometry. *Acta Otol.* **49**, 453.

Holden, H. (1975). *Cryosurgery* Pitman, London.

Holdorff, B. (1975). Radiation damage to the brain. In *Handbook of clinical neurology* (ed. P. V. Vinken and G. W. Bruyn), p. 639. North-Holland, Amsterdam.

Hooper, R. (1969). *Patterns of acute head injuries.* Edward Arnold, London.

Hough, J. V. (1973). Diseases of the middle ear. *Oto-laryngology.* Vol. 2, W. B. Saunders, Philadelphia.

House, W. (1963). Middle cranial fossa approach to the petrous pyramid. *Arch. Otolaryng.* **78**, 460.

——, and Hitselburger, W. E. (1976). Transcochlear approach to the skull base. *Arch. Otolaryng.* **102**, 334.

Hydén, H. (1960). The neuron. In *The cell.* (ed. J. Brachet and A. E. Minsky) Vol. IV, p. 292. Academic Press, New York.

Jongkees, L. (1965). Facial paralysis complicating skull fracture. *Arch. Otolaryng.* **81**, 518.

——, (1972). On peripheral facial paralysis. *Arch. Otolaryng.* **95**, 317.

Kettel, K. (1946). Discussion remark. *Acta Otol. (Stockh.)* **34**, 381.

——, (1950). Peripheral facial paralysis in fractures of the temporal bone. *Arch. Otolaryng.* **51**, 25.

——, (1959a). *Peripheral facial palsy; Pathology and surgery.* Thomas, Springfield, Illinois.

——, (1959b). Management of peripheral nerve paralysis due to trauma. *Proc. roy. Soc. Med.* **52**, 1069.

Krekorian, E. (1971). The repair of combat-injured facial nerves. *Laryngoscope* **81**, 1926.

Lassman, L., McIver, I., Thompson, C., and McLeod, I. (1958). The role of respiratory insufficiency in the mortality of brain-stem injuries. *Lancet* **i**, 90.

Lathrop, F. D. (1946). Facial nerve surgery in the European theatre of operations. *Laryngoscope* **56**, 665.

Laumans, E. (1962). Facial paralysis by perforating trauma through the external auditory meatus. *J. Laryng.* **76**, 127.

Lea, D. (1946) *Actions of radiations on living cells.* Cambridge University Press, Cambridge.

Leek, J. (1974). An anomalous facial nerve: the otologist's albatross. *Laryngoscope* **84**, 1535.

Lele, P. (1963). Effects of focused ultrasonic radiation on peripheral nerve, with observations on local heating. *Exp. Neurol.* **8**, 47.

Leonard, J. R., and Belafskey, M. L. (1973). Temporal bone fractures. Three identical cases of lateral middle ear fractures, with facial nerve injury, and conductive hearing loss. *Laryngoscope* **83**, 587.
Lieberman, A. (1971). The axon reaction. A review of the principal features of perikaryal responses to axon injury. *Int. Rev. Neurobiol.* **14**, 49.
Love, J. G., and Svien, H. J. (1954). Results of decompression operation for trigeminal neuralgia. *J. Neurosurg.* **11**, 499.
Lytton, B., and Murray, J. G. (1954). Effects of the peripheral pathway on the regeneration of nerve fibres. *J. Physiol.* **126**, 627.
Manning, J., and Adour, K. (1972). Facial paralysis in children. *Pediatrics* **49**, 102.
Mawson, S. (1974). Diseases of the ear. 3rd edn. Edward Arnold, London.
Maxwell, J. H. (1975). In *Salivary glands and the facial nerve* (ed. J. Conley). Thieme Stuttgart.
McCabe, R. (1970). Management of hyperfunction of the facial nerve. *Ann. Otol.* **79**, 252.
——, (1972). Injuries to the facial nerve. *Laryngoscope* **82**, 1891.
McGovern, F. (1968). Facial nerve injuries in skull fractures. Recent advances in management. *Arch. Otolaryng.* **88**, 536.
McGuirt, W. F., and McCabe, R. (1977). Facial nerve cable autografts. *Laryngoscipe* **87**, 415.
McHugh, H. (1959). The surgical treatment of facial paralysis and traumatic conductive deafness in fractures of the temporal bone. *Ann. Otol.* **68**, 855.
——, (1963). Facial paralysis in birth injury and skull fractures. *Arch. Otolaryng.* **78**, 443.
McLellan, M. S., and Vautier, T. (1973). Neonatal seventh nerve palsy in the absence of haemotympanum. *Amer. J. Obstet. Gyn.* **117**, 572.
Miehlke, A. (1969). Typical sites of facial nerve lesions. *Arch. Otolaryng.* **89**, 122.
——. (1975). *Surgery of the facial nerve.* W. B. Saunders, London.
Morrison, A. W. (1971). In: *Diseases of the ear, nose and throat* (ed. J. Ballantyne), p. 387. Butterworth, London.
Nathaniel, E., and Pease, D. (1963). Collagen and basement membrane formation by Schwann cells during nerve regeneration. *J. Ultrastructure. Res.* **9**, 550.
Nissl, F. (1892). Über die Veränderung der Ganglionzellen am Facialiskern des Kanichens nach Ausreissing des nerven. *Allg. Z. Psychiat.* **48**, 197.
Olsson, Y. (1968). Mast cells in the nervous system. *Int. Rev. Cytol.* **24**, 27.
——. (1971). Mast cells in human peripheral nerve. *Acta Neurol. Scand.* **47**, 357.
Paine, R. (1957). Facial paralysis in children. *Pediatrics* **19**, 303.
Palva. T., Karta. J., and Palva, A. (1977). Immediate and short term complications of chronic ear surgery. *Arch. Otolaryng.* **102**, 137.
Panse, F. (1970). Electrical lesions of the nervous system. In: *Handbook of clinical neurology* (ed. P. V. Vinken and G. W. Bruyn), p. 344, Vol. 7. North-Holland, Amsterdam.
Pinner, B., and Campbell, J. B. (1965). Alkaline phosphatase activity of incision and modes during degeneration and regeneration of peripheral nerve fibres. *Exp. Neurol.* **12**, 159.
Pollard, J. D., Gye, R. S., and McLeod, J. G. (1971). An assessment of immunosuppressive agents in exp. peripheral nerve transplantation. *Surg. Gyn. Obs.* **132**, 839.
Pollman, L. (1937). Fazialsparesen. *Mschr. Ohrenhk.* **71**, 1068.
Portman, M., Sterkers, J., Charachon, R., and Chourad, C. (1975). *The internal auditory meatus.* Churchill Livingstone, London.

Potter, M., and Braakman, R. (1976). In: *Handbook of clinical neurology* (ed. P. V. Vinken and G. W. Bruyn), p. 105, Vol. 24. North-Holland, Amsterdam.
Proctor, B. (1956). The ear in head trauma. *Laryngoscope* **66**, 16.
Ramadier, J. A., and Chaussé, R. (1937). *Traumatismes de l'oreille.* Masson, Paris.
Ranvier, L. (1871). Recherches sur l'histologie et la physiologie des nerfs. *Arch. Physiol. I*, Ser. **4**, 129.
——. (1872). Des étranglements annulsaires et des segments interannulaires chez les Raies et les Torpilles. *C.R. Acad. Sci.* (*Paris*) **75**, 1129.
——. (1875). *Traité technique d'histologie.* Savy, Paris.
——. *leçons sur l'histologie du systeme nerveux.* Savy, Paris.
Rhoton, A. (1974). Microscopy of the internal auditory meatus. *Surg. Neurol.* **19**, 981.
Richards, A. (1973). Traumatic facial palsy. *Proc. roy. Soc. Med.* **66**, 556.
Riskaer, N. (1946). The course of otitic facial palsy under adequate treatment of the ear. *Acta Otol.* (*Stockh.*) **34**, 380.
Rohrt, T., and Lorentzen, P. (1976). Facial nerve displacement in the middle ear. *J. Laryng.* **110**, 12.
Russell. (1973). In: *Textbook of neurology* (ed. H. H. Merritt). p. 369. Lea and Febiger, Philadelphia.
Scholtz, W., and Hsu, Y. K., (1938). Late damage from roentgen irradiation of the human brain. *Arch. Neurol. Psychiat.* **40**, 938.
Schwann, T. (1839). *Mikroskopiche Untersuchungen über die Ubereinstimmung in der Struktur und dem Wachstum der Tiere und Pflanzen.* Berlin.
Shambaugh, G. (1967). *Surgery of the ear.* Saunders, Philadelphia.
——. (1975). In: *Surgery of the facial nerve* (ed. A. Miehlke), p. 237. Saunders, Philadelphia.
Silverside, J. (1964). The neurological sequelae of electrical injury. *Can. Med. Ass. J.* **91**, 195.
Singer, M. (1959). In: *Regeneration in vertebrates* (ed. C. S. Thornton), University of Chicago Press.
Sjöstrand, J. (1965). Morph changes in glial cells during nerve regeneration. *Z. Zell. Forsch. Mikrosk. Anat.* **68**, 481.
Sotelo, C., and Palay, S. L. (1971). Altered axons and axon terminals in the lateral vestibular nucleus of the rat. Possible example of axonal remodelling. *Lab. Invest.* **25**, 653.
Spallanzani, C. (1729–99). *Prodroma di un opera sopra la Reproduzioni animali.* Modena.
Stahle. (1976). Personal communication via Angell-James.
Stroebe, H. (1893). Experimentelle Untersuchungen über degeneration Nerven nach Nerletzungen. *Beit. Path. Anat.* **13**, 160.
Sunderland, S. (1968). *Nerves and nerve injuries.* Livingstone, Edinburgh and London.
——. (1970). Anatomic features of nerve trunks in relation to nerve injury and nerve repair. *Clin. Neurosurg.* **17**, 38.
Sutherland, J. M. (1974). *The epilepsies. Modern diagnosis and treatment.* 2nd edn. Churchill Livingstone, Edinburgh.
The Lancet (1976). Any hope for the cut central axon? and references therefrom: *Lancet*, **i**, 1224.
Thomas, P. K., Dyck, P., and Lambert, E. (1975). *Peripheral neuropathy*, p. 743. Saunders, Philadelphia.
Torvik, A., and Skjösten, F. (1971). Electron microscopic observations on nerve cell regeneration and degeneration after axon lesions. *Acta Neuropath.* (*Berlin*) **17**, 248.

Tos, M. (1971). Fractures of the temporal bone: course and sequelae of 248 fractures of the petrous temporal bone. *Ugeskr. Laeg.* **13**, 1149.

Virchow, R. (1858). *Die cellular Pathologie in inhrer Begrundung auf physiologische und pathologische Gewebslebre.* August Hirschwald, Berlin.

Waller, A. (1850). Experiments on the section of the glossopharyngeal and hypoglossal nerves of the frog, and observations of the alterations produced thereby in the structure of their primative fibres. *Phil. Trans. roy. Soc. Lond. B* **140**, 423.

——. (1852). Sur le reproduction des nerfs et sur la structure et les functions des ganglions spinaux. *Arch. Anat. Physiol. Wiss. Med.* 392.

Ward, L. M. (1975). Injury to the facial nerve during surgery of the parotid gland. *Brit. J. Surg.* **62**, 401.

Weiss, P. (1944). *In vitro* transformation of spindle cells of neural growth into macrophages. *Anat. Rec.* **88**, 205.

——. (1969). Neuronal dynamics and neuroplasmic (axonal) flow. In: *Cellular dynamics of the neuron* (ed. D. H. Barondes). Academic Press, London.

——, and Hiscoe, H. B. (1948). Experiments on the mechanism of nerve growth. *J. exp. Zool.* **107**, 315.

Young, J. Z., and Henneman, E. (1961). Reversible blocks of nerve conduction by ultrasound. *Arch. Neurol.* **4**, 83.

Zühlke, D. (1956). *Die peripherie Facialisparesis ihre Bedeutung in der Ohrenkeilkinde under besonderer Berucksichtigung kindlieher Gerichtslakmungen.* Dissertation, Munich.

6 Investigations of facial nerve function

6 Investigations of facial nerve function

AN ACCURATE history is important in the diagnosis of facial nerve dysfunction. We have shown in preceding chapters that a seventh nerve lesion is often part of a systemic disease. Therefore a complete physical examination, especially of the nervous system is required. An ophthalmological examination could demonstrate papilloedema or other relevant afflictions of the eye, and an otological examination, using a microscope if necessary, should not be forgotten.

Sections of this chapter will deal with the main areas of specialized investigation which may be required. However, we must remember the value of other tests; for example, the examination of sputum in chest diseases may help in the diagnosis of tuberculosis, or a bronchial neoplasm. Bacteriology for pathogenic organisms in ear disease, and cytology in general, are both useful forms of investigation.

Laboratory investigations

Laboratories have limited time and resources. It is important to try and select those estimations which are relevant to the problem under investigation.

Blood Examination of the blood can give a great deal of information in bacterial infections, but is less valuable in the investigation of viral diseases. These investigations are also useful to determine the non-infective causes of facial paralysis.

(1) A full red blood cell count should be performed on all patients. Anaemia itself may be associated with many diseases which could involve the facial nerve.

(2) The serum vitamin B_{12} level is occasionally useful. Folic acid deficiency can cause neuropathies.

(3) Changes in the white cell total, or differential count, are seen in leukaemia, infective mononucleosis, and some generalized infective conditions. A considerable decrease may occur during treatment with cytotoxic drugs, for example vincristine. Eosinophilia occurs in

parasitic infections such as toxoplasmosis. In some patients with collagen disease the eosinophil increase may be thought to resemble that seen in eosinophilic leukaemia. Lupus erythematosus cells should be watched out for where disseminated lupus erythematosus is suspected.

(4) The erythrocyte sedimentation rate, if raised, may indicate more generalized disease, and thus indicate that investigation of the plasma proteins should be carried out.
(5) A fasting blood sugar level will help to eliminate diabetes mellitus.
(6) Blood cultures for bacteria may be necessary.
(7) Blood urea, liver function tests, and electrolyte studies are required to assess kidney and liver function. Dehydration will also affect the amounts of individual chemical constituents, and thus will be reflected in electrolyte changes.
(8) Serum levels of calcium, phosphate, and magnesium may help to eliminate rare conditions associated with neuropathies.
(9) Zoster titres should be estimated in any possible herpetic lesions.
(10) Serological tests are required for the detection of syphilis.

Urine A full urinary examination can give useful information in patients with a facial paralysis. Most out-patient departments carry out routine screening of urine on all patients.

(1) Glycosuria may indicate the presence of diabetes mellitus.
(2) Albumen and casts could suggest renal disease, causing hypertension and associated facial paralysis.
(3) Bence-Jones protein is found in neuropathies associated with myeloma.
(4) Haematuria occurs in hypernephroma. A secondary deposit from the tumour may cause facial paralysis.
(5) Toxic drugs such as barbiturates are excreted in the urine.
(6) Porphyrias can be detected.
(7) Lead, mercury, and other heavy metals may be excreted in the urine. Although they can produce neuropathies, such metal poisoning is now rare in this country.

Cerebrospinal fluid This provides the fluid medium which surrounds the brain and spinal cord, also filling the ventricular system. Formed in the ventricles from the choroid plexuses, it is absorbed, mainly via the arachnoid villi, into the venous sinuses. In addition to secretion and absorption there is also a constant process of dialysis with the blood stream. Exchange of chemicals between the cerebrospinal fluid and blood occurs across the arachnoid membrane. This has been confirmed by recent studies using labelled cells.

Disease in the brain or in other parts of the nervous system may produce changes in the composition of the fluid. Many such diseases affect the facial nerve. Fortunately, it is relatively easy to obtain samples of the cerebrospinal fluid for examination. The following parameters can then be measured.

(1) Pressure is measured at the time of puncture.

(2) Bacterial content is important in meningitis and some brain abscesses.

(3) Excessive numbers of red and white cells may be present in meningitis or sub-dural haematoma.

(4) Protein content may increase in posterior fossa neuromas or other tumours.

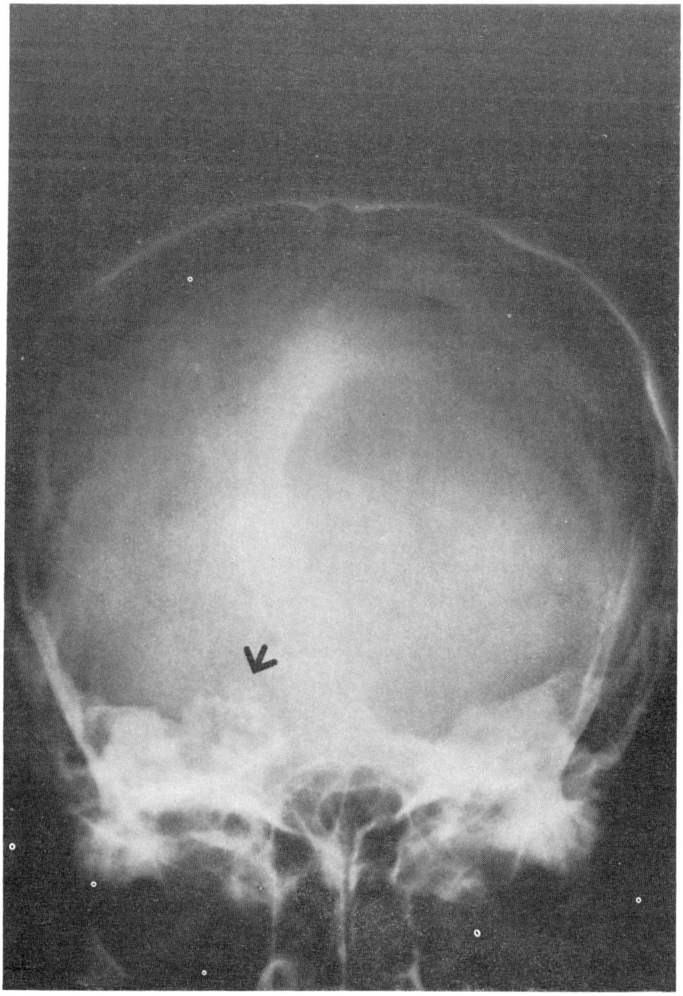

Fig. 6.1. Radiograph showing a meningioma of the petrous apex (arrow).

(5) Gold colloidal, or Lange curve abnormalities can occur, in multiple sclerosis, for example. There may be changes in gamma-globulin, and immuno-globulin content. A full description of the mechanisms, and differences, in various diseases is discussed by Walton (1977).

(6) Serological tests such as Wasserman, Kahn, V.D.R.L., and the treponema immobilization tests are important to exclude venereal disease.

(7) Virology studies usually give information at too late a stage to be useful in diagnostic procedures.

(8) Contrast studies of the cerebrospinal fluid can assist investigations of central nervous and occasionally peripheral nervous system disorders.

Faeces An examination of the faeces should be made where gastro-intestinal causes of a neuropathy are suspected.

(1) Occult blood suggests a primary neoplasm may be present.

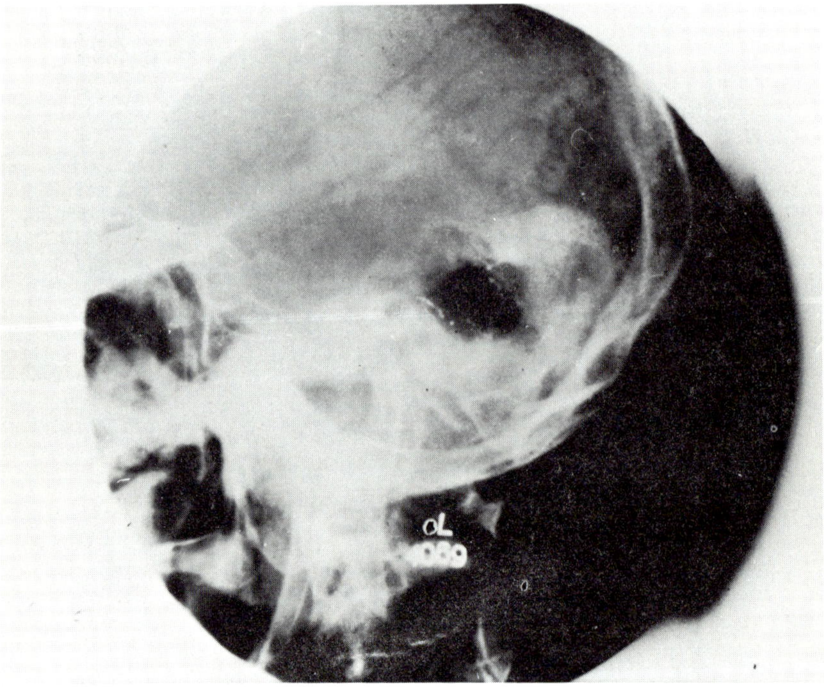

Fig. 6.2. Radiograph in which a neoplasm of temporal bone has resulted in an extensive area of bone destruction.

(2) Patients with steatorrhoea or other intestinal disease could have vitamin deficiency neuropathies. Investigation of these diseases is discussed in medical textbooks.
(3) Examination of the faeces allows virus identification in cases of meningitis or encephalitis.
(4) In some countries the presence of parasites may suggest the origin of upper motor neurone facial paralysis (Chapter 3, p. 88).

Radiological investigations

(1) Plain films of the skull are helpful in the diagnosis of acoustic neuromas or meningiomas (Fig. 6.1). Narrowing of the bony canals, or

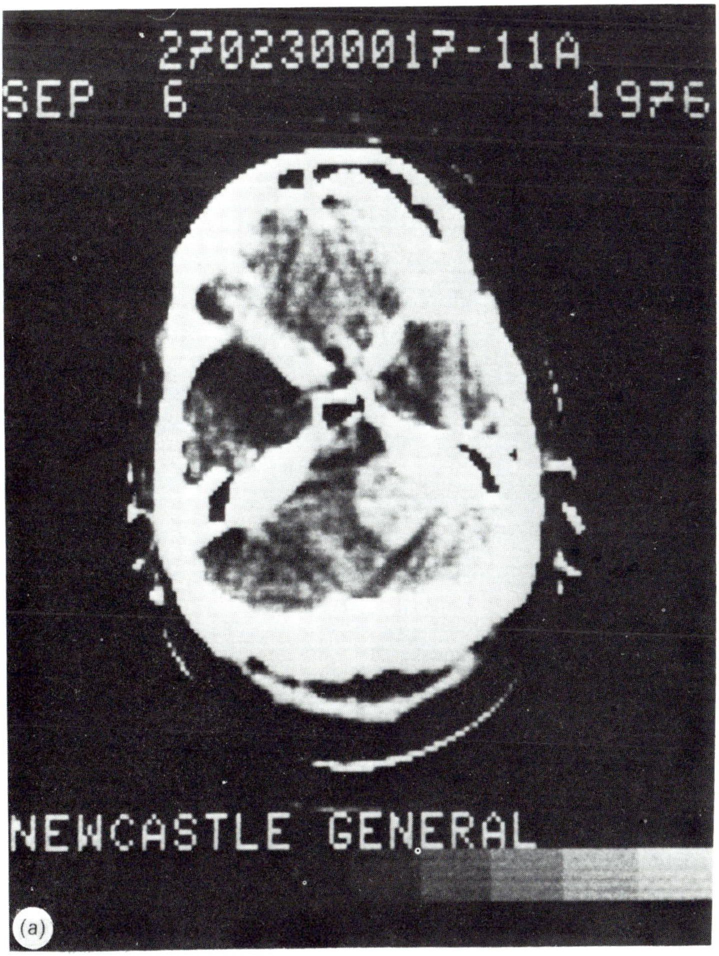

Fig. 6.3. (a) E.M.I. scan showing a large acoustic neuroma.

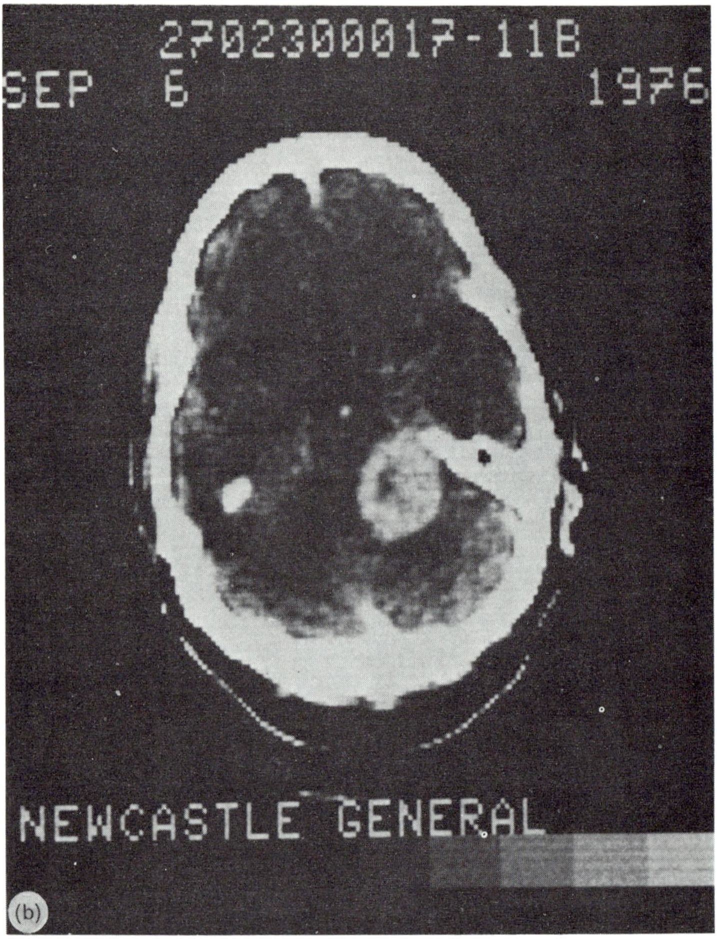

Fig. 6.3. (b) E.M.I. scan showing a large acoustic neuroma with central cystic degeneration.

evidence of Paget's disease can also be demonstrated. Cholesteatoma and tumours of the middle ear and temporal bone are recognizable by the bone destruction they produce (Fig. 6.2). Fractures of the skull are not always easy to identify.

(2) Tomograms often serve to give a more accurate location of pathology than plain X-ray studies.

(3) Brain scans using radio-active isotopes are used for the investigation of intracranial lesions. Patients with seventh nerve damage of upper or lower motor neurone type may require this examination.

(4) Where it is available computerized axial tomography greatly facilitates the diagnosis of intracranial lesions (Fig. 6.3 (a) and (b)).

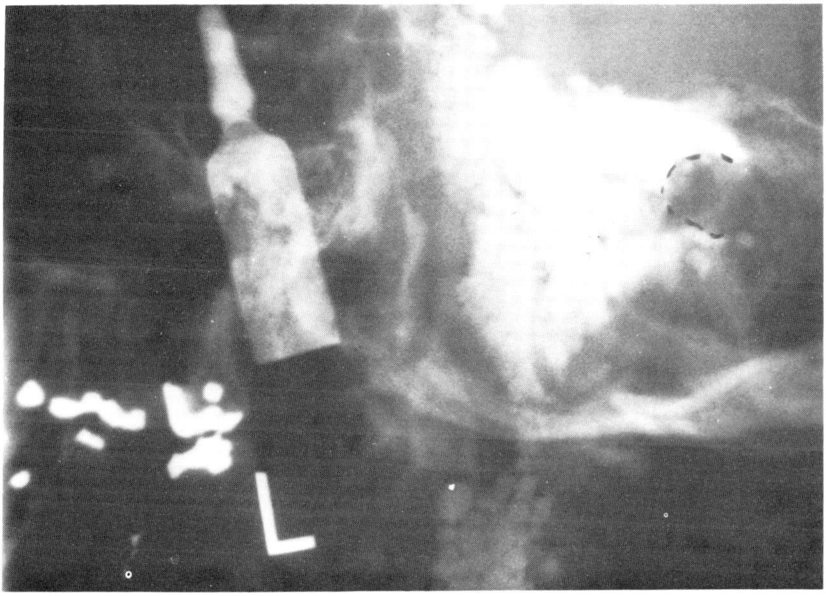

Fig. 6.4. Contrast radiography. Dye fails to enter the internal auditory canal.

(5) Angiography can outline a glomus jugulare tumour or a meningioma. Displacement of cerebral vessels by tumours may be demonstrated.
(6) A retrograde jugular venogram often localizes a glomus jugulare tumour much better than conventional angiography.
(7) General skeletal surveys may be required to search for a possible neoplasm.
(8) Radiology of the renal tract can be useful. We have seen at least three cases of facial paralysis caused by a secondary deposit from a hypernephroma in the cerebellopontine angle.
(9) Contrast studies via the cerebrospinal fluid, using air or myodil, are very useful. Their value in the posterior fossa is well shown in Fig. 6.4.
(10) In the pre-operative assessment of congenital middle ear defects, temporal bone tomography is essential. Abnormal routing of the facial canal is readily demonstrated, particularly in external meatus atresia, and will help to avoid nerve damage at any subsequent operation.

The electrical activity of the cortex

Electro-encephalography It is possible to record the brain's continuous electrical activity, either directly from the brain or in patients with intact bony skull coverings. Disease in the brain may alter these electrical potentials, and electro-encephalography plays a very important part in the study of intracranial pathology, including upper motor neurone facial paralysis.

Echo-encephalography If an ultrasonic beam is passed across the brain it is reflected off certain structures, and the resultant pattern can be recorded on an oscilloscope. The pulses arise not only from the skull walls on both sides, but also from the ventricles and central mid-line structures. Should these mid-line structures be displaced to one or other side, then the pulse will be reflected either earlier or later than expected, depending on whether the displacement is towards, or away from, the side of the stimulus. Unfortunately, the method has many limitations. A positive result may be helpful but a negative result means nothing. Tumours or abscesses, associated with a facial paralysis, can cause a detectable shift.

Nerve biopsy and electron microscopy

In some facial nerve disorders it is necessary to decide whether to perform a biopsy. In certain conditions this may be taken from the facial nerve itself, but in more generalized disease, a biopsy from any nerve will suffice. The biopsy may have to be taken from the motor portion of a nerve, for example in a motor neuropathy, and it must be borne in mind that the biopsy itself may produce some paralysis and result in increased sensory and motor loss in the area supplied by the nerve. Because of this risk, nerve biopsy is little used in facial nerve studies. However, a biopsy from the sural nerve may be helpful in polyneuropathy, and biopsy of the chorda tympani nerve is also quite feasible. This nerve is easily accessible by the permeatal approach. The risk of loss of taste is more acceptable than the possible increase in facial paralysis by direct biopsy of the main nerve. Perhaps more use will be made of this nerve in future investigations of patients with lower motor neurone facial paralysis. Removal of a nerve biopsy is relatively easy using the operating microscope. Techniques of histological preparation and examination are to be found in books of neuropathology.

Karatay *et al.* (1976) removed a portion of the chorda tympani from six patients with Bell's paralysis, all of whom had been paralysed for at least two months. As a control they used a section of nerve from a patient who was submitted to stapedectomy. The authors give their findings in detail, with electron micrographs. These latter were difficult to interpret, and utilize as a guide to aetiology. There were areas of degeneration together with areas of regeneration, but no definite pattern of nerve change was revealed. In particular no evidence of any viruses was found. May and Schlaepfer (1975) have also used the chorda tympani nerve biopsy as part of a study of Bell's palsy. There were 15 patients with Bell's palsy, and a control group of 9 patients. The latter were having operations on non-infected ears. In the opinion of the investigators, nerve biopsy allowed better assessment of prognosis and could also determine the value of methods used in treatment. This is an excellent article, with a full discussion not only of nerve biopsy, but of various modern therapies including surgery. There is also a good list of references.

Immunofluorescence

This is used for bacterial identification and also as an aid in the localization of cellular antigens. It can also be used to detect viral antigens. As this technique develops it should be possible to expand medical knowledge considerably. Studies of viral antigens and methods of viral reproduction may produce future advances in an understanding of the causation and in the treatment of facial paralysis of viral origin.

Neuro-otological tests

Full audiometric and vestibular function tests may be required in patients with facial paralysis due to an acoustic neuroma or other posterior fossa tumour. Details of these tests can be found in standard textbooks of otolaryngology.

Electrodiagnosis

Although the interpretation of the results of electrical tests of facial nerve function is often difficult, the tests themselves are straightforward enough and may usefully be described here.

Electromyography The electromyograph (EMG) records the electrical activity of muscle. Three patterns are seen, which identify (a) normal muscle, (b) denervated muscle, and (c) muscle suffering from a myopathy. Concentric electrodes, which are hollow needles with a core of insulated wire bared at the tip, are inserted directly into the facial muscles. The electrodes are connected via an amplifier to a cathode ray oscilloscope and a loudspeaker. The potential difference between the core and the shaft of the needle is demonstrated both visually and acoustically (Fig. 6.5).

(a) *Response from normal muscle* At rest normal muscle shows no electrical activity. On weak voluntary contraction action potentials of single motor units appear. These are sharp, biphasic waves with an amplitude of up to about 2 mV and a duration of several milliseconds.

As the force of voluntary contraction increases, further motor unit discharges appear and their rate of firing and their amplitude both increase until they can no longer be distinguished from one another. A complex 'interference pattern' is obtained but the biphasic or sometimes triphasic character of the waves is maintained (Fig. 6.6). There is only a small proportion of polyphasic waves in normal muscle. When the concentric electrode is first inserted into

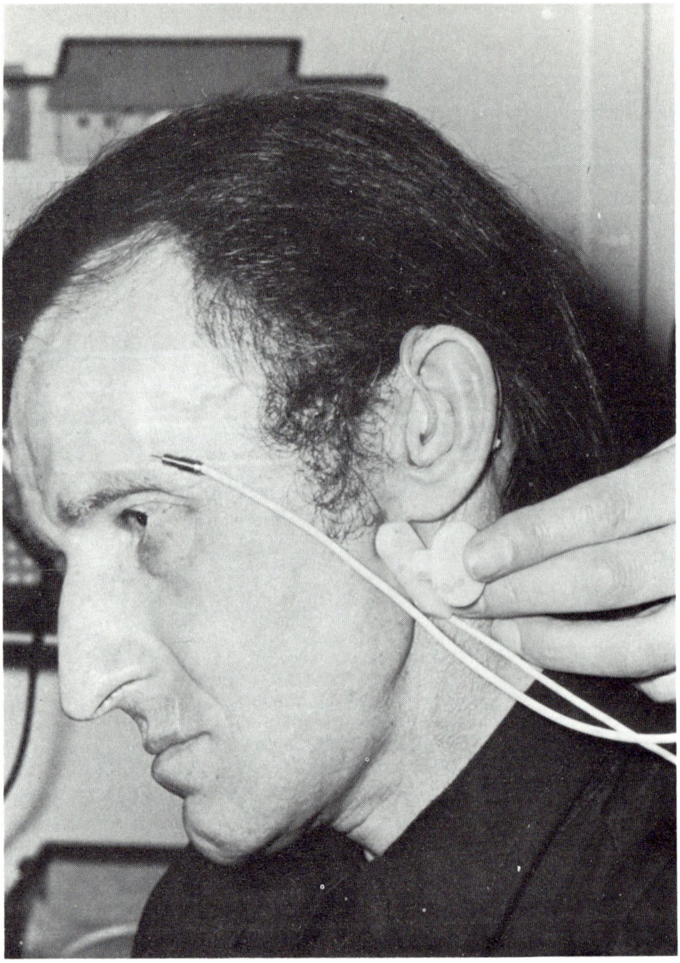

Fig. 6.5. An EMG facial nerve stimulator and needle electrode in position.

the muscle a short burst of electrical activity is provoked. This normal 'insertion activity' is of brief duration.

(b) *Response from partially or completely denervated muscle* Fibrillation potentials occur when the muscle is at rest. These are spikes of low amplitude (about 100 μA) and of about 1 ms duration. They produce a characteristic clicking noise in the loudspeaker. Fibrillation potentials appear 7–21 days after denervation. The underlying mechanism of fibrillation is unknown, but the time course of its appearance corresponds to the Wallerian degeneration in the damaged nerve.

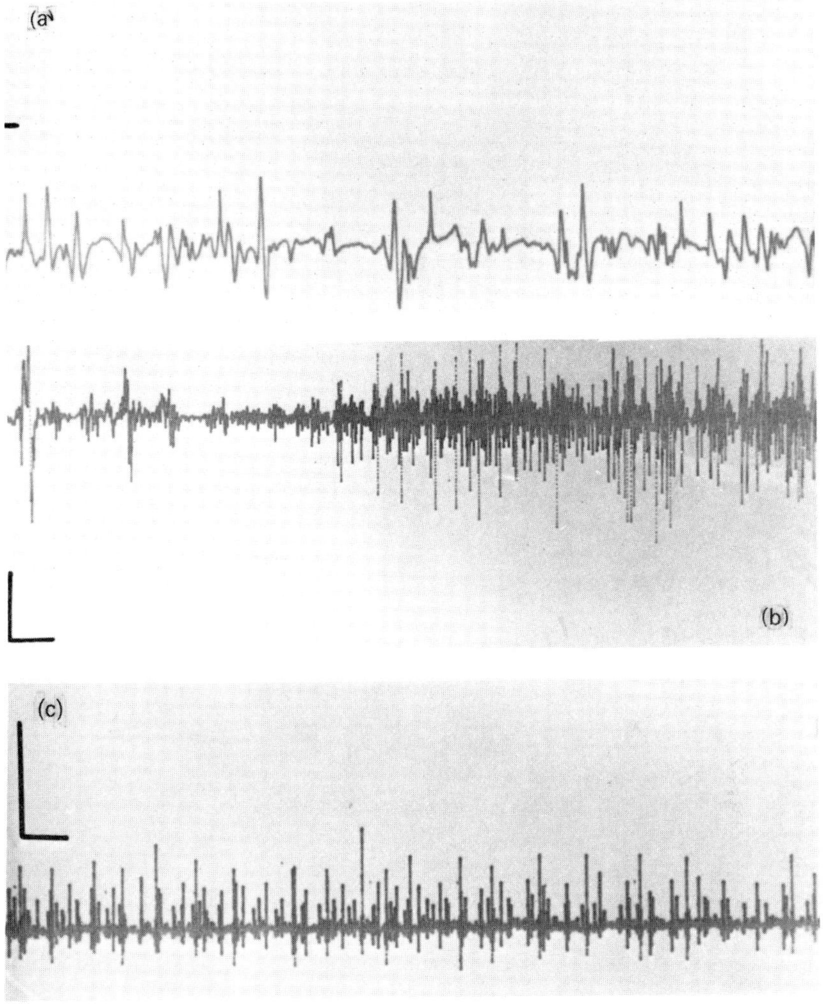

Fig. 6.6. (a) Biphasic sharp waves on E.M.G. (Calibration 100 μV:5 ms). A concentric needle electrode in the orbicularis oris. Weak contraction results in the recruitment of separately identifiable motor units.

(b) Normal interference pattern on E.M.G. (Calibration 50 μV:10 ms). As the force of the muscle contraction increases (left to right) individual motor units cannot be identified separately. The superimposition of large numbers of asynchronously recruited potentials produces an interference pattern.

(c) Fibrillation pattern on E.M.G. (Calibration 50 μV:5ms). Profuse spontaneous fibrillation occurring at rest in the orbicularis oris muscle. The facial nerve had been damaged during a posterior fossa exploration 21 days prior to this examination.

Fasciculation may occur. This is the spontaneous rhythmic firing of motor units when the muscle is at rest.

The normal interference pattern is altered as a result of the reduced number of motor units activated.

(c) *Response in myopathies* The interference pattern produced by active contraction is altered by the appearance of numerous polyphasic action potentials of varying amplitude and duration.
Electromyography of the facial muscles is commonly used in clinical practice as a test of facial nerve function. It is very helpful in the diagnosis of abnormal facial movements such as myokymia and hemifacial spasm (Chapter 4, pp. 130 and 128). Its value in cases of facial paralysis is more limited.

Nerve excitability tests It has been known for over a century that innervated muscle will respond to brief pulses of faradic (a.c.) current applied to the nerve, while denervated muscle ceases to respond to faradism. Its response to galvanism (d.c.) is slow and prolonged compared to the fast twitch of innervated muscle. When the muscle has undergone severe atrophy it fails to respond to either faradism or galvanism. In practice these tests have been replaced by the use of a stimulator capable of delivering square pulses of known amplitude and duration. By plotting the threshold of muscle excitability in response to stimuli of varying strengths and duration, characteristic 'strength–duration curves' are obtained. These can indicate normal innervation of muscle, early denervation, and also signs of reinnervation.

In facial nerve testing the stimulator is placed over the facial nerve between the ramus of the mandible and the mastoid process and a pulse of 1 ms duration is usually employed. The minimum strength of stimulus required to produce a visible twitch in any part of the face is normally found to be 2–5 mA. The measurement for both facial nerves is approximately the same in each individual. A difference greater than 3·5 mA between the two sides is regarded as pathological. The severe limitation of this test is that during the first three days of muscle paralysis the distal part of the nerve remains normally excitable. Even if one facial nerve has been completely severed, the difference in threshold excitability between the two facial nerves will not be detectable until the fourth day after injury. Thereafter a steadily increasing stimulus is required on the paralysed side to obtain a muscle contraction. The maximum tolerable stimulus is 10–15 mA.

Skill and experience are required by the observer to distinguish between contraction of the masseter muscle via the trigeminal nerve and stimulation of the facial muscles by the facial nerve.

Conduction time tests By combining electromyography with nerve stimulation tests, it is possible to measure the time taken for the electrical impulse to travel from the point of stimulation to reach its muscle and excite a contraction. In nerve disease due to axonal degeneration the conduction time or conduction velocity is surprisingly little reduced. In those disorders characterized by segmental demyelination, e.g. diabetic neuropathy or the Guillain–Barré syndrome, the conduction velocity is markedly reduced. These tests are more easily applied to nerves which travel for a long distance near the surface of a limb before they reach their muslces, e.g. ulnar and median nerves.

By using an electrode in the orbicularis oris muscle and stimulating the facial nerve behind the ramus of the mandible, it is possible to study conduction time in the facial nerve. The normal value obtained is about 4 ms. In practice the conduction time in facial nerve paralysis has not been found a very useful test since most facial nerve lesions are axonal (with Wallerian degeneration) and the conduction time is therefore seldom markedly increased.

Electrogustometry If the facial nerve is inflamed or damaged above the point where the chorda tympani leaves it, the sense of taste will be impaired and this can be tested electrically as well as chemically. Electrical testing is performed by applying a small anodal galvanic current (less than 100 μA) to the surface of the tongue. The minimum current which is detectable by the patient (usually as a metallic taste) is called the electrogustometric (ELG) threshold. This is usually similar in right and left halves of the tongue. Differences of up to 22 per cent between the two sides are considered within the range of normal variation by Alford *et al.* (1973). However, as a result of extensive testing, Mogens (1976) has come to the conclusion that the difference between the two sides must be of the order of 100 per cent before it can be considered pathological.

The test is a simple and effective way of revealing the functional differences between the two chorda tympani nerves in a case of unilateral facial paralysis. As a method of measuring the pathological alterations in taste thresholds which do occur in diseases not involving facial paralysis, it has been found insufficiently dependable for routine clinical use.

Electrically induced blink reflex Electrical stimulation of the supraorbital nerve produces a reflex contraction of the orbicularis oculi. This can be recorded through electrodes placed on the lateral aspect of the muscle.

Kimura *et al.* (1976) have studied the loss of this reflex and its recovery in patients with Bell's palsy. They found it helpful in predicting the course of recovery. In their series the earlier the reflex returned to normal, the more complete was the recovery of facial nerve function.

Acoustic stapedius reflex In recent years impedance audiometry has become a standard means of investigation in otolaryngology clinics and has made the testing of the stapedius reflex a brief and simple procedure. Conventional pure tone audiometry is concerned with the sound waves that are transmitted by the tympanic membrane, through the ossicular chain, to the inner ear. Impedance audiometry, on the other hand, studies the sound waves that are impeded by (reflected from) the tympanic membrane. If the stiffness of the tympanic membrane and its attached ossicular chain is increased, a greater proportion of the sound waves which strike the tympanic membrane is reflected back and the impedance is increased. An acoustic probe is inserted into, and seals, the external auditory meatus of the ear being tested. The probe can deliver a test tone at a constant intensity and is designed to detect any change in impedance encountered by the tone. A loud acoustic signal of around 90 db is then presented to the non-test ear. Under normal circumstances, a bilateral contraction of the stapedius muscle takes place to diminish the transmission of such a loud noise through the stapes to the cochlea. The contraction of the stapedius muscle stiffens the ossicular chain and increases the impedance at the tympanic membrane. A less technical explanation is that the contraction of the stapedius muscle causes the tympanic membrane to be drawn inwards or medially. This indrawing of the tympanic membrane increases the volume of the sealed external auditory canal and thereby reduces the pressure in the canal. This change of pressure is detected indirectly by the acoustic probe.

The afferent path of the reflex is the auditory nerve and the efferent path is the facial nerve via its branch to the stapedius muscle. The pathway from the cochlea through the brain stem nuclei to the facial muscles is frequently referred to as the 'sonomotor reflex arc'.

The stapedius reflex test is valid only if

(a) the tympanic membrane and middle ear are normal on the test side, and
(b) the non-test ear has sufficient hearing to detect the acoustic signal as a loud sound.

Under these circumstances, the absence of a recordable stapedius response in a patient with ipsilateral facial palsy indicates that the lesion is proximal to the origin of the branch to the stapedius muscle. Return of the stapedius reflex may be detectable before visible recovery of the facial paralysis. Unlike tests of taste function and lacrimation, the stapedius reflex test gives an unequivocal answer in patients with normal ears. As soon as the loud acoustic signal is presented to the non-test ear the acoustic impedance is increased and remains increased for the duration of the signal. Immediately the signal ceases the impedance returns to normal. If the nerve to the stapedius is not functioning, however, no contraction of the muscle occurs and no change in acoustic impedance takes place. Provided the ears are normal no false-positive or false-negative results are encountered. It is a completely objective and painless test and requires only standard audiology equipment.

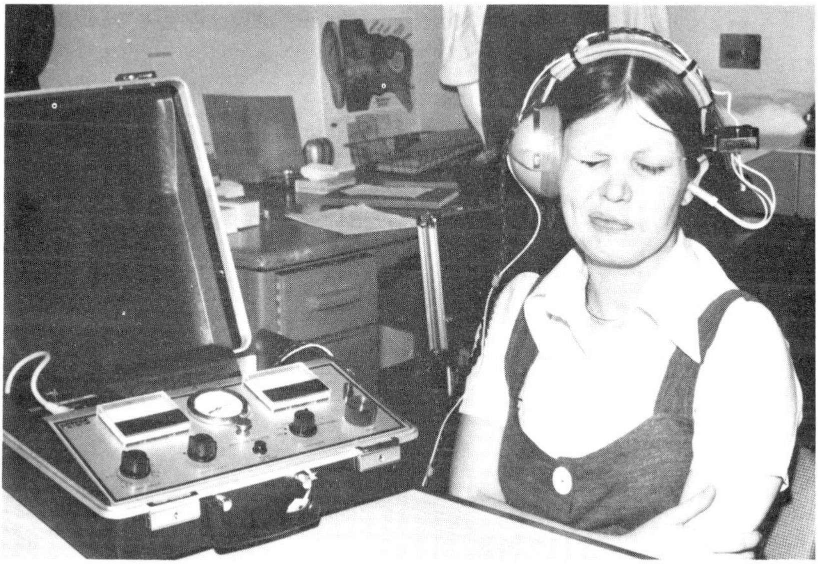

Fig. 6.7. Impedence audiometry in progress on patient with incomplete left facial palsy.

The impedance audiometer is in everyday use in ENT clinics for the investigation of conductive deafness. In traumatic lesions of the facial nerve the stapedius reflex test will accurately determine whether the lesion is proximal or distal to the branch to the stapedius muscle. In diffuse lesions of the facial nerve, e.g. Bell's palsy, the return of the stapedius reflex may be an early sign that recovery is taking place.

We use this test frequently, but seldom use lacrimation or taste tests. The stapedius reflex test deserves to be more widely known outside the field of audiology, and we recommend it to our readers (Fig. 6.7).

Electrocochleography No other audiological tests apart from the stapedius reflex are currently used in facial nerve testing although Bochenek and Bochenek (1976) suggested that electrocochleography might be used in future. This is an objective audiological test using the same sonomotor reflex arc that is used in the stapedius reflex test (afferent auditory nerve–efferent facial nerve). Wide-frequency clicks of around 110 db intensity are presented to the ear at a rate of 10 per second. If the reflex arc is intact, a myogenic response is detected by post-aural electrodes after a latency of 11–15 ms. The myogenic response arises in the post-auricular muscles and appears to be mediated through the post-auricular branch of the facial nerve. This leaves the nerve trunk distal to the stylomastoid foramen. It is necessary to use an averaging computer to record the myogenic response because it is small and would otherwise be submerged in the many other changes in electrical potentials which can be picked up from the scalp.

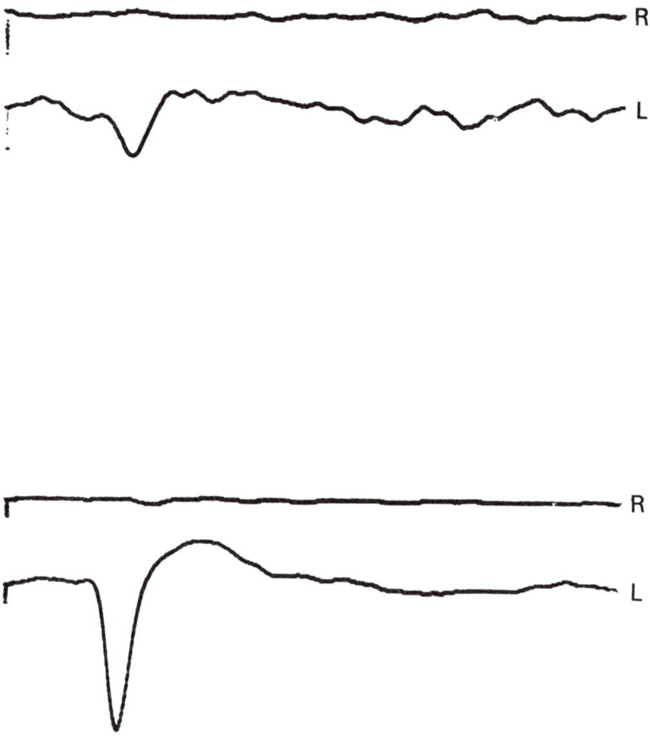

Fig. 6.8. Reflex postauricular myogenic response: medium intensity stimulus (upper tracings) and high intensity stimulus (lower tracings). Patient has a right-sided Bell's palsy. Note absent R postauricular response to both medium and high intensity stimuli.

Bochenek and Bochenek studied 23 patients with unilateral peripheral facial paralysis. Twenty-one of the patients had lesions proximal to the stylomastoid foramen and 2 had lesions distal to it. The reflex myogenic response was present only in the 2 patients with distal lesions. Although the purpose of their paper was not to compare electrocochleography with current tests of facial nerve function, their suggestion that this would help to divide facial nerve lesions into infraforaminal and supraforaminal groups is very interesting and worthy of further study. Electrocochleography requires much more sophisticated equipment than impedance audiometry and at present is found only in specialized audiology centres (Fig. 6.8).

The applicability of electrical testing The clinical features of facial paralysis are so obvious that these tests are not required to confirm the diagnosis. They are used primarily in an attempt to determine the prognosis and, to a much lesser extent, in an attempt to localize the site of the facial nerve lesion. Prognosis depends on whether the nerve

(a) has a simple conduction block without loss of axonal or nerve sheath continuity—neuropraxia,

(b) is severed with loss of axonal and nerve sheath continuity—neurotmesis, or,

(c) has suffered loss of axonal continuity only, following which Wallerian degeneration occurs—axonotmesis.

(a) Neuropraxia occurs in a small percentage of patients with Bell's palsy. These will recover completely within a few weeks. Electrical nerve excitability tests and strength-duration curves remain normal throughout the whole period of the paralysis. Electromyography reveals no fibrillation potentials.

(b) Neurotmesis occurs when a nerve is severed by surgical or non-surgical trauma. Nerve excitability tests remain normal for the first three days but nerve excitability becomes progressively reduced thereafter. After 1–3 weeks electromyography demonstrates the presence of fibrillation potentials in the denervated muscle, and after a year or more fibrillation potentials disappear as the muscle atrophies and becomes fibrosed.

(c) Axonotmesis occurs in the majority of cases of Bell's palsy and in lesser degrees of trauma. Nerve excitability remains normal for the first three days but becomes progressively reduced thereafter, the reduction being directly proportional to the amount of degeneration. If nerve excitability is only slightly reduced during the first few weeks, then little degeneration has occurred and the prospect of good recovery is increased. After 1–3 weeks electromyography reveals the presence of fibrillation potentials. The number of these is proportional to the amount of degeneration. If few fibrillation potentials are present a month after the onset of the paralysis the prognosis is considered to be good. Conversely numberous fibrillation potentials as early as ten days after the onset of the paralysis suggests that recovery will be poor. The disappearance of fibrillation potentials after three months or so suggests that reinnervation is taking place. This can precede any clinical evidence of recovery. It also suggests that surgical interference with the nerve is not indicated.

The presence of action potentials on volitional movement of the face indicates that some muscle fibres are innervated even if no movement is detected clinically. Their continued presence in the early weeks proves that the paralysis is incomplete. The appearance of these action potentials after a period of absence indicates that reinnervation is taking place. In both circumstances, they confirm that the nerve is in physical continuity.

In Bell's palsy patients Sarala Devi *et al.* (1978) found that serial testing of the nerve excitability threshold helped to establish the prognosis. They also found the tests helpful in regulating the dosage of prednisone used in treatment. However Rogers (1978) found that the combination of electromyography and conduction time tests gave a more accurate assessment of the facial nerve state than nerve excitability tests alone.

Summary

(1) None of the electrical tests give evidence of nerve damage before the third day.
(2) The electrical tests only indicate those degenerative and regenerative changes that have taken place.
(3) To forecast future changes in the nerve on the basis of these tests involves considerable speculation.

Taste test

The simplest way of testing this is by chemical agents. (We already have described the more complex electrical test.) The patient is asked to protrude his tongue and the examiner places some salt or sugar on the papillae at the edge of the dorsum of the tongue. The patient is asked to determine the taste before withdrawing the tongue into the mouth where saliva might carry the test substance to the opposite side or to the posterior third of the tongue. This test is useful in detecting the presence or absence of taste in the areas of the tongue supplied by the chorda tympani and glossopharnygeal nerves on each side. It is not sufficiently accurate to detect reduced taste sensation in an area of the tongue. Although it is possible to determine the taste threshold chemically by using progressive dilutions of a salt solution, the threshold values are of academic interest only. Not only do thresholds vary enormously between individuals but each individual's threshold shows quite marked diurnal variations.

Schirmer's test of lacrimation

This simple technique for measuring lacrimal gland secretion is named after the German ophthalmologist who first described it in 1903. A strip of fine filter paper (5 mm × 35 mm) is sharply bent at 5 mm from one end. This end is then hooked into the lower conjunctival sac without applying any anaesthesia. The length of the filter paper which is soaked by the lacrimal fluid is measured after a fixed interval of 3 minutes or so. The strips from the right and left eyes are compared with each other. A marked reduction of lacrimal flow on one side suggests a paralysis involving the secretomotor fibres of the greater petrosal nerve, which leaves the facial nerve at the geniculate ganglion.

In a well-balanced study of 140 normal individuals Hanson *et al.* (1975) recorded differences of more than 300 per cent between the lacrimal flow on each side. In unilateral facial paralysis they suggest that a difference of around 400 per cent or greater is diagnostic of a supraganglionic lesion.

The interpretation of Schirmer's test is more complicated in acoustic neuroma patients where involvement of the trigeminal nerve can produce conjunctival anaesthesia. In addition, the tumour may have an irritative rather than a paralytic effect on the facial nerve, at least initially. Morrison (1975) records that four of his patients suffering from acoustic neuroma had a consistently *increased* lacrimation on the affected side, severe enough to be considered a symptom.

Submandibular salivary flow test

The rate of secretion from the submandibular salivary glands after stimulation by lemon juice can be measured by inserting a fine polythene cannula into Wharton's duct on each side. In unilateral facial paralysis, a very marked reduction in the salivary flow on the affected side, compared with the normal side, is held to indicate a severe lesion of the facial nerve with a consequently poor prognosis. May *et al.* (1976) claim that a severely diminished salivary flow can be detected within two days of the onset of paralysis, in Bell's palsy cases which are likely to develop nerve degeneration. If this is true, then the salivary flow test is capable of predicting denervation before it begins. May *et al.* concluded that if any treatment is capable of preventing nerve degeneration, this test would select those patients likely to benefit from it. Saito *et al.* (1978) prefer to measure the pH of the collected submandibular gland secretion rather than the volume. They point out that pH is directly proportional to the volume of saliva secreted. A low pH therefore indicates diminished activity of the chorda tympani nerve.

Topognosis of facial nerve lesions

Locating the level of the lesion in peripheral facial paralysis is of considerable value in lesions due to trauma and tumours. Variations in the level at which the chorda tympani joins the facial nerve can limit accuracy. In Bell's palsy the validity of topographic tests is disputed. May (1978) claimed that serial tests during the early stage of the disease confirmed his view that Bell's palsy is an ascending paralysis. His tests indicated that neuropathic changes involved taste, salivary flow, acoustic reflex, and lacrimal flow in ascending sequential order. This view is not shared by Adour *et al.* (1978) who believe that there is a generalized involvement of the whole nerve in Bell's palsy and that the lesion is not limited to specific levels. They record that in a group of 19 patients who had a normal acoustic reflex throughout the duration of their paralysis 9 (47 per cent) had a concommitant decrease in lacrimal function. Many clinicians have come to regard topographic tests as an indication of the severity rather than of the level of the lesion in Bell's palsy. Thus a patient with loss of taste and lacrimation is considered to have a more severe paralysis, and a consequently poorer prognosis, than one in whom these two functions have been preserved. Tschiassny's (1953) Table provides a useful summary of the topognostic tests (Table 6.1).

Table 6.1

Topognostic classification of facial nerve lesions based on the anatomy and function of the nerve (after Tschiassny 1953)

Level	Forehead movement	Bell's phenomenon	Emotional movements	Blink reflex	Stapedius reflex	Tears	Taste
Supranuclear	yes	no	yes	yes	yes	yes	yes
Nuclear	no	yes	no	no	no	yes	yes
Supragenicular	no	yes	no	no	no	no	yes/no
Transgenicular	no	yes	no	no	no	no	no
Suprastapedial	no	yes	no	no	no	yes	no
Infrastapedial	no	yes	no	no	yes	yes	no
Infrachordal	no	yes	no	no	yes	yes	yes
Infraforaminal	no	yes	no	no	yes	yes	yes

References

Adour, K. K., Byl, F. M., Hilsinger, R. L., Kahn, Z. M., and Sheldon, M. I. (1978). The true nature of Bell's palsy: analysis of 1,000 consecutive patients. *Laryngoscope* **88**, 787.

Alford, B. R., Jerger, J. F., Coats, A. C., Peterson, C. R., and Weber, S. C. (1973). Neurophysiology of facial nerve testing. *Arch. Otolaryngol.* **97**, 214.

Bochenek, W., and Bochenek, Z. (1976). Postauricular (12 ms latency) responses to acoustic stimuli in patients with peripheral facial nerve palsy. *Acta Otolaryngol. (Stockh.)* **81**, 264.

Diamant, H. (1963). Electro-physiological studies on human taste nerves. *Proceedings of the 1st International Symposium on Olfaction and Taste.* Pergamon, Oxford.

Hanson, J., Fikentscher, R., and Roseburg, B. (1975). Schirmer test of lacrimation. Its clinical importance. *Arch. Otolaryngol.* **101**, 293.

Karatay, S., Katircioglu, S., and Erbengi, T. (1976). Ultrastructural investigations on the degenerative and regenerative processes in the chorda tympani in Bell's paralysis. *Acta Otolaryngol. (Stockh.)* **81**, 304.

Kimura, J., Giron, L. T., and Young, S. M. (1976) Electrophysiological study of Bell's palsy. Electrically elicited blink reflex in assessment of prognosis. *Arch. Otolaryngol.* **102**, 140.

May, M. (1978). Bell's palsy: progressive ascending paralysis, therapeutic implications. *Laryngoscope* **88**, 61.

——, and Schlaepfer, W. M. (1975). Bell's palsy and the Chorda Tympani nerve.

——, Hardin, W. B., Sullivan, J., and Wette, R. (1976). Natural history of Bell's palsy. The salivary flow test and other prognostic indicators. *Laryngoscope* **86**, 704.

Mogens, F. (1976). Electrically evoked taste threshold. *Ann. Otol. (St. Louis)* **85**, 359.

Morrison, A. W. (1975). *Management of sensorineural deafness.* p. 68. Butterworths, London and Boston.

Robertson, M. (1970). Simple instrument for measuring the sense of taste. *Brit. med. J.* **ii**, 109.

Rogers, R. L. (1978). Nerve conduction time in Bell's palsy. *Laryngoscope* **88**, 314.

Saito, H., Higashitsuji, H., Kishimoto, S., Miyamoto, K., and Kitamura, H. (1978). Submandibular salivary pH as a diagnostic aid for prognosis of facial palsy. *Laryngoscope* **88**, 663.

Sarala Devi, Challenor, Y., Duarte, N., and Lovelace, R. E. (1978). Prognostic value of minimal excitability of facial nerve in Bell's palsy. *J. Neurol. Neurosurg. Psychiat.* **41**, 649.

Tschiassny, K. (1953). Eight syndromes of facial paralysis and their significance in locating the lesion. *Ann. Otol. (St. Louis)* **62**, 677.

Walton, J. N. (1977). *Brain's diseases of the nervous system*, 8th edn. Oxford University Press.

7 Treatment of facial nerve disorders

7 Treatment of facial nerve disorders

Introduction

FACIAL nerve disorders can be alleviated by:

(a) pharmaceutical or other specific treatments, such as megavoltage therapy;
(b) surgery;
(c) a combination of the above methods;
(d) no treatment at all.

In addition, there are conditions for which there is no known therapy.

Pharmaceutical treatment (including irradiation)

The modern principles of pharmacological action of drugs are important when dealing with disorders of the facial nerve. The following are well-recognized areas of drug action:

1. Pharmaco-dynamics.
2. Pharmaco-kinetics.
3. Pharmaco-genetics.

The potential advantages and disadvantages (toxic effects and drug interactions) of pharmaceutical treatment have to be carefully weighed before starting any course of drug treatment. Nowadays drugs are subjected to extensive clinical trials (double-blind cross-over) before they are released onto the market. Information on drug safety can be obtained via the Committee on the Safety of Medicines (Calne 1975).

Many patients are taking, or at least carrying, a veritable polypharmacy, making the task of identifying an adverse reaction very difficult. In a patient with facial paralysis it is important to examine all the drugs being prescribed. Only in this way can you exclude possible toxic effects being produced on peripheral nerves by the medication. Treatment of facial nerve damage is discussed under separate headings in this chapter. Most of the drug treatment is directed towards an underlying disease or injury, and will thus influence recovery of the associated facial paralysis. Megavoltage treatment, perhaps in conjunction with cytotoxic drugs, will be supervised by a specialist.

A combined clinic of all the disciplines involved is the usual follow-up regime.

Surgical treatment

Exposure of the facial nerve

When the facial nerve is dissected in the temporal bone laboratory it is easy to see all its vascular connections. This is not the case during an operation, when even gentle elevation of the nerve can produce bleeding, and inadvertent rough handling may produce a haematoma in the sheath. The facial nerve exposed by surgery is unlike the already exposed nerve as seen in cholesteatoma or neoplastic conditions. In the latter case, the nerve seems less vascular in its connections, and is apparently less traumatized by handling. Presumably some protective fibrosis has been acquired.

During the post-war years great advances have been made in devising new methods of access to this long cranial nerve. These methods can be divided into two groups.

1. To expose the nerve during its course from brain stem to stylomastoid foramen.
2. To provide access to the nerve in its facial portion.

Between the brain-stem and the stylomastoid foramen (a) A posterior craniotomy gives access to the posterior fossa and its contents. Microsurgery is required to deal with tumours involving the facial nerve in this region. The patient can usually return home two weeks after surgery. However, the complications of fifth nerve damage, and possibly brain-stem infarction can occur. For example, one of our patients had a complete unilateral upper limb paralysis, following successful removal of an acoustic neuroma. Recovery took several days. This was due to compression by the cerebellar retractor during the operation. Access to the facial nerve can, therefore, produce considerable morbidity. This must be considered before advising operation.

(b) The translabyrinthine approach to the internal auditory meatus again provides excellent access to this region of the facial nerve. Using this approach, damage that has occurred during the course of surgery to the facial nerve can be repaired, but not as easily as in the following method.

(c) The middle fossa approach to the internal auditory meatus is now the generally accepted method of access to the middle fossa, and the intrameatal portion of the seventh nerve. It is quite feasible for the procedure to be continued into an exploration of the middle ear, and vertical segments of the facial nerve, down as far as the stylomastoid foramen. A brief outline of one method follows.

A skin incision is made just anterior to the pinna, at the level of the zygomatic arch, and extended vertically to the upper margin of the temporalis muscle. In most patients it is possible to keep this incision within the hairline. The muscle is now incised to expose the bone, and a craniotomy is carried out using a cutting drill. The opening should be of sufficient size to allow optimum visibility. Its lower margin should be on a level with the floor of the middle cranial fossa.

The operating microscope is then used for the elevation of the middle fossa dura inwards over the arcuate eminence, then medially and anteriorly. This exposes the facial hiatus and the neighbouring large petrosal nerve. It should be remembered that the geniculate ganglion lacks a bony cover in 5–10 per cent of people. It is not advisable to elevate the dura as far as the foramen spinosum, as troublesome bleeding can occur. Once haemostasis has been obtained, a suitable spatula is inserted to elevate the temporal lobe, positioning it so that there is a good view of all the necessary landmarks. All bone is removed from the geniculate ganglion, and dissection follows the canal of the facial nerve to reach the internal auditory meatus. During this stage of the operation great care must be taken to avoid the cochlea, which lies close to the ganglion. The bone has to be elevated very gently, as the facial nerve can very easily be damaged at this stage of the operation. Once all is clear, it remains only to incise the dura over the internal auditory meatus to inspect its contents. Now the seventh nerve is in view across the middle fossa, from the internal auditory meatus to the middle ear tegmen. Having completed repairs to the facial nerve and any other surgical requirements, the exposed structures are repaired as much as possible. A muscle graft will close the internal auditory meatus. Fascia, or a piece of bone from the craniotomy can be placed over the tegmen if necessary. There are numerous techniques, and we have only described one of them, mainly in order to draw attention to the various landmarks (House 1963; Pulec 1966; Fisch 1972b).

Good anaesthesia and an operating microscope are essential for this complex operation. Opening up the internal auditory meatus gives a surprisingly good view of its contents. We have used this approach for many years in gaining access to the facial nerve. It should, however, be emphasized that even if the patient has a known pre-operative paralysis, it can be very difficult, or even impossible, to note any changes under the microscope which would allow the part damaged by an infective disease or trauma to be identified.

(d) Exposure of the nerve from the middle ear to the stylomastoid foramen will complete visualization of the facial nerve. There are numerous techniques for this part of the operation. If the middle fossa has already been explored, the original incision can be extended backwards and downwards, then by using the conventional modified radical operation, good access can be obtained to the lateral semicircular canal (Fig. 7.1). A narrow part of the

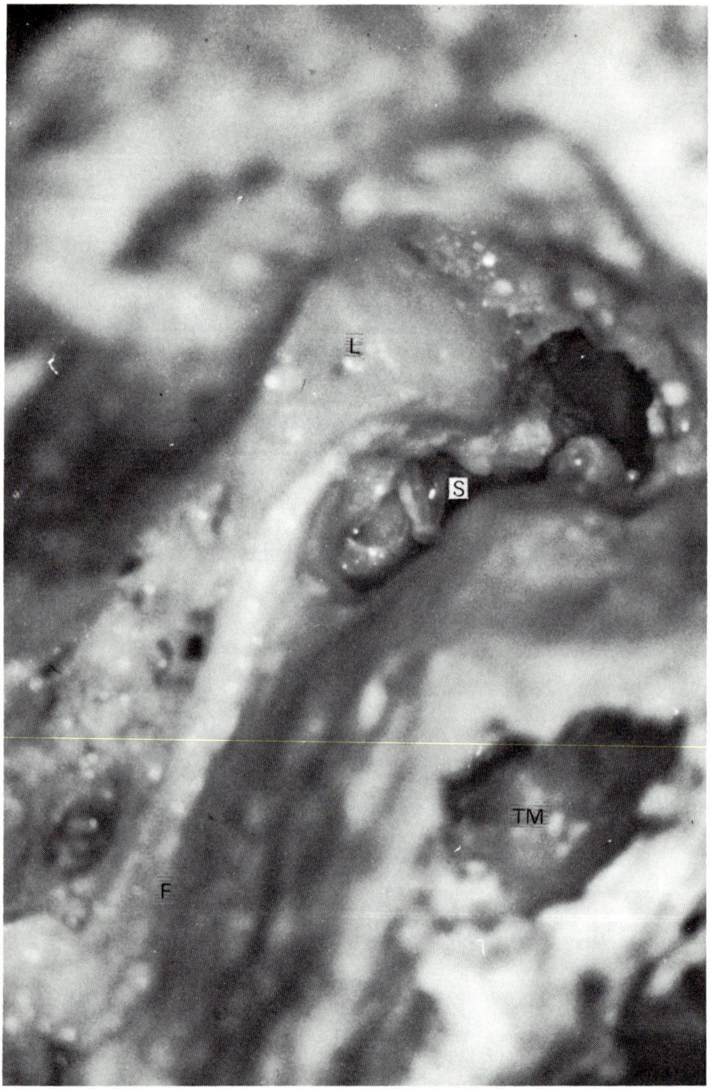

Fig. 7.1. Relation of facial nerve to lateral semicircular canal. The middle ear with the stapes is seen clearly. F verticle segment of facial nerve; L lateral semicircular canal; TM tympanic membrane; S stapes.

posterior meatal wall can be left as the bridge, in order to support the tympanic membrane (Fig. 7.2). Having exposed the nerve in this portion of the canal, it is quite easy to work forward and then upward through the tegmen to expose the upper portion. The vertical part is followed down to the stylomastoid foramen. Careful drilling under magnification, gentle bone

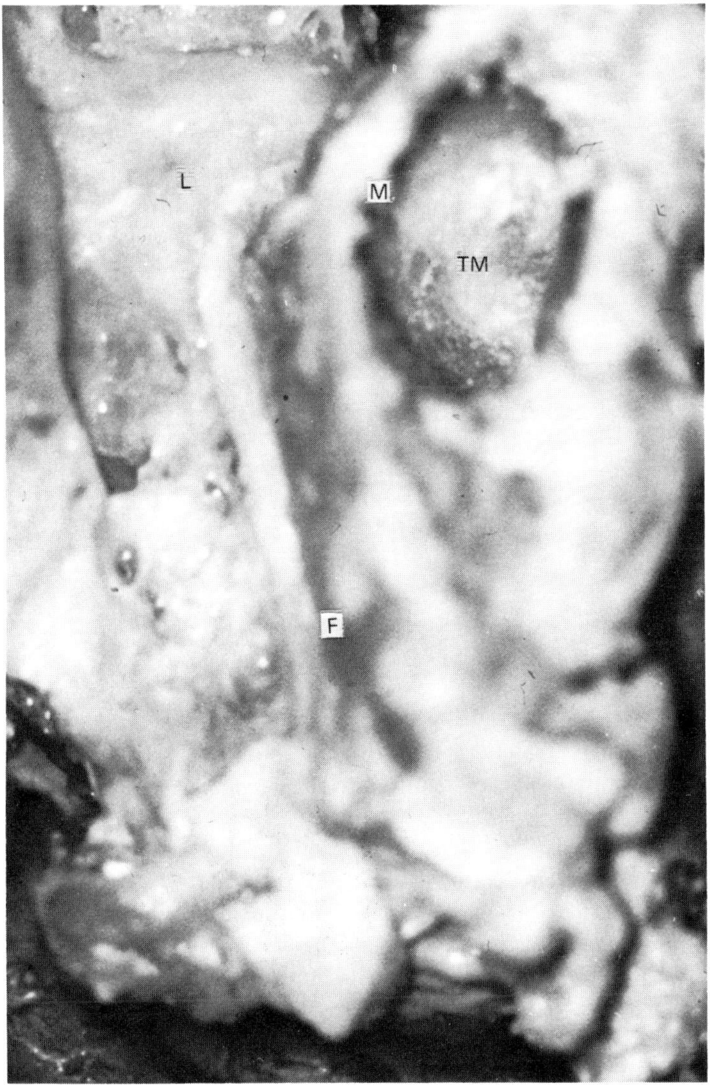

Fig. 7.2. The verticle segment of the facial nerve is exposed. A narrow margin of meatal wall is left to support the tympanic membrane.

elevation, and continuous suction are necessary in order to avoid damaging the nerve in its canal.

Some surgeons prefer endaural incisions to expose the nerve in its vertical segment, in the manner described by Wullstein (1957). The method used in a combined approach tympanoplasty, leaving the posterior canal wall intact, can also be used (Jansen 1967; Sheehy 1968, 1970; Wullstein 1957). Following skull trauma, or if decompression is undertaken, the procedure must not only be safe, but it should permit reconstruction of damaged ossicles, and if necessary avoid damage to intact ossicles and ear drum.

The facial portion Techniques are described in textbooks of parotid surgery (Conley 1975). Adequate cadaver practice should be obtained before starting on patients. Disease and scarring can make this operation extremely difficult, and complete familarity with the area is absolutely vital for successful results. An excellent account of his method is by Conley (1978).

Repair of damage to the facial nerve

Having exposed the nerve, in whole or in part, any damage can be assessed and repaired. The following classification is suggested for the repair of the damaged facial nerve.

Simple decompression A length of the nerve is found to be swollen, and surrounding haematoma can usually be easily removed. Some authorities deem this sufficient treatment to relieve pressure on the nerve, and allow of potential recovery. However, others (Jongkees 1970; Kettel 1975) insist that to leave the nerve thus is not adequate surgical decompression. They imply that there are two areas of pressure: the original source from within the nerve, probably oedema; and the compounding effect of its confinement in the bony canal. Results show that in addition to the removal of a haematoma, releasing the bony cage is of immense value in relieving pressure. Opening the nerve sheath remains more controversial. The large number of clinicians, in favour of only minimal facial nerve surgery, feel that incision of the nerve sheath is unnecessary and might indeed produce more damage.

Occasionally following trauma, small pieces of bone may be found penetrating the nerve. Removal is quite simple. If the nerve sheath has had to be incised it must be re-covered at the completion of the operation. Various materials have been suggested to seal the nerve sheath: silastic, amnion, or vein, with a final cover of Gelfoam, fascia, or muscle. We favour the use of a seal of thrombin.

End-to-end anastomosis When the nerve is severed, the extent of recovery depends on the amount of damage. A good result is fairly certain only if the sheath remains intact. When the nerve has been divided, the cut ends may retract, leaving a gap. No function will return unless the nerve ends remain very close together, or if, where they part significantly, a graft is inserted. Whatever method of repair is used, success depends on a complete lack of tension in the nerve.

It is potentially harmful to attempt strenuous efforts at approximation: pulling on the cut nerve ends can damage vascular attachments. End-to-end anastomosis should not be carried out unless it is quite certain that safe extension can be achieved. In our experience of 10 such severed nerves in the middle fossa, 6 could be brought together without damage. Only in a recent injury is it possible to make sure there is minimal rotation of the nerves at their new junction. If the injury is long standing, anastomosis should not be attempted, as wrong re-routing occurs, with the usual results of facial incoordination. A graft will give better functional results.

Once it has been decided that end-to-end anastomosis is feasible the cut ends must be freshened, and, under magnification, a suture or two can be used to approximate the ends. Some surgeons prefer to allow the nerve ends to remain in apposition without suture. Thrombin can then be positioned around the anastomosis to seal it.

There are several ways of gaining extra mobility, and therefore minimizing tension. Lathrop (1956) suggested dissection of the nerve from the stylomastoid foramen to the parotid gland. However, there is no guarantee of lack of tension by this method, and future scarring could exert traction on the healing nerve. Mündnich (1967) mobilizes part of the parotid gland, and this would appear to be a more reasonable method of gaining a few millimetres. A technique of re-routing the nerve from its canal, across the middle ear, was described by Bunnell (1927) and Martin (1931). Although this does indeed provide extra length it has the severe objections of leaving the nerve unsupported in the middle ear and, more important, disturbing many vascular connections in the original canal. We have no experience of this method, and prefer autogenous grafting. There is no doubt that in cases where the anastomosis can be made without tension, it is preferable to leave the nerve stable in its own Fallopian canal. In fact, many surgeons rely on the nerve ends anastomosing of their own accord, and do not insert any sutures.

Anastomosis with a neighbouring nerve It is possible to anastomose the facial nerve with another nerve in the vicinity. Korte (1903) is reported to have carried out the first successful anastomosis between a divided facial nerve and the hypoglossal nerve. Stookey (1922) then advocated using the accessory nerve. The disadvantage of this method is of course that there is whole or partial loss of function of the other nerve. Loss of a hypoglossal nerve may cause subsequent difficulty in eating, drinking, and speaking. Nowadays the accessory nerve can be split (Bragdon and Gray 1962), and there is less loss of function. Ballance and Duel stated in 1932 'recovery after the union of one nerve with another, and even after direct suture of a divided nerve, though often wonderfully satisfactory as compared with the preceding paralysis, is never functionally perfect', a statement which is still true today.

Although suture of a cut nerve was mentioned by de Chauliac (1363), there was little subsequent mention of the subject until much later (Fauré cited by Bréavoine 1901; Kennedy 1911; Munch 1904; and others). However, in

1895, Sir Charles Ballance united the facial and accessory nerves end-to-side, in a patient whose seventh nerve had been damaged by mastoid surgery. Apparently the paralysed muscles eventually responded to faradic stimulation but follow-up is not recorded. Cushing (1903) reported a similar case of anastomosis with eventual facial symmetry, reasonable eye closing, and a level mouth.

Evans (1974) discussed 13 patients on whom he performed facial-hypoglossal anastomosis. The operations were carried out between 1966 and 1970, and were all followed up for two years or more. Twelve patients had paralysis due to previous acoustic neuroma surgery, and one was as a result of herpes zoster oticus. Evans's experience showed there was little to be gained either by early operation, say at 6 months, or by waiting up to 14 months before surgery. The disadvantages of this operation, such as increased difficulty in eating, drinking, and speech have been widely quoted. For prophylaxis Evans advocated the use of the split accessory nerve instead of the hypoglossal if much pre-operative dysfunction was apparent in the mouth. He concluded that there is a definite place for this operation.

We have had experience of seeing only 5 patients following facial-hypoglossal anastomosis. Of these, 3 were restored to normal symmetry, but there was not a great deal of improvement in purposeful movements. Two did not benefit at all, and indeed found that difficulty with eating and drinking had increased. Facial glossopharyngeal anastomosis was suggested to Ballance in about 1900 by Professor Schafer, then occupying the Chair of Physiology at University College, London. After the surgeon had carried out a number of the operations he remarked on how little morbidity there was as regards taste. Recovery of that sense in the tongue was very rapid, and there was no apparent motor disturbance. Smith (1972) appears to consider that nerve cross-over operations do not restore much controlled movement to the paralysed side. However, the tone of the muscles is improved.

Autogenous nerve grafts This may be the only way of establishing continuity when a piece of nerve is damaged, or missing. There are various cutaneous nerves readily available for grafts.

(a) the lateral cutaneous nerve of thigh.
(b) the greater auricular nerve.
(c) the ilio-inguinal nerve.

When taking the graft it is important to take a greater length than is required, not only to avoid initial tension, but also to allow for any future shrinkage. The new section should be as close in diameter as possible to the damaged sections. There are two disadvantages of autogenous nerve grafts.

i. the length required for repair may not be available, and
ii. the neurological deficit that could result from its removal to act as a graft might inconvenience the patient.

We have carried out autogenous grafts using the lateral cutaneous nerve. It is easily accessible in the thigh, and causes little deficit to the patient. The graft is easily handled. Two epineural sutures were used to join it to the seventh nerve, and the ultimate recovery was satisfactory as far as the patients were concerned, although there was evidence of some wrong routing, with involuntary movement and inco-ordination.

Ballance and Duel (1932) described their technique. They exposed the damaged facial nerve, and cut away the injured area with a sharp knife, taking care not to disturb the cut ends any more than was necessary. As a graft they used the external respiratory nerve of Bell, now called the nerve to the serratus anterior, in the axilla. This graft must have been quite short as they were able to re-suture the nerve after obtaining the graft. It is of great interest that they did not use sutures for the facial nerve repair, but allowed the nerve graft to lie in the canal, in close contact with the original nerve ends. They noted a rapid collection of plasma around the junctions.

Krekorian (1971) gave an excellent account of repair to facial nerves injured during combat in the Vietnam War. This is a useful article which attempts to classify some of the problems encountered in these patients. Similar trauma can arise from civilian missile injury and from urban warfare. His comments are still of topical interest. He discussed 16 patients, most of whom had extensive local trauma. The longest delay between injury and repair was 8 months, and one patient had a bilateral facial paralysis. In all cases, the paralysis was of the lower motor neurone type.

Following operation 5 patients were classified as good recoveries, that is only minimal evidence of previous facial paralysis. Five were classified fair recoveries, that is a noticeable limitation of facial muscle movement, and the remainder showed poor recovery, or no recovery at all. Presumably the last group of patients could be helped by plastic surgery in the future. Krekorian's results are admirable.

Homografts The first recorded nerve homograft was carried out by Alberti (1878). Homografts have not been successful because of the unfavourable immune responses of the host to foreign tissue. Any success must eventually be due to changes in the antigenic properties of the graft during preparation and storage. Methods of possible reduction in antigenicity have included immersion in low temperature saline, formalin or alcohol fixation, freeze-drying, and irradiation (Marmor 1964). Gye *et al.* (1972) wrote on the use of immunosuppressive agents in human nerve grafting. They used freeze-dried irradiated human nerve homografts in large defects of peripheral nerves in 8 patients, who were also treated with azathioprine. In 4 cases to repair trauma, and in 4 because of leprosy damage. There was evidence of sensory return in 7 cases, but no sign of small muscle re-innervation in any patient.

Such methods lie in the realms of immunology, and might be usefully applied to facial nerve repair where long segments of the nerve have been damaged. Many investigators have stopped work on homografts because of the intense foreign-body reaction produced, reducing the graft to fibrous tissue, and effectively blocking onward neuronal transmission. However, difficulties in bridging large gaps have continued to stimulate research to try and reduce antigenicity.

Inlay grafts Inlay grafts can be used to repair a partially damaged nerve. However, few surgeons hold the view that a portion of the nerve should be sectioned and grafted as an alternative to plastic repair to the face by modern methods. Patients who have recovered from a glomus jugulare tumour often show a limited type of facial defect which could be surgically treated by an inlay graft. We have five such patients at the present. None will submit to any further surgery, and we agree with their decision.

Plastic surgery involving the facial nerve As we have seen, some reactivation of the face can be obtained by direct nerve anastomosis or the use of a graft. However, there remains a group of patients in whom such means of repair are not practicable, or in whom attempts at re-innervation have been unsatisfactory. Many of the static or dynamic types of operation lead to a reasonable functional result, but no restoration of normal mimic expression. The fascial sling operation is a good example.

In 1971 two entirely new applications of methods for re-animation of unilateral facial paralysis were presented. Thompson (1971) demonstrated that free autogenous transplants of skeletal muscle could survive and function in recipient sites, even at some distance from their origin. The principles he adhered to were:

1. The muscle must be transplanted as a complete unit, including the tendon of insertion.
2. The muscle must have been denervated at least two weeks prior to its transfer. It is well known that one of the physiological results of denervation in muscle is to reduce metabolic requirements greatly. This will help the muscle to become established in the new site.
3. The graft must be applied in direct contact with normally innervated skeletal muscle when transplanted. Basic studies on this were made by Erlacher (1915), Hogan (1965), and Thompson (1961). The commonly used skeletal muscles are the palmaris longus from the arm, and the extensor digitorum brevis from the foot. Technical details are given by Thompson (1971). He used the palmaris longus in 11 patients, and the extensor digitorum in 4 patients.

The period of surveillance then was three months to two years. Only 2 cases were not successful out of the original 15 patients. This technique is especially indicated after complete facial muscle dennervation. Smith (1971) described the use of an autograft of sural nerve to connect the nerve on the paralysed side of the face to the normal nerve on the other side, using an operating microscope. Connections were made using the zygomatic and buccal portions of the nerve on each side. Improvement in facial symmetry took 3–6 months.

Millesi *et al.* (1971) wrote an account of fascicular nerve grafting in rabbits. They concluded that one of the main causes for failure of nerve grafting was undue tension, a factor we have mentioned previously. They also emphasized the value of operative magnification.

Freilinger (1975) combined the two new methods to form a new technique to correct facial paralysis. By using a crossed sural graft, and free autogenous muscle grafts, these workers produced new muscular innervation. So far 2 cases have been reported, both successful. These patients had post-traumatic facial paralysis, and one had already been submitted to a decompression operation. The surgery was performed about 6 months after the injury.

Anderl (1976) reiterated the important groups of muscles in the face which have to be considered in restoration of function. We repeat the list here:

(1) the temporal,
(2) the orbital,
(3) the buccal; and
(4) the mandibular.

Anderl suggests a two-stage operation. First, using the operating microscope, crossed sural grafts are inserted. After an interval of 6 months, the union is made with branches of the corresponding divisions on the paralysed side. Obviously for this method to be successful, the facial muscles have to be capable of return to function, and he suggests it must be carried out within two years of the original injury or disease. He quotes a 50 per cent success rate from 15 patients. Using the technique of Millesi *et al.* (1971) no sutures are required.

Where the muscles are atrophied, the same principle of cross-face nerve transplantation can be combined with a free muscle graft. Full details are given in Anderl (1976). It is of interest that this surgeon considers physiotherapy an important part of the subsequent treatment. He also gives electrical stimulation from the completion of the operation, and continues until recovery is complete. Anderl (1976) once again mentions the fifth nerve in cosmetic surgery. Many attempts have been made in the past to utilize the power of muscles supplied by this nerve to re-animate the face. His article describes the methods he is now using.

In all these operations, the eye on the affected side must be protected, and in Britain tarsorrhaphy is the commonest operation for this purpose. Morel-Fatio and Lalardie (1964), Mühlbauer *et al.* (1973), and Anderl (1972) have all described various other techniques using springs, magnets, and silastic membranes. They can all be removed once normal function has been restored. Surgical methods are fully described in the relevant articles.

Discussion

In general, facial paralysis characterized by rapid onset and equally complete recovery is usually the result of localized demyelination. Subsequent remyelination produces a good recovery of function without treatment. On the other hand, when neuropathies involve axonal destruction, recovery, if feasible, can take place only if there is axonal regeneration. Restoration of function is therefore slow, and often incomplete.

We have described all the recent methods of surgical access to the facial nerve. With modern techniques any part of the nerve can be repaired. Various methods of repair have been mentioned, but none of these is ideal. The techniques available must be assessed by the surgeon at the time of operation.

In the majority of patients who develop seventh nerve paralysis of lower motor origin, the underlying aetiology is known, and treatment directed to the underlying disease will often lead to a resolution of the paralysis. In diseases of unknown, or untreatable aetiology, such as in multiple sclerosis, or certain virus infections, only supportive measures can be taken.

Areas of conflict over treatment are for Bell's paralysis and the treatment of traumatic lesions of the facial nerve. Industrial and road accidents, together with missile injuries, produce the vast majority of the latter type of damage.

The objectives of surgical correction in unilateral facial paralysis are as follows:

1. To re-establish the symmetry of the face in repose.
2. Having achieved this, to restore as much of the principle elements of expression as possible.
3. To avoid uncontrolled movements, such as involuntary eye winking, which would make some expressions embarrassing.

The old established methods of nerve suture and autografts can produce excellent results, and we have also described recent methods of plastic surgery for facial paralysis. Have we now reached the stage when we should stop and re-orientate our thinking about residual unilateral facial paralysis? For example, should we ever consider decompression operations in Bell's paralysis? Most recover fully, and the few that remain with a deficit can now have the benefit of plastic surgery, by sural graft, muscle transplant, or a combined operation. We hope no surgeon would disagree that re-exploration is still desirable in immediate post-operative injury, in order to give the patient the best possible chance of recovery. However, we would suggest that lesions which tend to leave minimal deformity should be treated conservatively, and the patient offered plastic surgery later on if necessary. Drugs such as cortico-steroids would still be used by those physicians or surgeons who are convinced of their values. In the rare cases of bilateral facial paralysis we will describe new uses of muscle to produce some facial control by Edgerton *et al.* (1975).

It is important to balance the following considerations. When should plastic reconstruction take place, and how does it interfere with the normal process of regeneration?

Obviously it is not easy to determine the optimal time for attempting surgery to achieve re-innervation in facial paralysis. Normal recovery must not be hindered, nor must the muscles be allowed to atrophy, or they will not react to re-innervation. Anderl (1976) is willing to commence the first stage of his procedure after 18 months, if no sign of regeneration is evident from EMG studies. However, our own experience has shown complete recovery up to two years after onset of paralysis. Some compromise solution is obviously necessary.

Conditions causing upper motor neurone facial paralysis

Traumatic disorders

Operative details are found in neuro-surgical textbooks. The formation of burr-holes for the removal of sub-dural haematoma, and the elevation of bone splinters or fractures are very important procedures in the management of head trauma. In these patients relief of the seventh nerve damage is likely to be only part of the treatment of an upper motor neurone injury, varying in degree up to a complete hemiplegia.

Neoplastic disorders

The extent of a benign or malignant neoplasm usually determines the central nervous system involvement. Remedial surgery can result in damage to previously unaffected areas, including the face. High voltage therapy may produce some relief, temporary or permanent, but the resultant damage to the surrounding cortical matter may itself produce further damage, and possibly extensive neurological deficit. The amount and form of treatment must be assessed in individual cases, and the patient must be kept under constant observation, in case avoidable damage occurs. These are difficult cases to deal with.

Degenerative disorders

In this group we include cerebral thrombosis, haemorrhage, and embolic episodes, commonly grouped under the term 'strokes'. Attention to the primary cause may be the only treatment, as in endocarditis, hypertension, or carotid artery stenosis. Prognosis seems to depend little on treatment in the truly degenerative group of disorders which may affect the facial nerve. Initial management with steroids and dexamethasone may reduce cerebral oedema, and thus avoid harmful cerebral anoxia (*British Medical Journal*, 1977b). Respiratory insufficiency leads to anoxia and further brain damage (Lassman *et al.* 1958; Frew 1961; Cooper 1961). Micro-surgery can be used to initiate cerebral re-vascularization in the prophylaxis of further degenerative cerebral vascular incidents (*The Lancet* 1976). In particular, Yanekawa (1976) reported his results in anastomosing the superficial temporal artery to the middle cerebral artery in cases of stroke. Apparently, those patients with an established stroke were not greatly benefited, but patients with transient ischaemic attacks were greatly improved. Such work offers hope to patients in whom facial paralysis due to cerebral injury is reversible.

Infective disorders

Bacterial Meningitis, brain abscess, and thrombo-phlebitic infections with subsequent damage to the facial nerve are now much less common in this country than they were 20 years ago. The majority of all infective cranial cases seen at the Regional Neurological Centre, Newcastle General Hospital, are of otitic origin. Better investigations, especially with the E.M.I. scan (computerized axial tomography) are very helpful in the early diagnosis of such disorders, and bacterial studies, including the isolation of the anaerobic *Bacteroides fragilis*, have improved the ultimate prognosis. Intrathecal and intraventricular, as well as the usual intravenous, intramuscular, and oral routes for the administration of drugs are now used. Facial nerve recovery depends entirely on the site and extent of the cerebral infection, and the residual damage once the infection has been cleared. With the recognition that anaerobic organisms such as Bacteroides were a main source of morbidity has come more effective treatment to control them, and both mortality and morbidity have now decreased. Recently we have been using metronidazole (Flagyl), 0·4 g every 8 hours until the infection is controlled. It is important to remember that high and continued dosage of metronidazole can itself produce a sensory peripheral neuropathy (Ingham 1975). Tuberculoma can be treated either medically, surgically, or by a combination of both. Supranuclear facial paralysis will be seen if the tract is involved. In recently described cases there has been full recovery of the face after medical treatment (Tandon 1975; Ramamurthi 1970).

Viral Viral disease of the nervous system is receiving greater attention, and more knowledge is being gained of the various forms it may take. The prognosis of facial nerve involvement will depend entirely on the general management of the patient. Progress with anti-bacterial therapy has undoubtedly been more successful than attempts at anti-viral treatment. There are at least two factors which hinder the development of anti-viral therapeutic measures.

(a) Virus infections often tend to have a very rapid clinical course, so that there is seldom any time for the use of specific treatment.

(b) Virus multiplication takes place within cells. This means that any possible treatment aimed at the virus may well have ill-effects on the host. In the case of disease caused by the 'slow' viruses, time is available if the means of treatment could be developed. Methidazone has been shown to be effective in the prophylaxis of smallpox, the first demonstration of a drug effective against virus disease in human beings (Bauer *et al.* 1963).

For a number of years an alternative approach to therapy, viral interference' has been tested. The name 'interferon' was coined by Isaacs and Lindemann (1957) for anti-viral proteins, which suppress viral replication. These substances are produced by the cells which are infected, and appear non-toxic and non-antigenic to the host cells. Remarkably, they also render the cells resistant to further virus infections.

There now appears to be little doubt of the importance of interferon in checking many virus infections. The part that it plays in acquiring general cellular immunity and the mechanism by which it is produced in virus diseases are less certain. Pyrexia is said to stimulate its production; and it can also be produced by other means, including bacteria, malarial parasites, and some chemicals. Walters and Israel (1974) give more detailed information on interferon. The action of interferon is specific for the animal from which it originates, and, to treat facial nerve disorders of a viral origin in man, must therefore be derived from a human source. Despite all the advantages in the use of interferon, it has remained in the background of therapeutics for years. However, more clinical applications are becoming possible. One of the best known is its use for the treatment of chronic hepatitis B (Jordan *et al.* 1974; de Somer *et al.* 1973), and recently for the treatment of a patient with Green Monkey disease (*British Medical Journal* 1977c). The seventh nerve is often involved in nervous system virus disease, and improved prognosis will depend on the success of progress in viral technology.

Toxic disorders

Progressive dialysis encephalopathy resulting from renal dialysis was described by Alfrey in 1972. The focal neurological deficits very commonly include facial weakness, which tends to become worse as the dialysis continues. There is no specific treatment available for the facial paralysis. Prognosis depends entirely on the future course of dialysis, and any possible transplantation. A similar encephalopathy has been described in normal people who have been exposed to aluminium (McLaughlin *et al.* 1962).

Summary

The treatment of upper motor neurone facial paralysis is in general directed towards the underlying pathology, for example towards the neoplasm which has produced a metastatic lesion in the central nervous system. Whatever the cause, cosmetic deformity of the face is much less in upper than lower motor neurone damage, mainly because forehead movement is retained. Other aspects, such as disturbed limb movements, usually grossly outweigh any facial asymmetry. Local plastic surgery, as described in the section on repair can always be used to correct minor residual facial damage. It also seems that some cortical action helps to give mouth control, preventing many of the difficulties seen in lower motor seventh nerve paralysis.

Conditions causing lower motor neurone facial paralysis

An alphabetical list of systemic disorders

Actinomycosis The response to penicillin and to the tetracycline group of antibiotics is very good. Many conditions which are treated by these drugs are thus prevented from being infected by the Actinomyces. However, long-term penicillin or antibiotic therapy may be required to eliminate small, and remote areas of residual infection. Penicillin has to be administered by intra-muscular injection, whereas the tetracyclines are effective orally.

Surgical drainage may be necessary for established collections of infection, as in a mastoiditis. However, facial paralysis secondary to infection produced by Actinomycosis in the ear or mastoid, should have a favourable spontaneous recovery rate.

Amyloidosis Once the diagnosis has been established, a careful search must be made to determine any familiar tendency, concomitant inflammatory disease, or multiple myeloma. Although knowledge of the pathology of this condition has broadened considerably, there is still no effective means of treatment, either generally, or as regards seventh nerve involvement. Steroids are not of any value. Amyloid tissue can completely replace nerve tissue. If this occurs a graft or plastic surgery may be required (Meretoja and Teppo 1971).

Blastomycosis This type of infection responds to two drugs:

(1) Amphotericin B is curative in both North and South American types of blastomycosis, and is given by slow intravenous drip, working up to a maximum dosage of 75 mg per day in adults.
(2) North American blastomycosis also responds to 2-hydroxystilbamidine, but the South American variety is quite resistant to this drug, which has to be given in higher doses, up to a maximum of 250 mg per day, also given via a slow intravenous drip.

Clinical remissions can be achieved by the sulphonamides, but relapses occur unless the treatment is maintained continuously. Mastoid surgery for drainage may be required, but no decompression of the facial nerve is necessary unless it becomes involved in healing fibrosis. In severe cases, excision of the involved nerve segment, and grafting, may be required. Should the deficit be less severe, plastic surgery to the face may be preferred by both patients and surgeons. Recently the usefulness of miconazole therapy in South American blastomycosis has been reported (Negroni 1977).

Diabetes Mellitus Diabetes can produce some peripheral neuropathy, but fortunately the progress of the nerve involvement can often be halted and even improved by correction of the underlying abnormality. If the causal metabolic disturbance is kept under control, then a degree of prophylaxis may be obtained against peripheral neuropathy. Treatment depends on the severity of the disease.

1. Dietary control, with restriction of carbohydrates.
2. By insulin.
3. Sulphonylureas. These act by lowering the blood glucose in patients capable of producing endogenous insulin.
4. The biguanides. A readily absorbed biguanide is phenforminhydrochloride; this has the advantage that it can be given in a sustained-release preparation.

These measures will usually, between them, produce some control of diabetes mellitus. Thus neuropathy may be prevented, or, if present, be arrested, and finally resolve. Details on the treatment of the disease can be found in the appropriate textbooks.

Malignant otitis externa This is a severe, and possibly fatal condition, complicating diabetes mellitus, and involving the seventh and other cranial nerves. It is absolutely essential to bring the underlying diabetes under control.

It is doubtful that surgery to the granulomatous area of the condition in the ear has a useful place in treatment; indeed surgery does not appear to influence recovery of the facial nerve function. A recent review by Prasad (1976) suggests the use of intravenous carbenicillin, together with intramuscular gentamicin.

Some good results in diabetic neuropathy have been reported with the use of clofibrate (Berenyi 1971). Vitamins are really only of value if a deficiency exists. The control of pain in this type of neuropathy requires much care; the effectiveness of analgesic drugs varies greatly between patients. In general, the return of function in facial paralysis associated with diabetes mellitus is good, and we do not think that surgery is necessary.

Diphtheria This is essentially a preventable disease. Should it be contracted, any lower motor neurone facial paralysis, which is a rare complication, will resolve spontaneously as the patient responds to therapy. Anti-toxin must be given in the first 48 hours; otherwise it does not seem to mitigate the illness. Drug treatment is with penicillin or clindamycin, in a dosage appropriate to the age and weight of the patient. Surgical exploration of the facial nerve is not necessary.

Ear neoplasms The seventh nerve can be involved directly in two ways.

1. If the neoplasm arises in the external auditory canal, especially on the posterior wall and floor, or in the middle ear or mastoid, the facial nerve is immediately at risk.
2. The nerve may also be invaded directly if the upper cervical nodes are involved (Fig. 3.8).

Treatment is by excision of the primary neoplasm if possible. Radical mastoidectomy should be performed to give access. A full course of megavoltage therapy, which must include the gland-bearing areas, is also given. Recovery of a facial nerve which has been directly involved in a neoplasm is unlikely, but, if the neoplasm is successfully cured, plastic surgery can be used to give complete facial recovery. It is very difficult indeed to find the nerve surgically in the post-irradiation fibrosis, and we suggest that attempts to repair the nerve by a free graft are likely to be less successful in these patients than the results of good plastic surgery. Once again it is important to remember that infection may have helped to produce the initial facial nerve damage, and that some improvement can result from concurrent antibiotic therapy.

Echinococcosis-hyatid disease There is so far no medical treatment which is effective against infestation with the unilocular cysts of the causative tapeworm. A new technique of dealing with the cysts by cryo-surgery is described by Saidi (1977). Perhaps this may eventually be useful for cysts which involve the seventh cranial nerve in its upper or lower motor neurone areas.

Geniculate neuralgia The varying distribution of the origin of the sensation of pain in the area of the fifth and seventh nerves arises from the changes which have taken place in the course of evolution. In lower vertebrates, such as the fish, the seventh is an important sensory nerve. However, in man, the fifth nerve is the main sensory source in the face and head.

The medical treatment of geniculate neuralgia is very limited indeed. Sedatives, analgesics, and phenytoin can be tried, and many patients show spontaneous remissions. However, should the condition become severe, surgery should be considered. If the nervus intermedius is sectioned intracranially, there should be a permanent cure, as the ganglion cells will have been isolated from the central nervous system. Kunc (1965) suggested that the pain fibres of the seventh, ninth, and tenth nerves form a bundle running between the Bardach bundle and the trigeminal tract in the medulla, and his article gives details of tractotomy operations and their results.

Pulec (1976) gives a historical review, and then discusses the surgical treatment of 15 patients with geniculate neuralgia. He describes the middle fossa approach for removal of the geniculate ganglion and division of the nervus intermedius. He reports that the inclusion of the anterior 20 per cent of the diameter of the motor portion of the facial nerve, with geniculate ganglion excision, caused no facial weakness, and resulted in a more complete excision of ganglion cells. In some patients previous selective section of the fifth cranial nerve had also been performed. Geniculate neuralgia and its source is difficult to define. Surgical treatment has not yet been perfected. Reports of other series may help us to make better decisions on treatment.

Glomus jugulare tumours Small tumours in the middle ear are accessible to surgery, especially cryo-surgery. It is seldom, however, that these tumours involve the seventh nerve. Paralysis always indicates a more widespread lesion and surgery is liable further to damage the nerve. Despite hypotensive techniques it is impossible to obtain a clear operative field, or to define landmarks, especially the seventh nerve.

It was first shown by Frew and Finney (1963) that these very vascular tumours respond to mega-voltage therapy. The effect is to produce fibrosis, and thus slow their progress for many years. Some resolution of facial paralysis often follows a course of treatment (Frew 1965).

Although we have never seen this, it has been reported that post-irradiation fibrosis may itself produce facial weakness. If the indications are that no tumour remains, then exploration of the nerve can be undertaken, and a nerve graft inserted. Should the facial defect be slight, then cosmetic surgery is preferable.

One of our patients has a facial paralysis initially produced by a glomus jugulare tumour in the middle ear in 1956. Progress of both tumour and paralysis were halted by a tumour dose of 5·5 kR. She still has some slight weakness of the side of her mouth, but does not wish to have cosmetic surgery. Another patient who presented with a complete right lower motor neurone seventh paralysis in 1966 was found to have a similar tumour of the middle ear and mastoid. A full course of megavoltage therapy was administered over five weeks. Improvement of the paralysis started about one month after completion of treatment, and continued until she was left with a minimal defect. None of us, including the patient, feel that any improvement could be obtained by plastic surgery. We have five such cases being followed up as outpatients. The nerve is probably involved by pressure of the tumour, or a mild degree of infiltration. The latter is more likely, because of the persistent degree of slight loss of function after treatment. We have never seen a patient have absolute recovery, but none have required any remedial surgery. More important, no patient's facial damage has ever been increased by therapy.

Histiocytosis X This comprises the following disorders: Letterer–Siwe disease, Hand–Schuller–Christian disease, and eosinophilic granuloma. Treatment of Letterer–Siwe disease is both of the general disease and of associated conditions such as a seventh nerve paralysis. Irradiation of lesions and treatment of microbial infections can be effective.

The use of steroids and vinblastine have been shown to be helpful in the local and general manifestations of Hand–Schuller–Christian disease. If the seventh nerve is involved by an eosinophilic granuloma, the response to irradiation is excellent. Any residual defects can be treated as required, by exploration and grafting or by cosmetic surgery. Mastoid exploration is usually only for the purpose of obtaining a biopsy. Decompression of the nerve is not recommended. Tos (1969) reviewed 500 patients and gave suggested forms of treatment.

Infective mononucleosis—glandular fever This is mostly a self-limiting disease, and many patients receive no treatment. Oral penicillin or sulphadimidine will help to prevent secondary infection. There is no specific treatment for an established seventh nerve paralysis due to glandular fever, but spontaneous recovery is usual. No prophylaxis is as yet available for the disease (Allison 1950; Michel *et al.* 1975).

Infective polyneuritis (Guillain–Barré syndrome) Apart from the use of steroids there is no specific treatment. However, in a recent retrospective study no difference was noted between patients treated with cortico-steroids, and a similar untreated group (Goodall *et al.* 1974). The use of cytotoxic drugs has been suggested (Yuill *et al.* 1970), but no definite indications are apparent as yet. Bilateral facial paralysis occurs as part of a symmetrical polyneuropathy. There is no indication for seventh nerve decompression, and in our experience the prognosis has been satisfactory and facial recovery is good. Cases of Guillain–Barré syndrome may require tracheostomy and supportive treatment from a well-equipped respiratory unit.

Leprosy The infecting bacteria are *Mycobacteria leprae*. Fortunately, there is a specific antimicrobial agent, Dapsone, in addition to a longer acting agent, Acedapsone. Since the latter requires an intramuscular injection only once every two months it is the drug of choice in developing countries. These drugs are both of the sulphone group. For patients who do not respond, or show adverse reactions, various other drugs can be tried, rifampicin (Rees *et al.* 1970) and clofazimine (Karat *et al.* 1971). The former is rapidly bactericidal in leprosy. Thiosemicarbazone is also available.

Treatment is continued until a general clinical improvement occurs, including resolution of the seventh nerve paralysis. Patients may require treatment for 1–8 years, depending on the type of infection. Large numbers of patients throughout the world have seventh nerve paralysis due to leprosy, but surgical treatment is not yet available to many of them. However, as facilities improve in what are usually isolated communities, surgical repair of damaged nerves, or plastic surgery will become possible. Work on nerve homografts has included some patients with leprosy (Gye *et al.* 1972). If the facial nerve is involved, a sufficiently long graft of autogenous origin is usually available.

The success of future treatment lies in detection at an early stage, before the permanent and crippling lesions occur. Mobile clinics can now allow treatment at, or near the patient's home, and thus avoid moving them from familiar surroundings (The Leprosy Mission 1976).

Experienced specialists in leprosy are of the opinion that prognosis in seventh nerve paralysis is poor. The magnitude of the effect depends on the number of axons damaged, or eventually destroyed (Pettit 1975). Neural pain due to intra-neural pathological swelling can be a great problem, and the injection of local anaesthetic and the use of analgesics are suggested. Opening up the nerve sheath appears to have little beneficial effect, and it can lead to herniation through the opening, thus leading to further nerve damage.

Leptospiral infections In a disease which is usually both mild and self-limiting it is difficult to assess the therapeutic value of drugs. Leptospira anti-sera, and penicillin will remove the bacteraemia. However, the effect on any seventh nerve paralysis is probably only coincidental, and recovery from both the illness and a peripheral nerve involvement is usually spontaneous. The damage which may occur to kidney and liver is the usual cause of mortality in severe cases.

Leukaemia Since the facial paralysis of lower motor type is usually caused by the pressure of the tumour, no surgery is indicated. General treatment of the disease is required by a specialist oncologist. Haemorrhage into the facial nerve has been reported, and residual defects may require plastic surgery. Our experience of such cases has been that complete recovery is usual once the disease has been controlled. Presumably even local infiltration of the nerve by leukaemia or lymphoma can be controlled by general treatment (Henson 1970).

Intracranial hypertension can occur in children with leukaemia, and this may cause lower motor neurone paralysis, either by intra-neural haemorrhage, or the formation of a haematoma compressing the nerve. Complete regression with treatment is rare, but is occasionally seen. In one case it was reported by Poppi and Morganite (1961). Treatment was with cortisone therapy. Sklansky *et al.* (1974) discuss in detail the management of patients with peripheral nerve lesions in leukaemia. Fourteen patients had a seventh nerve paralysis, and 4 of them showed bilateral involvement. A satisfactory response following radio-therapy was obtained in 9 patients.

Lymphocytic choriomeningitis There is no known treatment for such diseases. Dick (1975) discusses the possible uses of immuno-suppression, and describes the animal experiments that have been carried out using cyclophosphamide. General supportive measures are required. Any recovery of facial nerve function depends on total recovery from the infective process.

Malaria The complete treatment of this disease is described by Wilcocks (1972). No facial nerve surgery such as decompression or grafting is indicated.

Marble bone disease The recurrent facial paralysis should be treated surgically only as a last resort. Contrary to previous views, decompression is required in the full length of the nerve, not only of the vertical segment (Hamersa 1973). Better radiological techniques have shown narrowing of the long canals involving most cranial nerves, including the seventh. A similar reduction in diameter of its long bony canal occurs along its whole length. The reason for the intermittent lower motor neurone paralysis, which may affect the child before any more permanent involvement sets in, is not clear. One case has been observed by the authors. Only a single attack of unilateral facial paralysis has occurred so far, and as yet there is no indication for surgical intervention. Since the disease produces its damage on the seventh nerve by eventual narrowing of the canal, some surgeons may feel that plastic surgery offers better long-term results.

Measles Facial paralysis is usually associated with a concomitant otitis media in measles. In these days of prophylactic penicillin or sulphonamides, seventh nerve damage has almost completely disappeared from the list of complications of measles in developed countries. Where it does occur, treatment as for acute otitis media should result in complete facial nerve recovery. If response to antibiotics is inadequate, mastoiditis with seventh nerve involvement is a clear indication for surgical drainage. Nowadays post-auricular abscesses are treated with penicillin or sulphadimidine until only a small collection of pus remains, when all that is required is a small incision down through the periosteum to enable the purulent material to be sucked out. Formal mastoidectomy in places where continuous antibiotic treatment is possible should seldom be required if this procedure is followed. The facial paralysis will gradually completely recover. Active and passive immunization are available for measles, and the disease with its complications may eventually be eliminated. A recent review article on the treatment of measles in the tropics is in the *British Medical Journal* (1976b). Modern references are available.

Melkerrson–Rosenthal syndrome Several patients have been submitted to facial nerve decompression. Kettel (1947) described areas of necrotic bone, but no convincing evidence of aetiology. Steroids have been tried with some initial success. No other drugs or antibiotics seem to be of any value. Canale and Cox (1974) also carried out facial nerve decompression in a 7 year old girl. Both sides were submitted to surgery, and there was full recovery on each side after the operations. However, previous attacks of paralysis had responded to cortico-steroids.

We do not see any convincing evidence in favour of decompression. Treatment with steroids appears to encourage the facial oedema to subside, and the seventh nerve paralysis should resolve spontaneously.

Middle ear neoplasms In squamous cell carcinoma of the middle ear, which is the most common of these tumours, a regime of treatment is now well established. Preliminary mastoidectomy is performed to give access and exposure thus allowing of future observation. It is not necessary to remove the facial nerve even should it appear to be involved in tumour. Preliminary mastoidectomy is followed by a full tumour dose of megavoltage therapy. It is our experience that early involvement of the seventh nerve by a neoplasm is seldom improved by irradiation. The paralysis may be halted, but even minimal improvement rarely occurs. Should the disease eventually be cured, then exploration of the nerve can be undertaken, and a graft inserted between the damaged ends, either in the middle ear or temporal bone. This will have to be done to both sides in those rare cases of bilateral middle ear carcinoma.

Other types of middle ear tumours such as sarcomas are suitable only for irradiation and associated cytotoxic therapy. Surgery merely produces widespread metastases. The management of secondary deposits in the temporal bone which may involve the seventh nerve will depend on the likely outcome of the primary neoplasm, wherever, and whichever type it may be. Facial nerve involvement and prognosis will vary from case to case, and each will have to be judged on its merits.

If a middle ear neoplasm is not controlled by mastoidectomy, cytotoxic drugs, and megavoltage treatment, then petrosectomy may be the only solution. In such extensive surgery (Fig. 2.4), the facial nerve has to be cut (Fig. 5.7). There are two options available for treating the resultant paralysis. Direct anastomosis with another nerve is feasible if the seventh nerve has only been damaged close to the stylomastoid foramen. Then hypoglossal, or split accessory nerve suture can be carried out. If the facial nerve has been sectioned at any other location reconstructive plastic surgery with crossed sural grafts can be initiated once the patient has recovered. The eye must be protected between the operations.

Having on two occasions failed to find the facial nerve whilst attempting a graft in patients with controlled middle ear neoplasms, we now consider that plastic surgery is more likely to produce a successful result.

Migraine The transient facial paralysis does not require any treatment, and will resolve spontaneously without residual deficit. Reassurance is necessary, and the already somewhat anxious type of patient may well need treatment to reduce anxiety. Hemiplegia, a rare occurrence, also has a good prognosis. This is also true of the facial weakness, which will be of upper motor neurone type.

Many opinions exist as to the best treatment for migraine itself. Ergotamine tartrate is the drug of choice for the actual attack. In very severe cases clonidine hydrochloride is now being used as a prophylactic (Shafar *et al.* 1971).

Moebius's syndrome and agenesis of nuclei The facial paralysis is usually bilateral and often fairly symmetrical. Few reports of attempts to correct the deformities are to be found in the literature. One of the most recent is by Edgerton *et al.* (1975). This article quotes two patients in whom repair of the paralysed face was undertaken, using in both cases transfer of functioning striated muscle to support and animate the face. In the first instance, using a wide collar incision, and a vertical one on each side of the neck, they were able to raise the platysma muscle bilaterally onto the cheek region. The sites of insertion were the parotid fascia just anterior to the tragus. One beneficial outcome was to change the direction of the muscle pull so that they elevated the corners of the mouth, and prevented the drooling which had been so embarrassing to the patient. Speech was improved, as was the smile. The nerve supply utilized would be the anterior cutaneous nerve of the neck. In the second case temporalis muscle was used to produce a smile—as requested by the patient. Edgerton *et al.* give full details of the technique of transference of strips of innervated muscle to the upper margins of the mouth. Fascia lata grafts were placed circum-orally to help mouth closure. The post-operative result appears to have been satisfactory.

It is encouraging to see articles about the treatment of facial paralysis in these congenital syndromes. The children, who may be quite intelligent, are hampered not only by lack of facial expression, but also by indistinct speech. Drooling and the catching of food in the mouth are also troublesome. Combinations of these plastic operations will greatly reduce this morbidity, and raise the standard of life.

Hemifacial atrophy has been described as occurring with a seventh nerve paralysis, as in Moebius' syndrome, but it can, however, be found with intact nerves. Wells (1977) describes a means of correcting the deformity. He uses a flap from the lower abdominal wall. Details are given in the article.

Multiple sclerosis Until a cure can be found, treatment must of necessity be supportive. Fortunately, the facial paralysis subsides without any treatment. Possible residual defects could be dealt with by plastic surgery.

ACTH has a beneficial effect on the exacerbations of multiple sclerosis, including facial nerve paralysis, although there is no apparent alteration in the long term course of the disease. Various dosages have been suggested. An example of a dose regimen is as follows: 60 units of ACTH gel twice daily for 1 week, then 40 units of ACTH gel twice daily for 1 week, followed by a gradual reducing dosage over the next 6 weeks to complete the course. Potassium supplements and checks on serum electrolytes are also included. It now appears that prednisone does not produce comparable results in its effects on acute relapses.

Mumps In the few patients we have seen with a seventh nerve paralysis, associated with deafness and vertigo, as a result of contracting mumps, the only symptom to recover was the paralysis, leaving the patient with a sensorineural deafness, and a non-functioning labyrinth. Steroids are usually given, but no convincing evidence is available of their effectiveness on the face. Certainly they have no effect on the ear and labyrinthine symptoms, or on the prognosis of inner ear recovery. There is no evidence of any indication for facial nerve surgery.

Neurilemmomas Careful dissection using a microscope is required in extra-temporal and intra-temporal tumours. Conley and Janecka (1974) describe the surgical treatment of 23 tumours in 17 patients. In their group 9 tumours were intra-temporal and 14 were extra-temporal in origin. Details of technique and repair are described. Immediate anastomosis, autogenous graft, and hypoglossal anastomosis were all utilized. These authors also dealt with two malignant schwannomas, using a combination of surgery and radiotherapy. The results were not very good in these two patients. Further benign tumours are discussed by Neely and Alford (1974) and Pulec (1966). The latter described 100 consecutive cases of decompression for Bell's palsy, out of which he found 2 patients with benign neurilemmomas.

Noma A recent article by Durrani (1973) describes the treatment of 12 patients between 1966 and 1972. Surgery included considerable soft tissue repair, and anastomoses of facial nerves in the vertical mastoid segment, and in the face.

Nutritional neuropathy In theory the only necessary treatment is to supply the specific deficiency. However, it is not always possible to identify the dietary lack, and usually a number of vitamins are given in a high calorie diet. Supplements of thiamin, niacin, riboflavin, ascorbic acid, pantothenic acid, and pyridoxine are recommended. A number of patients will require treatment for the underlying condition, such as alcoholism, or intestinal disorders.

Osteitis fibrosa cystica (von Recklinghausen's disease) General treatment of the hyperparathyroidism, with removal of the parathyroid adenoma is required. No local treatment for seventh nerve involvement is indicated.

Otitis media 1. *Acute infective otitis media.* About 0·5 per cent of all cases of acute otitis media are said to be complicated by a lower motor neurone facial paralysis. Our own experience makes us doubt this high estimate, and we have found spontaneous recovery in all cases, see also Cawthorne (1963) and Riskaer (1946). We have never needed to have recourse to surgical intervention. The advent of antibiotics has revolutionized the treatment of otitis media, and reduced its complications (McGovern and Fitz-Hugh 1956).

2. *Chronic otitis media.* This can be divided into three main groups.

(a) Patients who have a persistent drum lesion in the pars tensa, but in whom the ear normally remains dry, and in whom no cholesteatoma is evident. Such cases, when they present with a seventh nerve paralysis during an acute infective episode can be treated conservatively. Both infection and paralysis should subside completely with antibiotics. No surgery is required. A congenital dehiscence of the Fallopian canal accounts for the facial paralysis in acute infective episodes.

(b) Those patients with a long history of otitis media, in whom evidence of cholesteatoma is present, and who develop a facial paralysis. It is our opinion that immediate exploration of the mastoid and middle ear should be performed. Infection and pressure are the usual aetiological factors. Antibiotics should, therefore, supplement the surgery. Removal of the cholesteatoma is usually sufficient treatment to allow the facial nerve to recover rapidly. Granulations can be gently removed from around the nerve if necessary, and it is unlikely that any further surgical repair will be necessary. This is our own experience, and that of other authors, over many years (e.g. Jongkees 1970).

(c) Another very important group of patients may present with either seventh nerve paralysis and a running ear, or alternatively, unilateral facial spasm and no ear symptoms. These patients have a congenital cholesteatoma (Fig. 3.12). In many cases the disease is very extensive, and may have to be followed into the middle cranial fossa, and even to the internal auditory meatus. We have not found the prognosis for recovery very good in these patients. Re-exploration and a nerve graft may be required later. Less severe cases will only require moderate cosmetic surgery.

Discussion. Should a patient not show recovery 24 months after the resolution of an acute otitis media, then exploration, and possibly grafting are required. Plastic surgery may be an acceptable alternative.

Apart from those patients with congenital cholesteatoma it is not necessary to decompress the nerve. The nerve may be already exposed, and great care should be taken to avoid further damage by manipulation. The treatment of infection, and removal of sequestra and the pressure of debris are often sufficient to allow of recovery. Even when the paralysis is of long-standing duration the nerve should be left alone at the initial operation. Allowing the nerve naturally to recover is always the best approach in these patients after the causative disease has been cured. Decompression and grafting can always be carried out later on if it becomes evident after at least 2 years that no recovery is going to take place. The presence of residual infection does not appear to hamper successful grafting results.

We have seen one patient in whom removal of a simple inflammatory polyp resulted in an immediate post-operative facial paralysis. Surgery had been very gentle, and bleeding was minimal. Fortunately, recovery was rapid and complete, and the ear also healed. Our view is that the polyp had become attached to the nerve sheath via a dehiscence in the middle ear canal area, and that removal of the polyp had produced damage by traction. We have not seen this recorded in the literature. This case underlines the fact that great care is necessary during all operations in the region of the facial nerve, no matter how simple the procedure may appear to the surgeon.

Paget's disease The only treatment of value for facial nerve paralysis is the general treatment of the disease. Calcitonin should provide some prophylaxis against seventh nerve involvement. Established paralysis will probably fare better with cosmetic surgery than decompression. Progress of the disease is likely to destroy the original benefits of any bone surgery.

Poliomyelitis The prophylaxis of this disastrous illness has been one of the great advances of the post-war years. However, cases still occur in our own country as well as abroad. There have been many attempts made to find an anti-viral agent to treat the acute phase of the disease. At levels which will not damage the body as a whole, guanidine inhibits the increase of sensitive viruses. About three groups of poliomyelitis virus are included in this group. The action of this drug is not yet fully understood, but it has been known for many years that it can influence neuro-muscular transmission. Other possible anti-viral substances are discussed in books of virology dealing with the nervous system (Illis 1975).

Recovery from the seventh nerve paralysis will depend entirely on the general progress of the disease. Any residual defects must be treated with plastic surgery. There is no place for surgical decompression. Paine (1957) reports one case in which the facial nerve was paralysed following immunization against poliomyelitis. In this case the nerve was decompressed, but nothing abnormal was found.

Porphyria An early, rapid, and accurate identification of the biochemical deficit in the patient or the family is essential. Prophylaxis is against the precipitation of acute attacks by drugs, one of the best known of which is the barbiturate group. Recovery from the facial nerve lesion is usually complete. No surgery is required (Ridley 1969; Aubert and Ginshoarg 1970).

Ramsay Hunt syndrome, herpes oticus At present, our method of treatment depends at which stage of the disease the patients are first seen. If they present some weeks after the onset, then no specific treatment is of any value, only the usual supportive measures of eye protection and cheek supports together with re-assurance. Patients who are seen within 48 hours of onset can be treated with either ACTH gel, 120 units daily, on a decreasing dosage, or on prednisone 30 mg daily, also on a decreasing dosage, both over a period of six weeks. We now give alternate patients these two parallel methods of treatment, using patients who are seen at a later stage, and therefore not treated, as controls. No antibiotics are given. Hydrocortisone cream 1 per cent is useful if the vesicles are irritable. Mostly, however, they dry up quickly leaving small scars. We have only once seen a patient with post-herpetic neuralgia in this syndrome. Any incidental vertigo may require treatment with a labyrinthine sedative. Decompression is not favoured in our department for the treatment of this disease at any stage. Fisch (1975) favours early decompression, citing good results in four patients who were operated on within two weeks of onset.

Recovery may take as long as two or three years in these patients, and even then may leave small areas of deficit, most often around the corner of the mouth, which may require cosmetic surgery. As regards drugs, cytarabine has been claimed as being of use in herpes virus involvement in general, and amantadine is of great value in the treatment of any post-herpetic neuralgia (Galbraith 1973). Juel-Jensen and McCallum (1972) claim to reduce the incidence of such neuralgia by the early use of steroids. The setting up of some controlled trials, or at least definitive groups of patients as we have described, may lead to a better idea of the correct treatment, and probable prognosis in these patients. A recent article (*British Medical Journal* 1976a) gives a useful and up-to-date summary of the present knowledge on the use of chemotherapy in varicella–zoster infections. In 2 of our patients complete recovery of the face has occurred in just one week, after a paralysis of two years. They were initially treated with ACTH.

Sarcoidosis This is a disease with a high rate of spontaneous remission. As a result, controlled observations of drug therapy have been difficult to obtain. The drug used most frequently is prednisone. The duration of treatment depends on the clinical course of the illness. The recovery of the involved cranial nerves is quite unpredictable. We cannot see any place for surgical intervention by decompression: the majority of reviewed cases have responded to steroids, and obtained return of facial function in about six months.

Lambert and Richards (1964) reviewed a large number of cases of sarcoidosis of the upper respiratory tract, including six cases with unilateral or bilateral seventh nerve paralysis. Out of 179 cases showing evidence of sarcoidosis, 24 were described as Heerfordt's syndrome. The authors suggested decompression of the facial nerve if early recovery with steroids was not obtained. We have fortunately not seen any such resistant cases, and still advise a policy of 'wait and see'.

Other drugs which have been used include the antimalarials, chloroquine and hydroxychloroquine, as well as oxyphenbutazone (Munt 1975). Although they are effective enough during the course of treatment, relapses are common when these drugs are discontinued. All anti-tuberculous therapy is ineffective.

Syphilis Treatment of the facial paralysis in syphilis is entirely that of the disease itself. Any deficit from upper or lower motor neurone seventh nerve damage will require plastic surgery. No facial nerve surgery such as decompression is indicated.

Tetanus Active or passive immunization are available. Large doses of penicillin are effective in established cases. Supportive measures may be necessary, including muscle relaxants, tracheostomy, and controlled respiration. Prognosis for facial recovery is good providing the general infection is controlled.

Thrombotic thrombocytopenic purpura (Moschcowitz's disease) Medical treatment of the underlying disease includes the use of cortisone. Surgery is confined to splenectomy. The response of the upper or lower seventh nerve paralysis depends on the outcome of the disease. No local therapy exists (d'Eramo and Levi 1972).

Toxoplasmosis Drugs that appear to have some therapeutic effect in this disease are as follows:

(1) Pyrimethamine (Daraprim), an anti-malarial drug. It appears to work with

(2) sulphonamides, which potentiate its action. However, pyrimethamine can have toxic effects on the haemopoetic system, and blood counts are necessary during treatment.
(3) Spiramycin is a much less toxic drug, and can either be used alone, or in combination with the above two drugs.

Toxoplasmosis is usually a mild illness, and the above therapies would only be suggested for complications such as a unilateral seventh nerve involvement. Recovery of the face should then be rapid and spontaneous without surgery. There has been only one recorded case of toxoplasmosis complicated by a bilateral seventh nerve paralysis (Duc 1969).

Tuberculosis Treatment may be required only for the involved ear, or ears, and any consequent facial paralysis. In some countries, the disease may also be associated with chest infection.

Management of thoracic tuberculosis will also remedy any otological manifestations, and nowadays complete recovery of the facial paralysis should occur. It is wise to remember that the original neuropathy may have been due to infection, and will thus be cleared by an antibiotic, following which specific antituberculosis therapy can be initiated. Indeed, it is most probable that the patient will be diagnosed initially as having infective otitis media, acute or chronic, with a seventh nerve involvement. Only resistance to the usual treatment, and the results of a swab will establish the correct diagnosis. Surgery is required only for the removal of bone sequestra, or the appearance of a resistant mastoiditis. Drugs which are at our disposal for the treatment of tuberculosis, including its otitic form, are as follows:

(1) isoniazid, the most effective drug, and relatively non-toxic. The dosage is 5 mg per kg body weight daily;
(2) ethambutol, highly effective;
(3) the antibiotics streptomycin and capromycin, which can cause vestibular and cochlear toxicity;
(4) rifampicin, highly active and well tolerated;
(5) para-amino-salycylic acid (PAS), which is now much less favoured since new drugs with better patient tolerance have been produced;
(6) cortico-steroids; although they have been shown to produce reactivation of quiescent cases, they may also be life-saving in very ill tuberculous patients; other forms of chemotherapy can be used subsequently.
(7) thioacetazone, a cheaper substitute for PAS, commonly used in combination with isoniazid;
(8) pyrazinamide, a powerful drug which may, however, produce liver damage;
(9) ethionamide which commonly produces side-effects of nausea and malaise.

Multi-drug therapy is used in case a given strain has native resistance to one drug. However, when the bacterial population is low, isoniazid alone may be used. In other cases a combination of isoniazid and rifampicin, or isoniazid and ethanbutol may be used. There are varying opinions on the possible combinations of drugs, and the duration of treatment.

It is our opinion that all patients with otitic tuberculosis, whether it is isolated to the ear or not, should be under the care of a specialist otologist and an experienced physician. Although the prognosis for any associated facial paralysis is good, a few patients may be left with varying deficits. Some may require minimal plastic repair; others more extensive procedures. One of the present authors (I.F.) has exposed the facial nerve in two patients with otitic tuberculosis, and found it was involved in thick fibrous tissue. The anatomy was very distorted and made surgery difficult. Excision of the nerve in its vertical segment, and insertion of a femoral cutaneous graft produced moderate results in both cases. We would recommend exploration only when it is quite obvious that no recovery is going to take place, and following consultation with a plastic surgeon. A recent and authoritative account of the treatment of tuberculosis in our own and developing countries is by Fox (1977).

Tumours in the carotid body These relatively rare tumours respond well to radiotherapy. Surgery is not recommended, especially in older patients, in case the common or internal carotid artery has to be ligated. Recovery of facial nerve damage is unlikely. Any facial deficit should be repaired by cross-nerve anastomosis (McGuirt 1975).

Tumours in the cerebellopontine angle and brain-stem Such tumours have been described in detail in Chapter 3. Treatment may be surgical, by megavoltage therapy, or by cytotoxic drug therapy. Combinations of treatments may be necessary.

Ependymomas of the fourth ventricle involving the facial nucleus are rarely amenable to complete surgical removal, and respond only slightly to radiation therapy. In general, the rare secondary deposits from distant sites are treated by megavoltage, and occasionally decompression operations may be required. Only if the primary tumour became controlled as well, is facial nerve repair considered.

Neurilemmoma The most common tumour to be discovered in the cerebellopontine angle is the neurilemmoma. Removal without damage to the seventh nerve will allow the previously pressurized facial nerve to recover, and restore normal function to the face.

The choice of surgical approach depends on the size of the tumour, (the translabyrinthine approach is not feasible for the removal of a large neurilemmoma), and the personal preference of the surgeon. We prefer the posterior craniotomy approach. Retraction of the cerebellum medially provides an excellent view of the area (Fig. 5.4). It is essential to identify the facial nerve in order to preserve it, and prevent further damage. In large tumours which do not extend into the internal canal, surgery is best commenced by drilling away sufficient of the posterior canal wall to visualize the nerves, and to identify the facial nerve. The tumour is then dissected away from the nerve without excessive manipulation or traction. If the tumour is both large and mainly intra-canalicular, then the seventh nerve must be identified from the medial or brain-stem side. The canal is then drilled out. Whatever method or approach is used, careful identification of the nerves is absolutely essential. This cannot be done without the use of an operating microscope, and facial nerve stimulator.

Toxic effects

(1) *Alcohol.* Despite the high incidence of alcohol dependency, it rarely produces a seventh nerve paralysis. Patients require vitamin supplements and appropriate psychotherapy. The prognosis for seventh nerve recovery is usually good, and recovery spontaneous.
(2) *Arsenic.* Treatment is either with British Anti-Lewisite, or penicillamine. Facial recovery is satisfactory.
(3) Heavy metal poisoning is now rare in this country. We have only seen one case of seventh nerve paralysis due to lead poisoning, and that was 20 years ago. Treatment would depend on the metal causing the damage.
(4) Rabies vaccination neuropathy responds well to cortico-steroids (Vejjajiva 1975).
(5) Trilene and gold. Facial nerve neuropathy has been seen during the use of Trilene in industry, and gold in medical therapy. Recovery is spontaneous once the causative factor has been recognized.

Surgical trauma

The brain stem and posterior fossa area The facial nerve can be damaged in these areas by section, traction, or occasionally by diathermy.

Section The facial nerve may be torn off the pons, and in this case no repair is possible in the cerebellopontine angle. Plastic surgery may be considered at a later date. Alternatively, anastomosis with another nerve in the neck may be possible. If the nerve is sectioned in the posterior fossa, leaving some pontine attachment there are several choices of method of repair. In 1958, Norman Dott described a method of combining an intracranial and extra-temporal repair of such a damaged seventh nerve which he maintained allowed a return to both voluntary and emotive facial expression. A description of his method follows. A length of sural nerve is sutured first to the cut end of the nerve in the angle region, or in the canal. It is then passed around the temporal bone through the craniotomy opening, and eventually anastomosed with the peripheral end of the facial nerve in the retromandibular area. There must be no tension if the autogenous sural graft is to be successful. Suture within the skull is carried out under microscopy, and the graft is threaded out between the sternomastoid and splenius capitis muscles, arriving just below the mastoid process. Dott then placed a silver clip on the end and left it in place for 90 days, to allow re-innervation. Then he dissected the facial nerve at the point where it leaves the stylomastoid foramen, divided it, and sutured the peripheral end to the freshened end of the transplant. Good results have also been reported from several other sources (Drake 1960; Fisch 1975).

Direct suture of the nerve is possible in the cerebellopontine angle if the ends can be brought into apposition without tension. Insertion of a graft in this area is extremely difficult, and the nerve is left totally unsupported after the operation. Fortunately, in our experience, this operation is becoming less common, due to more careful dissection of the seventh nerve at the time of removing the neuroma.

Kiuslitz (1974) and Rhoton (1974) give excellent accounts of their experience in facial nerve preservation during posterior fossa surgery. Drake (1972) describes his experiences with direct anastomosis of the damaged facial nerve within the posterior fossa. It is evident from his experiences that feasibility depends on the amount of nerve missing, and the ability to join the ends without tension. His article gives details of his techniques.

Traction Will produce varying degrees of seventh nerve damage according to the severity of the injury. Recovery is usually good. Deficits may require cosmetic surgery.

Diathermy Diathermy injury usually destroys the nerve, and either a Dott repair or insertion of a graft is required.

The temporal bone area

1. Injuries incurred during selective vestibular section for relief of Ménières disease. Severe damage will require anastomosis or a graft, but minimal damage should be left alone, as a good recovery can be anticipated (Smythe *et al.* 1976; *British Medical Journal* 1977a).

2. Injuries may also occur during operations on the Gasserian ganglion. The same principles apply as above.

3. Injuries incurred during procedures in the middle ear and mastoid areas.

(a) Operations carried out under local anaesthetic, more popular abroad than in the UK, allow intra-operative damage to be discovered immediately by its effects on the face. In the UK operations under local anaesthetic are probably limited to ultrasonic labyrinthectomy. During stapedectomy potential injury to the facial nerve ranges from over-heating by the drill to actual tearing of the nerve. Malposition of a prosthesis may also cause damage. If the injury is slight the prognosis is good without further interference. For example, the re-adjustment of the prosthesis may be sufficient. However, if the nerve has lost its continuity, or been severely torn, then it must be explored, and, if necessary, a graft must be inserted. It may, however, be sufficient merely to decompress the involved portion of the facial canal to prevent haematoma pressure.

In any type of mastoidectomy the facial nerve can be damaged in the portion involved in the operation. As we saw in Chapter 5, the vertical segment, and the part just below the lateral semi-circular canal are particularly vulnerable (Fig. 7.1). Treatment must depend once again on an assessment of the damage. Our opinion is that in these patients the nerve should be exposed over the traumatized area, and carefully inspected. Severe damage will require anastomosis and a possible graft. We prefer to do this at the original operation. Fortunately, the presence of infection does not appear to hinder graft success in these cases. There are exceptions to the policy of immediate exploration of a nerve which has been damaged during temporal bone surgery. One exception is damage due to ultrasonic labyrinthectomy. The opinion of most surgeons with experience of patients who have had the nerve so damaged is that it is best to leave it alone, whereupon recovery will be rapid and complete. Cryo-surgical damage caused during therapy for Ménières disease also seems to recover spontaneously.

(b) General anaesthesia is more commonly used in the UK, and some other countries, for procedures in the middle ear and mastoid areas. This means that unless the surgeon observes damage to the nerve during the operation, a facial paralysis will be noticed only when the effects of the anaesthetic wear off. With modern anaesthetic techniques, this occurs very soon after operation, and the surgeon should satisfy himself that all is well before the patient returns to the ward. In our opinion there should be no exceptions to this rule, and at least one competent check should be made to the face in the recovery room. The action to be taken if damage is discovered will depend on its extent, and the opinion of the surgeon. In our opinion slight weakness should be allowed to pass, and recovery be reasonably anticipated (Fig. 7.3). Repair can always be carried out later if necessary. Gross paralysis should be an indication for immediate re-exploration and repair.

(c) Delayed facial paralysis, that is some hours or days after operation, can occur due, for example, to pressure of a pack, or the toxic effect of a pack containing iodine. Removal of the pack should lead to recovery. When the nerve has been left exposed, as in cholesteatoma cavities, great care must be exercised in placing any post-operative pack. The notes should also be

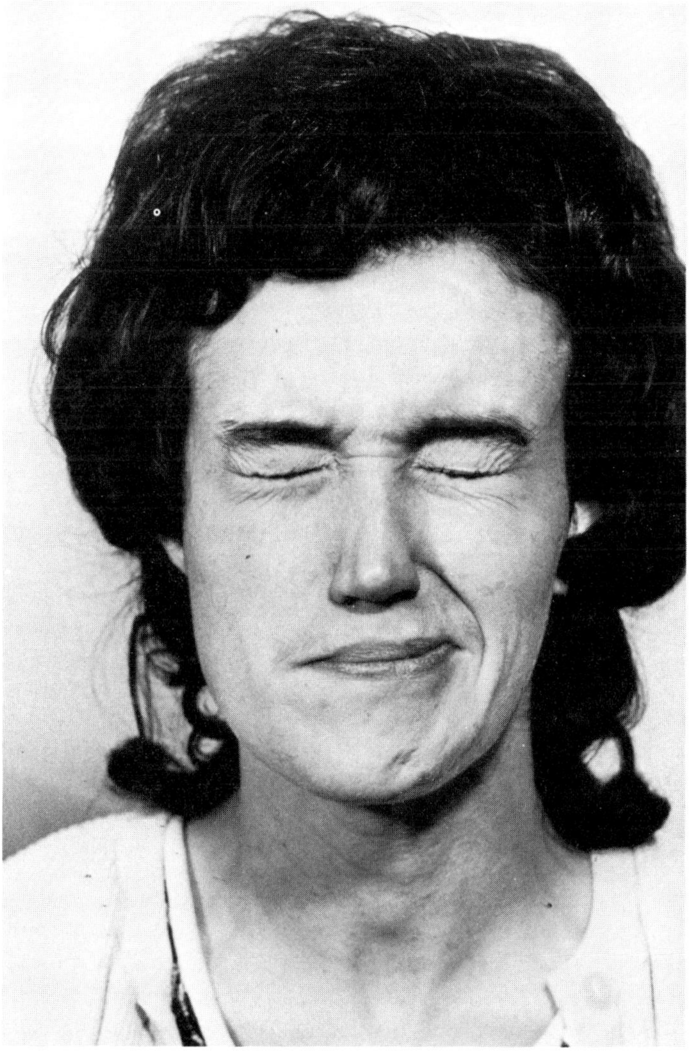

Fig. 7.3. This slight left facial paralysis occurred after a mastoidectomy for cholesteatoma. This patient recovered completely.

clearly labelled for the attention of future surgeons. The effects of inadvertent injection of local anaesthetic into the nerve, probably at the level of the stylomastoid foramen, should either have worn off completely, or show minimal effects when an operation has been completed.

(d) The applications of silver nitrate to granulations in a mastoid cavity, or overspill of alcohol during labyrinthectomy, and onto an exposed nerve, produce only a temporary paralysis. Surgery is not indicated.

The facial area

1. *Parotid gland surgery.* Here the facial nerve may have been infiltrated by a tumour, and so require excision during a parotidectomy. When the main nerve trunk is injured, then re-innervation of the whole face will be necessary, and a large graft must be used. Eneroth and Hamburger (1974) give very good advice about the treatment of parotid tumours, and we agree with them entirely. They state that one must decide from case to case whether immediate reconstruction of the facial nerve can be considered at the time of operation. They also describe the techniques which they use. We regard the most suitable donor as being the great auricular nerve, a branch of the cervical plexus. It has at least four branches which can be used for proximal anastomosis. Alberti (1962) gives an account of its use. Areas which do not eventually recover function can have further grafts at a later date.
2. *Surgery of the face, mouth, and mandible.* This may be for disease which has already damaged the facial nerve, and the surgeon may wish to repair the nerve at the time of the original operation. McGregor (1976) advocates an incision high up in the cheek when using a forehead flap (Fig. 7.4). This prevents the possible damage to the facial nerve which can occur using the retromandibular route to enter the mouth.
3. *Block dissection of the neck.* This should seldom cause damage to anything more than a cervical branch of the seventh nerve, but involvement by secondary nodes high up in the neck (Fig. 5.6) can damage the nerve. It is our experience in the latter that treatment with megavoltage therapy seldom produces any improvement in the paralysis. Surgery with repair is indicated only if the underlying disease is eventually controlled. A graft, or alternative nerve anastomosis may be possible.

Non-surgical trauma

1. *Obstetrical trauma.* Fortunately we have never seen a case which required any form of surgery, and our experience has been that recovery is spontaneous and rapid. It is not reasonable even to contemplate interference unless delivery has been so traumatic that intra-cranial damage has occurred. Shambaugh (1959) recommends operation when the infant reaches 4·5 kg and Müller (1962) at 3 months of age. Prophylaxis must obviously be the recommended ideal.
2. *Soft tissue facial injury.* Unless the damage is due to bruising of the nerve, exploration will be required when recovery is obviously not going to take place. Starting at the stylomastoid foramen and working anteriorly, the severed nerves are located and anastomosed. A stimulator is necessary. This is not a difficult operation and results are favourable. Conley uses silicone cylinders with a small window to allow fine approximation at the suture line. Allowance must be made for post-operative swelling. Long-standing injuries

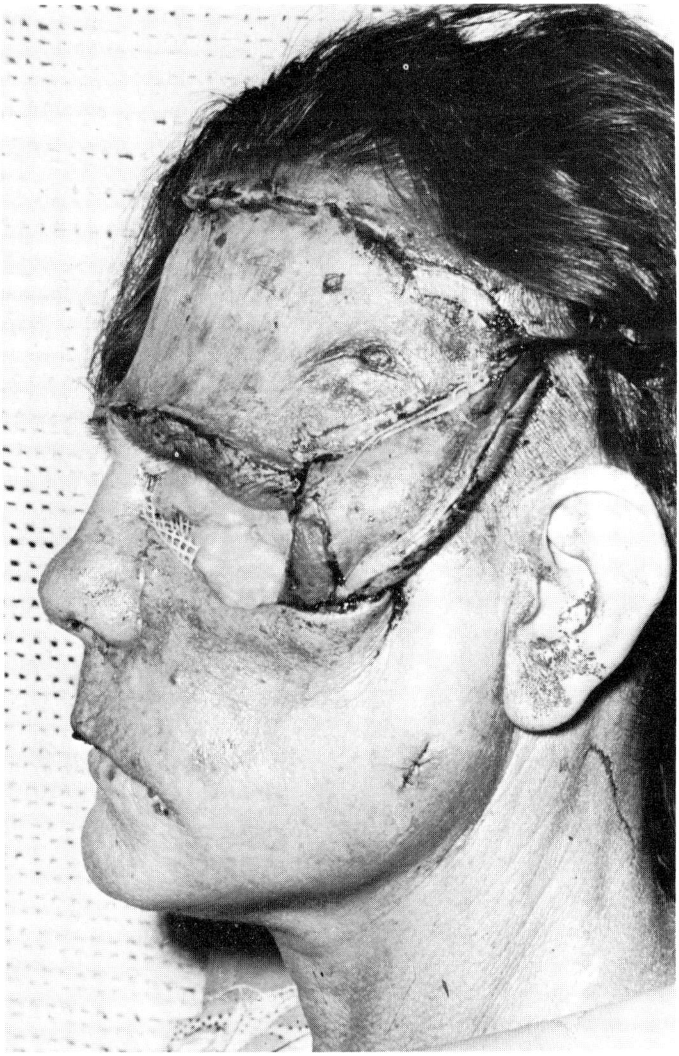

Fig. 7.4. Forehead flap inserted high up in order to avoid facial nerve damage.

with scar tissue may require a graft to bridge the gap and restore continuity (Campbell *et al.* 1955).

Morgan and Cramer (1974) write of their experiences in facial nerve repair. The patients were from the Vietnam war, and all damage was in the area distal to the stylomastoid foramen.

Twenty-nine patients are described, of whom 26 had multiple trauma. However, 20 cases showed a spontaneous return of function within four to five months. Great auricular nerve grafts were used in five cases, direct suture in three, and a graft utilizing a duplicated spinal accessory nerve in one case. Only one patient had no return of function. This excellent description of first-class work is relevant to missile injuries and civilian accident trauma of all types.

3. *Head injury*. One of the factors mitigating against increased knowledge about these cases is the difficulty of producing any controlled clinical trials of surgical treatment. Only the experience of years of work while associated with a large regional neuro-surgical centre enables us to make statements about what, in our opinion, is the correct treatment of facial nerve paralysis.

Patients in the UK have relatively quick access to individual and team specialists, as well as to considerable supportive measures. Our figures since 1965 show that over 90 per cent of cases of facial paralysis following injury will recover spontaneously. In the remainder, the vast majority are left with minimal cosmetic defects, easily remedied by cosmetic surgery. Very few are not restored to former health, with the exception of cases of complete lower motor neurone facial paralysis. It seems reasonable, therefore, to advise against surgery in these patients.

Our experience has not shown any great difference in prognosis between immediate and delayed seventh nerve damage, and recovery in the latter has also been about 90 per cent without treatment. In many cases, particularly those of delayed onset, the face is only partially involved, but this is not necessarily an indication of better or complete recovery.

Between 1950 and 1968, we explored surgically 20 patients with immediate facial paralysis, and 5 who showed delayed symptoms (Table 7.1). Apart from 4 patients who had bone splinters, and 10 who had complete division of the nerve, or damaged sections, no gross pathology was seen in the other nerves at operation. Patients who had no operation recovered just as quickly, and as well, during these years. Since 1968 we have not explored any nerve damage, and the results have been very satisfactory. Minimal cosmetic defects have responded well to plastic surgery, and no patient has been left with a major cosmetic defect. In any patient in whom a facial paralysis had had not improved at all after two years we would be prepared to explore the nerve and carry out a repair. Only 3 such patients have been seen over the past eleven years. This experience leads us to believe that most of the exploratory surgery of previous years was probably unnecessary. Indeed many of the apparent gaps found at operation may well have been produced by tensions exerted during the operation. Left alone, apposition would have been sufficient to allow of recovery. The traumatized areas which were excised would also probably have made a spontaneous return.

The only drugs of possible value in non-surgical trauma are ACTH or prednisone. An important article by Briggs and Potter (1971) discusses the possible prevention of delayed facial paralysis following head injury. Their

Table 7.1

Head injury patients with lower motor neurone facial paralysis submitted to decompression operation during the period 1950–68

Paralysis	Nerve injury	Number
Immediate	Bone splinter through the nerve in middle fossa	4
	Complete nerve section with repair by end-to-end anastomosis	6
	Nerve bruised and crushed	
	Excision and use of autograft	4
	No damage found to nerve	6
Delayed	No damage found to nerve	5
	Total	25

nability to provide controls is a possible criticism, but the idea is admirable, and may save further damage in some patients. Its application to any patient showing evidence of an injury which could implicate the facial nerve is thus quite acceptable. Our own practice is to use prednisone, starting at 30 mg daily, and gradually reducing the dose over six weeks. Briggs and Potter used and continue to use ACTH, and eventually stated that it was their impression that the drug had offered some protection against delayed facial nerve paralysis after head injury in a well-documented groups of patients. We retain the same impression, using prednisone. We have deliberately used the word impression, and not opinion, as the value of these drugs is not proven, and we await the results of controlled trials. Adour *et al.* (1977) review the surgical and non-surgical management of facial paralysis with head injuries. Fisch (1974) lays down the following guidelines for treatment.

1. Early surgery is indicated if, after a fracture of the petrous pyramid, more than 90 per cent of the fibres degenerate within 6 days of the onset of the facial paralysis.
2. Delayed surgery may be carried out if there is no improvement within six months.

He gives details of operative techniques, both in the approach to the damaged nerve, and also his method of repair, which is anastomosis without sutures. We agree with this, provided that no undue handling is necessary to gain apposition. Fisch describes 40 patients. Of these, 30 had sustained longitudinal skull fractures, and 10 had transverse injury. Smith (1966), in discussing the factors which may influence nerve repair prognosis, drew attention to the blood-supply of nerves, pointing out that nerves have mesenteries similar to those seen in the abdomen. Any excessive stretching may well damage this fine filamentous network. Jongkees (1969) gave his views on the correct timing of surgical repair, or decompression of the facial nerve. This is a stimulating article, and provides thought-provoking reading for those surgeons who do not see much indication for facial nerve surgery. Puvanendran *et al.* (1977) give a prospective study of delayed facial paralysis after head trauma. They studied 6304 cases with head injuries. There were 39 patients who had bleeding from one or both ears. Of these, 16 patients developed a facial paralysis of delayed onset; while 3 were found to have an immediate paralysis. They give the incidence of head injury and bleeding ears as 0·6 per cent, and the incidence of delayed facial paralysis as being 0·3 per cent.

The paralysis was delayed in onset from between 2 and 21 days. Radiological findings in the 16 patients were as follows:

(a) Eight patients showed a fracture of the skull. In 7 it was longitudinal and in only 1 was it a transverse injury.
(b) The remaining 8 patients showed no fracture, despite extensive radiological investigation.
(c) Twenty patients with bleeding ears, but no facial paralysis, did not apparently show any radiological evidence of skull fracture.

The article gives details of recovery in each patient. In conclusion, they are of the opinion that the results of leaving patients with delayed facial paralysis are poor. To improve the prognosis they suggest that early decompression would be the method of choice. We do not agree that this is necessarily true. Further damage may occur to the nerve during surgery, and the results of grafting may not be any better than if the patient was left to make a spontaneous recovery.

McCabe (1970), in discussing the timing and type of facial nerve repair, dealt with direct anastomosis, or the use of autogenous grafts. He states, and we agree from our own experience, that tissue sheaths or vein tubes play no part in protecting the anastomotic sites. They do, however, provide a ready supply of fibroblasts, which hinder nerve repair continuity. In addition they certainly delay re-vascularization of the damaged nerve, or the new graft.

The greatest problems in facial nerve repair are:

1. To keep the regenerating axons within the sheath.
2. To prevent connective tissue from growing into the nerve.
3. To maintain an adequate blood-supply.
4. To avoid any tension.

Sadé (1975) has summarized the treatment now available for facial nerve repair within the temporal bone in an article which dealt initially with six patients. All had either direct anastomosis or an autogenous graft. Like ourselves Sadé does not regard prognosis as being dependent on the method of repair. Direct suture or insertion of a graft can both be successful. Any differences, such as whether sutures are used or whether simple placing in alignment or epineural stripping is employed, do not affect the outcome. The use of various glues and seals over the joints are not important. In our view the most likely reason for any eventual success lies in the normal anatomical network of nerve branches in the face which is so complex that good recovery is possible even should many not become re-innervated.

Discussion The fact that a patient can lose several branches of the facial nerve without much obvious loss of function is well known, and is due to the great proliferation of branches in the face. Without this, such good and spontaneous movements would not be regained. Various operations and injections for relief of spasms and tics destroy multiple branches in the face, without evidence of serious facial paralysis. Ludman (1976) has suggested that small injuries inflicted on the nerve in its middle ear course may produce relief of spasm, with little facial deficit.

Repair of a damaged nerve may not be possible for one or more of the following reasons:

1. The patient may have multiple trauma, in which case any repair operation must await improvement in the general condition. By the time the operation can be undertaken it will have been made more difficult due to scar tissue.

2. Should the condition of the patient deteriorate during the operation, it may have to be abandoned before anastomosis or grafting is complete. In these cases, if possible, small silver clips should be left on the nerve ends, in order to facilitate later identification, before closing the wound. Small pieces of thread will suffice as markers if clips are not available. Light sutures to surrounding tissues will also help to prevent retraction of the nerve. This applies to nerve damage in soft tissue wounds.

Disorders of the facial nerve

Bell's paralysis Treatment depends very much on the opinion of the individual physician or surgeon as to the aetiology of this disorder. We have expressed our views in Chapter 4, but other hypotheses of aetiology exist.

1. *Ischaemia.* If the hypothesis that ischaemia is the cause of Bell's paralysis is correct, the proper treatment would be with vasodilators. Nicotinic acid, betahistine hydrochloride, even intravenous histamine have been suggested. Cervical sympathectomy has been shown to be ineffective.

2. *Oedema.* If it is accepted that oedema is the aetiological factor, then the above treatment (1) is contra-indicated. ACTH or prednisone would be the correct choice of therapeutic agents to reduce compressing oedema. Careful history-taking is, as always, essential. The use of cortico-steroids could reactivate tuberculosis, or exacerbate a peptic ulcer.

3. *Vitamin deficiency.* Vitamins, as far as we know, have never had any beneficial effect on the paralysis, but they do not seem to do any harm either. However, advocates of hypothesis 2 above, would not be in favour of using vasodilators such as nicotinic acid.

Surgical treatment Our experience in this hospital has convinced us that operative interference plays no part in the treatment of this type of paralysis. Between 1954 and 1960 we carried out decompression operations in 7 patients, from the stylomastoid foramen to the middle fossa. No abnormality in the appearance of the nerve was discovered during operation. All the patients recovered satisfactorily, but no better, and no faster than a control group in which no operation was undertaken. Since 1960, we have not operated on any such patients, and results remain satisfactory. Giancarlo and Mattuci (1970) discussed all the cases of presumed Bell's paralysis that they saw between 1965 and 1968. They were all treated initially with ACTH or prednisone, and the course of treatment was followed by nerve testing. If this showed nerve degeneration in any patient, he or she was offered a decompression operation. Out of 76 patients, 27 were advised to have surgery. All the other patients were treated conservatively, as their prognosis was considered excellent. The results were as follows.

1. The operated group: 19 patients had accepted surgery and their recovery rate was 73 per cent.
2. Eight patients refused surgery, and their recovery rate was only 14 per cent.

However, since all the patients had had initial treatment with ACTH or prednisone the beneficial effects of treatment could at least in part be attributed to the drugs, but the group who refused surgery were also drug treated. Also, no quoted abnormal pathology of the facial nerve was found at operation. May (1978) describes localized swelling of the nerve at different sites, observed during decompression.

Alford *et al.* (1970), in a realistic study of 42 patients with Bell's paralysis, considered the limitations of electro-diagnostic tests in helping one to decide on various treatments, including surgery. This is a detailed article, and much of its accords with our own views expressed in Chapter 6. Mechelse *et al.* (1971) reported a study of 25 patients. Eleven had a decompression operation within 3 weeks of the onset of the facial paralysis, and 14 had no treatment. All the patients were followed up for one year, and no statistical difference in recovery was noted. Adour and Swanson (1971) also reported no difference between operated and non-operated cases in their series.

Crabtree (1972) writes about the re-exploration of four patients who had been submitted to decompression for Bell's paralysis. None of the patients had benefited from the initial surgery. At the second operation he found that two patients had a large neuroma in the descending part of the nerve, as well as some bony constriction close to the original stylomastoid foramen. The tumour was excised, and a graft inserted. It is of interest that both patients had a neuroma, as well as considerable fibrosis in the same situation. Excision and grafting were necessary. The third case also showed excess fibrosis, and had to be grafted, and the fourth case was found to have invasion of the nerve by a parotid neoplasm. Histological studies showed these neuromas to be of traumatic origin. Not only may injury to the nerve be caused at the original decompression operation by inadvertent damage to the blood supply or nerve sheath, but also subsequent fibrosis may delay recovery. Further research on this subject may give more information on the condition of a decompressed nerve after the operation.

Pulec (1974) presents a series of 100 consecutive cases of Bell's paralysis treated by decompression. He states that one could wait at least 18 months before considering an operation, to leave time for spontaneous recovery. We ourselves have seen complete recovery take place more than 2 years following the onset of a Bell's paralysis. An even longer time has elapsed before recovery of full movements in some of our cases of herpes zoster oticus. Conley (1974) discussed a group of 32 patients with severe facial paralysis, from many different causes, of 2 to 30 years duration. He remarked that facial muscles may show recovery potential once they have been re-innervated. This was also recently discussed by Anderl (1976). To sum up, we ourselves feel that decompression has no place in the treatment of Bell's paralysis. In patients who show no recovery, or only partial recovery after two years, we would then consider exploration of the nerve. Grafting if necessary could then be carried out. Alternatively, cosmetic plastic surgery may produce as good a result. Each case would be considered on its merits (Cawthorne 1963; Cawthorne and Wilson 1963).

Cortico-steroids and related drugs Much has been written about the use of these drugs in Bell's paralysis. Taverner (1971) compared the effectiveness of prednisolone given orally, and intramuscular ACTH gel. One or other treatment was given on a random basis, using 186 patients with Bell's paralysis. His results were as follows:

(a) ACTH gel: 94 patients, 62 (66 per cent) recovered.
(b) Prednisolone: 92 patients, 79 (86 per cent) recovered.

He re-affirmed (Taverner 1973) the efficacy of prednisolone over ACTH, and concluded that it significantly reduced the overall incidence of denervation, as well as virtually abolishing severe degeneration of the seventh nerve. Adour *et al.* (1972) made a similar study, but this trial according to some critics, did not meet all the requirements of the modern standard clinical trial. May *et al.* (1976) evaluated the effect of steroid treatment on the natural history of Bell's paralysis. They studied 51 patients between 1972 and 1974 in a prospective, controlled, double-blind study. Treatment was started within 3 days of onset (it had been shown previously, by chorda tympani biopsy, that degenerative nerve changes did not start until then). One group of patients was given vitamin supplement treatment, and another group was given both vitamins and a total of 410 mg prednisone, on a gradually reducing dosage over 10 days. All the patients were followed up for six months. Assessment of results was made by independent physicians, and the results then statistically analysed. Factors such as age, sex, and general medical conditions were also considered. The conclusion of this careful study was that it demonstrated no statistically significant beneficial effect of steroid therapy on the prognosis of Bell's paralysis, and May *et al.* concluded that Bell's paralysis remained without a proven, efficacious method of medical treatment. We would endorse this statement, but feel it is important to point out that steroid therapy is not harmful, and we think it still justifiable to continue using this therapy if the physician feels that occasionally it could be of some benefit. Wolf *et al.* (1978) found improvement with steroids in aspects such as crocodile tears.

Lathrop (1976) gives a critical review of current trends in the management of the condition up to the date of his paper. Both medical and surgical forms of treatment are fully discussed.

Crocodile tears syndrome In our opinion initial re-assurance of the patient, and a policy of inactivity will, in many cases, allow spontaneous resolution. Golding Wood (1962) advocates tympanic neurectomy using a middle ear approach, and claims good results in such cases. Rosen and Konak (1973) report on four patients whose recovery was satisfactory following this operation. Our own opinion is that Vidian neurectomy is a more logical and successful operation for any patient with persistent symptoms. Using the approach through the maxillary antrum on the same side, and with an operating microscope the operation is not difficult. Details are available in textbooks of ENT surgery. A transeptal approach as described by Minnis and Morrison (1971) can also be used. Golding Wood (1973) gave a review of Vidian neurectomy. Although it appears to be the most reliable treatment it has the disadvantage of losing the capacity for tearing (Boyer and Gardner 1949).

Frey's syndrome (gustatory sweating) Prophylaxis rather than treatment is advocated by Rauch (1959). The autonomic nerves around the facial trunk should be carefully avoided during operations. Coldwater (1954) resected the auriculo-temporal nerve and its main anastomotic branches from the facial nerve in two patients with Frey's syndrome. Both patients obtained marked relief, and he advocates the operation as a prophylactic method at the time of any original surgery. Friedman *et al.* (1974) found the results of tympanic neurectomy very satisfactory in four patients suffering from gustatory sweating.

Facial tic In our experience there is no specific therapy for the control or cure of this distressing condition. Sectioning of the main branch of the seventh nerve is seldom carried out in this country. Psychiatric advice, tranquillizing drugs, or both, should be considered, but these often seem to be ineffective.

Strangely enough, many patients appear to come to terms with their affliction, and cease to require any medical advice. Certainly, there is no advantage in their attending outpatient clinics merely to be seen, and if the consultant can offer no further treatment, then further observation can be carried out by the general practitioner, with an occasional review in hospital to ensure that no new symptoms appear.

Hemifacial spasm In a small percentage of patients, hemifacial spasm has no apparent organic cause, and in an even smaller group the known pathology has been treated, but there is some residual spasm. In our experience the latter group contains patients with controlled glomus jugulare tumours who previously had seventh nerve involvement and patients who have had extensive cholesteatoma with facial paralysis. Such residual defects are not usually very marked and are mainly associated with small flutterings around one eye and the corner of the mouth. Few wish to have any treatment. A small number have been treated by section of the appropriate facial nerve branches, with satisfactory results. It is, however, absolutely essential first to test with an injection of local anaesthetic to see that control of the spasm can be obtained. In cases where the aetiology is unknown, attitudes to treatment vary from patient to patient. Some manage well without treatment, but others feel that any operation would be worthwhile. Again, local anaesthetic will not only test the effect of nerve section, but will allow a patient to assess the results, which could be complete facial paralysis if a very marked spasm had to be controlled. Whether to have an operation in which the main trunk of the facial nerve is severed is a tremendous decision for the patient to make. Repair by plastic surgery will be necessary at a later date. Ludman (1976) described a permeatal approach to the facial nerve in the middle ear. He reported that random damage to the nerve by a small current diathermy produced satisfactory palliation of hemifacial spasm in some of his cases. We prefer treatment by local section in the face. Fisch (1972a) gives the following principles for the surgical treatment of facial spasm, including blepharospasm:

1. The aim should be to produce the selective section of the facial nerve branches which transmit abnormal impulses to the facial muscles.
2. At the same time, complete denervation of the involved muscles following surgery should be avoided, a compromise which is difficult to achieve in practice.

Fisch describes his technique in detail, and compares the long-term results of the treatment of hemi-spasm and of bilateral blepharospasm. The latter is a much more difficult condition to treat, and the relapse rate is higher. Fisch uses the conventional section, followed by a bipolar microcoagulation. In addition he places a silver clip on the proximal cut end of the nerve, to permit ready identification, should he wish to re-explore the area.

Wagasuki (1972) treated 600 cases of facial spasm by inserting a needle into the main nerve trunk. This produces some direct injury to the fibres, but is reported to control the facial spasm by reducing the activity of the nerves supplying the affected area. If needle damage does not produce sufficient results then a small amount of alcohol is injected, just distal to the stylomastoid foramen. When the initial, induced facial paralysis subsides, the spasm is found to have disappeared. The method can be repeated should any spasm return at a later stage. The article gives full details of technique. Wagasuki reported that 471 patients responded well to the needle injury block, and a further 70 patients required a chemical block. In 35 patients neither method was effective.

McCabe and Boles (1972) used a selective facial neurectomy to treat hemi-spasm and blepharospasm. The surgical approach was essentially that used for a parotidectomy. After careful tracing of the nerves to the orbicularis oculi and upper part of the face by means of a nerve stimulator, the branches are avulsed from the muscles. This can also be used as a staged procedure in bilateral involvement. Totsuka *et al.* (1972) also used selective facial nerve branch block to treat hemifacial spasm. They injected a solution of 5 per cent phenol in glycerine, using first a stimulating needle electrode to ensure that the injection was into the correct area. Davis (1976), writing about a case of spastic eversion of the upper lids, suggests the use of facial nerve block. He used 1 ml of local anaesthetic, and 0·25 ml of alcohol to produce a temporary facial paralysis. This enabled him to deal with the eye condition before the facial movements returned. Neagoy and Dohn (1974) describe their experiences with hemifacial spasm due to vascular compression in the posterior fossa. Jannetta *et al.* (1977) discuss the definitive microsurgical treatment of hemifacial spasm. The principle of their treatment is to decompress the facial nerve by moving away an aberrant vessel. It is essential to know that this vessel is causing a compression at right angles to the nerve, and must be sited at the root exit zone of the nerve from the brain-stem. After mobilization of the arterial loop, separation of the artery and nerve is achieved by using a piece of muscle, sponge, or Teflon. A full description of operative techniques is given in their article. They discuss 47 patients. Further studies on series of these patients may prove of great value in helping to relieve this distressing condition.

In our opinion individual surgeons must use whichever method they find produces the best results. Hemifacial spasm is a very difficult condition to treat, and relapses are common following any method of treatment.

Facial myokymia Treatment depends entirely on the causal pathology. No surgical intervention is suggested. Reference to textbooks of medicine is recommended.

General treatment of facial nerve and associated conditions

Although we are going to divide our summary into groups of patients, (a) with upper motor neurone, and (b) with lower motor neurone damage, much of the general treatment is applicable to all cases of seventh nerve paralysis.

Upper motor neurone damage This group, in which the facial damage is probably only part of a wider range of disability, takes up much paramedical effort.

1. Physiotherapy helps to restore function and confidence. This eventually allows the patient to utilize to the maximum residual muscular co-ordination and movement.

2. Speech therapy is also essential, not only for the general encouragement of the patient, but in aiding rapid re-acquisition of speech, and control of the facial muscles.

Lower motor neurone damage This is, of course, a much larger group, and a lot has been written on methods to encourage restoration of function. Most of this advice in the past was based on the old idea that following injury the muscles would stretch, and thus when they became re-innervated would not function properly as they did previously. We now know that the muscles of the face do not behave in the same way as other muscles, for reasons which are still obscure. Park and Watkins (1949), in a study of 500 patients with Bell's paralysis, came to the conclusion that adjuvant therapy did not produce any better recovery.

However, in many centres the following methods are still in use.

1. Faradic stimulation does not produce any beneficial results, and absorbs time for patients and therapists in busy hospitals. However, it does not appear to do any harm, and is now being recommended by Anderl (1976). It has been suggested that over-use of faradism might produce secondary facial spasm. No convincing evidence of this is apparent, but we would not advocate the use of faradism because it does not appear to be helpful.

2. Facial exercises, either in front of a mirror, or in group therapy can be performed after instruction by a physiotherapist. These are never harmful, and make the patient feel that at least some treatment is being given. There is usually a long time to wait patiently until spontaneous recovery of a cosmetic deformity occurs.

3. Support for the sagging cheek can be achieved by attaching a lump of stent to the upper dentures, or teeth on the affected side. Apart from the cosmetic effect, such a support also helps with eating and drinking, and improves speech. Mouth-to-ear hooks are now seldom used to support the cheek. They are very unsightly and most uncomfortable. For patients in

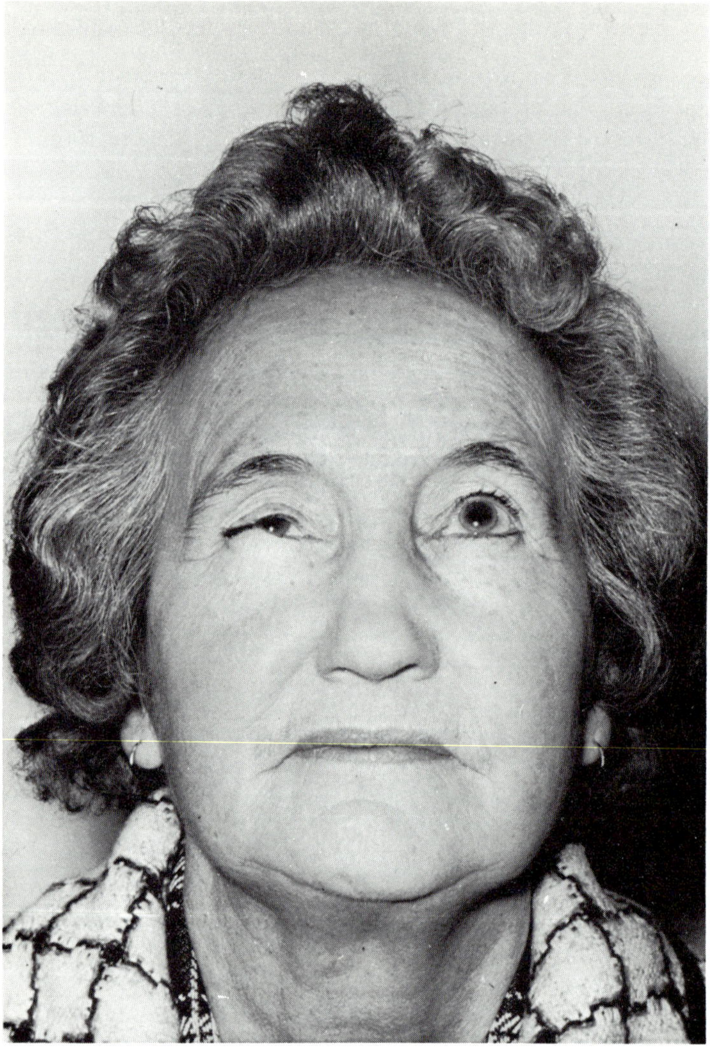

Fig. 7.5. Tarsorrhaphy to right eye.

whom dental support is not available, a piece of strapping on the cheek will help to pull it up. Again not ideal, but better than a sagging face.

4. The eye can be protected by tarsorrhaphy, or other aids to eye closure. If no surgery is available, a simple eye patch will suffice to protect the eye from any permanent damage. Artificial tears of methylcellulose are popular in some countries, especially America.

Most importantly the patient should be informed of the probable time that recovery will take. It is often very difficult to decide on exactly what to tell the patient. The wisdom of experience, based also on the aetiology, is needed. Many patients consider tarsorrhaphy to be a greater deformity than their actual facial paralysis (Fig. 7.5). Every case should be treated on its own merits, and no fixed rules can be laid down. It is, in our opinion, unwise to err on the side of optimism. Patients with facial paralysis, of upper or lower motor neurone type, respond very well to modest amounts of optimism and encouragement. It is absolutely essential that they are seen at reasonable intervals of time, about every three months, and preferably in hospital. Sufficient time should be devoted to their examinations, or they will soon consider such visits are a waste of time. In our opinion, backed up by discussion with our patients, such time is well spent.

Conclusions

The seventh cranial nerve is not the most important nerve which can suffer damage in a patient, nor is it necessarily the most frequently involved. It is nevertheless very obvious when it is involved in paralysis, or stimulation. Much embarrassment and even depression occurs in these patients.

Modern surgical techniques help to save the seventh nerve from damage, and are also used for repair. Of all the available literature, one article stands out: that by Balance and Duel (1932). Apart from being the first detailed description of a facial nerve graft, it contains comments relevant to modern surgery. Safety measures in all forms of industry help to mitigate, or eliminate, much head and face trauma. The use of protective helmets and suits, and car safety belts is on the increase.

Advances in the fields of immunization and prophylaxis may eliminate diseases which involve the facial nerve. Most of all, the improvement of medical facilities, readily available to all patients, must surely be one of the greatest achievements that we can hope to see in the future.

References

Adour, K. K., and Swanson, P. (1971). Facial paralysis in 403 consecutive patients. Emphasis on treatment response in patients with Bell's palsy. *Trans. Amer. Acad. Ophthal. Otolaryng.* **75**, 1284.

——, Winger, B. J., Bell, D. M., and Manning, J. (1972). Prednisone treatment for idiopathic Bell's paralysis. *New Eng. J. Med.* **287**, 1284.

——, Boyajian, J., Kahn, Z., and Schneider, F. (1977). Surgical and non-surgical management of facial paralysis following closed head injury. *Laryngoscope* **87**, 380.

Alberti, E. (1878). In: *Ber. Naturwissen Med. Nereines, Innsbruck*, **9**, 97.

Alberti, P. W. (1962). The greater auricular nerve. *Arch. Otolaryng.* **76**, 442.

Alford, B. R., Weber, S., and Senionis, R. (1970). Neuro-diagnostic studies in facial paralysis. *Ann. Otol.* **79**, 227.

Alfrey, A. (1972). Quoted in Dialysis Dementia. *Brit. Med. J. 1976*, **2**, 1213.

Allison, B. R. (1950). Infective mononucleosis in facial paralysis. *N.Y. St. J. Med.* **50**, 592.

Anderl, H. (1972). A simple method of correcting ectropion. *Plast. Reconstr. Surg.* **49**, 156.

——. (1976). Cross-face nerve transplantation in facial surgery. *Proc. roy. Soc. Med.* **69**, 781.

Aubert, M., and Ginshoarg, M. (1970). Polyneuritis associated with late cutaneous porphyria. *Rev. Neurol. (Paris)* **123**, 426.

Ballance, C., and Duel, A. B. (1932). The operative treatment of facial palsy. By the introduction of nerve grafts into the Fallopian canal, and by other intra temporal methods. *Arch. Otolaryng.* **15**, 1, and references therein.

Bauer, B., Vincent, St. L., Kempe, H., and Downie, A. (1963). Prophylactic treatment of small-pox contacts with N–ethylisation, β–thiosemicarbazone. *Lancet* **ii**, 494.

Berenyi, M. R. (1971). Treatment of diabetic neuropathy with clofibrate. *J. Amer. Geriat. Soc.* **19**, 763.

Boyer, F. C., and Gardner, W. (1949). Paroxysmal lacrimation (syndrome of crocodile tears) and its surgical treatment. *Arch. Neurol. Psychiat.* **61**, 56.

Bragdon, F. H., and Gray, G. (1962). Differential spinal accessory-facial anastomosis with preservation of function of trapezius muscle. *J. Neurol.* **19**, 981.

Bréavoine. (1901). *Trav. Neurol. Chir.*, 30th June, Paris. Quoted by Ballance and Dual (1932).

Briggs, M., and Potter, J. M. (1971). Prevention of delayed facial palsy. *Brit. Med. J.* **3**, 458.

British Medical Journal (1976a). Chemo-therapy for varicella-zoster infections. *Brit. Med. J.* **2**, 1466.

——. (1976b). Measles in the tropics. *Brit. Med. J.* **2**, 1339.

——. (1977a). Surgery for Ménières disease. *Brit. Med. J.* **1**, 124.
——. (1977b). Treatment of acute cerebral infarction. *Brit. Med. J.* **1**, 1.
——. (1977c). Interferon options. *Brit. Med. J.* **1**, 64.
Bunnell, S. (1927). Suture of the facial nerve within the temporal bone, with report of the first successful case. *Surg. Gynaec. Obstet.* **45**, 7.
Calne, D. B. (1975). *Therapeutics in neurology.* Blackwell, London.
Campbell, J. B., Bassett, A. L., Girado, J. M., and Seymour, R. J. (1955). Application of mononuclear filter tubes in bridging gaps in peripheral nerves, and for prevention of neuroma formation. *J. Neurol. Surg.* **13**, 635.
Canale, T. J., and Cox, H. (1974). Decompression of facial nerve in Melkersson's syndrome. *Arch. Otolaryng.* **100**, 373.
Casey, E. B., Jelliffe, A., Le Quesne, P., and Millett, Y. (1973). Vincristine neuropathy. *Brain* **96**, 69.
Cawthorne, T. (1963). Bell's palsies. *Ann. Otol.* **72**, 774.
——, and Wilson, T. (1963). Indications for intra-temporal facial nerve surgery. *Arch. Otolaryng. (Chic.)* **78**, 429.
Coldwater, K. B. (1954). Treatment of the auriculo-temporal syndrome. *Arch. Surg.* **69**, 54.
Conley, J. (1974). Long standing facial paralysis rehabilitation. *Laryngoscope* **79**, 2155.
——. (1975). *Salivary glands and the facial nerve.* Georg Thieme, Stuttgart.
——, and Janecka, T. (1974). Schwann cell tumours of the facial nerve. *Laryngoscope* **84**, 958.
——. (1978). Search for and identification of the facial nerve. *Laryngoscope* **88**, 172.
Cooper, E. A. (1961). Tracheostomy and controlled respiration. *J. Laryng.* **75**, 142.
Crabtree, J. (1972). Facial nerve decompression. *Arch. Otolaryng.* **95**, 395.
Cushing, H. (1903). The surgical treatment of facial paralysis by nerve anastomosis. *Arch. Surg.* **37**, 641.
d'Eramo, N., and Levi, M. (1972). *Neurological symptoms in blood diseases.* Miller and Metcalf, London.
de Chauliac (1363). *Chirurgica magna.* Tract III, doct 1, cap. 3.
de Somer, P., Billian, A., and Joniav, M. (1973). Mass production of human interferon in Diploid cells. Stim. by Poly-I:C. *J. Gen. Virol.* **19**, 1.
Davis, D. (1976). Spastic eversion of the upper eyelids. *Mayo Clin. Proc.* **51**, 85.
Dick, G. (1975). *Viral diseases of the nervous system.* (ed. I. S. Illis) p. 214. Baillière Tindall, London.
Dott, N. M. (1958). Facial paralysis—restitution by extra-petrous nerve graft. *Proc. roy. Soc. Med.* **51**, 900.
Drake, C. G. (1960). Acoustic neurinoma. Repair of facial nerve with autogenous graft. *J. Neurosurg.* **17**, 836.
——. (1972). Facial nerve function. *Arch. Otolaryng.* **95**, 420.
Duc, G. (1969). Bilateral facial paralysis and acquired Toxoplasmosis in a child aged 4 years. *Helv. Paediat. Acta* **19**, 207.
Durrani, K. (1973). Surgical repair of defects for noma. *Plast. Reconst. Surg.* **53**, 647.
Edgerton, M., Tuerk, D. B., and Fisher, J. C. (1975). Surgical treatment of Moebius syndrome by Platysma and Temporalis muscle transfers. *Plast. Reconst. Surg.* **55**, 305.
Eneroth, C., and Hamburger, C. (1974). Parotid tumours. *Laryngoscope* **84**, 1732.
Erlacher, C. (1915). Experimenteille Untersuchungen über plastik und transplantation von nerv und muskel. *Langenbecks. Arch. Klin. Chir.* **106**, 389.

Evans, D. M. (1974). Hypoglossal-facial anastomosis in the treatment of facial palsy. *Brit. J. Plast. Surg.* **27**, 251.

Fauré. Quoted by Bréavoine (1901).

Fisch, U. (1972a). The surgical treatment of hyperkinesia. *Arch. Otolaryng.* **95**, 400.

——. (1972b). Total intra-temporal exposure of the facial nerve. *Arch. Otolaryng.* **95**, 335.

——. (1974). Facial paralysis. *Laryngoscope* **79**, 2141.

——. (1975). In *Surgery of the facial nerve* (ed. A. Miehlke). Saunders, Philadelphia.

Fox, W. (1977). The modern management and therapy of pulmonary tuberculosis. Philip Ellman Lecture. *Proc. roy. Soc. Med.* **70**, 4.

Freilinger, G. (1975). A new technique to correct facial paralysis. *J. Plast. Reconst. Surg.* **56**, 44.

Frew, I. (1961). Tracheostomy and controlled respiration. *J. Laryng.* **75**, 136.

Frew, A., and Finney, R. (1963). Neoplasms of the middle ear. *J. Laryng.* **77**, 415.

Frew, I. (1965). The diagnosis of malignancy of the middle ear in later life. *Geriatrics* **20**, 759.

Friedman, W., Swerdlow, R., and Pomaris, J. (1974). Tympanic neurectomy. *Laryngoscope* **84**, 568.

Galbraith, A. (1973). Treatment of acute herpes zoster with amantidine hydrochloride. *Brit. Med. J.* **4**, 693.

Gardner, W. J., and McCubbin, J. (1965). Auriculo-temporal syndrome. Gustatory sweating due to misdirection of regenerated nerve fibres. *J. Amer. Med. Ass.* **160**, 272.

Giancarlo, M. R., and Mattuci, K. F. (1970). Facial palsy. Facial nerve decompression. *Arch. Otolaryng.* **91**, 30.

Goldberg, A. (1959). Acute intermittent porphyria. Effect of barbiturates in precipitating neuropathy in porphyria. *Quart. J. Med.* **28**, 183.

Golding Wood, P. H. (1962). Tympanic neurectomy. *J. Laryng.* **76**, 683.

——. (1973). Vidian nerve neurectomy. *Laryngoscope* **82**, 1673.

Goodall, J., Kosmidis, J., and Gedded, A. (1974). The effect of cortico-steroids on course of the Guillain–Barré syndrome. *Lancet* **i**, 647.

Grossberg, S. E. (1972). The interferons and their inducers: molecular and therapeutic considerations. *New Engl. J. Med.* **287**, 122.

Gye, R. S., Hargrave, J. C., Loewenthal, J., and McLeod, J. (1972). Use of immunosuppressive agents in human nerve grafting. *Lancet* **i**, 647.

Hamersa, H. (1973). Marble bone disease. *Oto-rino-lar. ital.* **36**, 21.

Henson, R. A. (1970). Peripheral neuropathy associated with malignant disease. In: *Handbook of clinical neurology* (ed. P. J. Vinken and G. W. Bruyn), North-Holland, Amsterdam.

Hogan, E. (1965). Enzymatic changes in denervated muscle. II. Biochemical studies. *Arch. Neurol. (Chic.)* **13**, 274.

House, W. (1963). Middle cranial fossa approach to the petrous pyramid. *Arch. Otolaryng.* **78**, 460.

Illis, I. S. (1975). *Viral diseases of the nervous system.* Baillière Tindall, London.

Ingham, S. (1975). Correspondence. *Brit. Med. J.* **4**, 39.

Isaacs, A., and Lindemann, J. (1957). Virus interference. I. Interferon. *Proc. roy. Soc. Med.* **147**, 258.

Jannetta, P. J., Abbasy, M., Maroon, J. C., and Ramos, F. M. (1977). Etiology and definitive microsurgical treatment of hemifacial spasm. *J. Neurosurg.* **47**, 321.

Jansen, C. (1967). Modern ear surgery on radical cavities. *J. Laryng.* **81**, 1187.

Jongkees, L. B. W. (1965). Facial paralysis complicating skull fracture. *Arch. Otolaryng.* **81**, 518.

——. (1969). Timing of surgery in intra-temporal facial palsy. *Laryngoscope* **79,** 1557.

——. (1970). Peripheral facial nerve paralysis and its surgical treatment. *Eye, Ear, Nose, Throat Monthly* **49,** 109.

Jordan, G., Fried, R. P., and Merigan, T. C. (1974). Administration of human leukocyte interferon in herpes zoster. *J. Infect. Dis.* **130,** 56.

Juel-Jensen, B. C., and McCallum, F. O. (1972). *Herpes simplex, varicella and zoster*. Heinemann, London.

Karat, A., Jeevaratnana, A., Karati, S. and Rao, P. (1971). Controlled trial of clofazimime in untreated lepromatous leprosy. *Brit. Med. J.* **4,** 514.

Kennedy (1911). *Phil. Trans. B.* **202,** 97. Quoted by Ballance and Dual (1932).

Kettel, K. (1947). Melkersson's syndrome: report of 5 cases, with special reference to the pathological observations. *Arch. Otolaryng.* **46,** 341.

——. (1975). In *Surgery of the facial nerve* (ed. A. Miehlke). Saunders, Philadelphia.

Kiuslitz, K. (1974). Perspectives and contra-indications of various nerve transplant techniques, in cases of facial paralysis after pontine angle trauma. *Chir. Plast. Berlin* **2,** 161.

Korte, W. (1903). Ein Fall von Nervenpfropfung des Facialis auf den N. hypoglossus. *Dtsch. med. Wschr.* **29,** 293.

Krekorian, E. A. (1971). The repair of combat-injured facial nerves. *Laryngoscope* **81,** 1926.

Kunc, Z. (1965). Treatment of essential neuralgia of the ninth nerve by selective tractotomies. *J. Neurosurg.* **23,** 494.

Laage-Hellman, J. E. (1958). Gustatory sweating and flushing, aetiological implications of latent period and mode of development after parotidectomy. *Acta Otolaryng. (Stockh.)* **49,** 306.

Lambert, V., and Richards, S. M. (1964). Facial palsy in Heerfordt's syndrome. *J. Laryng.* **76,** 684.

Lassman, L., McIver, I., Thompson, C., and McLeod, I. (1958). The role of respiratory insufficiency in the mortality of brain-stem injuries. *Lancet* **i,** 390.

Lathrop, F. (1956). Surgical repair of facial nerve: technique. *Surg. Clins. N. Amer.* **36,** 583.

——. (1976). A critical analysis of current trends in the management of Bell's palsy. *Laryngoscope* **8,** 1209.

Ludman, H. (1976). Facial dyskinesia. *Proc. roy. Soc. Med.* **69,** 576.

McCabe, B. F. (1970). Facial nerve grafting. *Plast. Reconst. Surg.* **45,** 70.

——. (1970). Management of hyperfunction of the facial nerve. *Ann. Otol.* **79,** 252.

——, and Boles, R. (1972). Surgical treatment of essential blepharospasm. *Ann. Otol.* **81,** 611.

McGovern, F. (1968). Fractures of the temporal bone involving the facial nerve. *Arch. Otolaryng.* **88,** 536.

——, and Fitz-Hugh, G. (1956). Diseases of the facial nerve. *Laryngoscope* **66,** 187.

McGregor, I. A. (1977). Semon Lecture. *J. Laryng.* **91,** 445.

McGuirt, W. F. (1975). Carotid body tumours. *Arch. Otolaryng.* **101,** 58.

McLaughlin, A., Kazantis, G., King, E., and Teare, D. (1962). Pulmonary fibrosis and encephalopathy associated with inhalation of aluminium dust. *Brit. J. Ind. Med.* **19,** 253.

Marmor, J. (1964). Regeneration of peripheral nerves by irradiated homografts. *J. Bone. J. Surg.* **46A,** 583.

Martin, R. (1931). Intratemporal suture of the facial nerve. *Arch. Otolaryng.* **13,** 259.

——. (1936). Surgical repair of the facial nerve. *Arch. Otolaryng.* **23,** 458.

May, M. (1978). Bell's palsy: progressive ascending paralysis, therapeutic implications. *Laryngoscope.* **88,** 61.

May, M., Wette, R., Hardin, W. B., and Sullivan, J. (1976). The use of steroids in Bell's palsy. A prospective controlled study. *Laryngoscope* **86**, 1111.

Mechelse, K., Goor, G., Huizing, E., and Hammelburger, E. (1971). Bell's palsy: prognostic criterion and evaluation of surgical decompression. *Lancet* **ii**, 57.

Meltzer, P., and Keleman, G. (1959). Pyocyaneus osteomyelitis of the temporal bone, mandible and zygoma. *Laryngoscope* **69**, 1300.

Meretoja, J., and Teppo, L. (1971). Histopathological findings of familial amyloidosis with cranial neuropathy as principle manifestation. *Acta Path. Microbiol. (Scand.) Section A* **79**, 432.

Michel, R. G., Popet, H., and Patterson, C. H. (1975). Infective mononucleosis, mastoiditis, and facial paralysis. *Arch. Otolaryng.* **101**, 486.

Millesi, H., Berger, A., and Meissl, G. (1971). Fascicular nerve grafting. In: *Transactions of the Vth International Congress for Plastic and Reconstructive Surgery*, p. 586. Butterworths. Australia.

Minnis, N. L., and Morrison, A. W. (1971). Trans-septal approach for Vidian neurectomy. *J. Laryng.* **85**, 255.

Marel-Fatio, D., and Lalardie, J. (1964). Palliative surgical treatment of facial paralysis. The palpebral spring. *Plast. Reconst. Surg.* **33**, 446.

Morgan, L. R., and Cramer, L. M. (1974). Treatment of facial paralysis produced by combat injury. *Plast. Reconst. Surg.* **53**, 647.

Mühlbauer, W. D., Segeth, H., and Hessman, A. (1973). Restoration of lid function in facial palsy with permanent magnets. *Chir. Plast. (Berlin)* **1**, 295.

Müler, H. (1962). Paralyses faciales non otiques. Indications chirugicales. *Ann. Otolaryng. (Paris)* **79**, 527.

Munch (1904). Semaine Med. (Paris) **24**, 73, quoted by Ballance and Duel (1932).

Mündnich, K, (1967). Zur problematik und zu einigen schweirigen situationen der reparativen facial schirurgie. *Chir. Plast. Reconst.* **3**, 86.

Munt, W. (1975). *Current therapy* (ed. H. F. Conn). W. B. Saunders, Philadelphia.

Neagoy, S. R., and Dohn, S. F. (1974). Hemifacial spasm secondary to vascular compression of the facial nerve. *Clev. Clin. Q.* **41**, 205.

Neely, J. G., and Alford, B. R. (1974). Facial nerve neuromas. *Arch. Otolaryng.* **100**, 298.

Negroni, R. (1977). Miconazole therapy in South American blastomycosis. *Proc. roy. Soc. Med.* **70**, 24.

Ozsahinoglu, C., and Harrison, M. S. (1975). A comparison of methods of extratemporal facial nerve repair. *J. Laryng.* **89**, 1095.

Paine, R. S. (1957). Facial paralysis in children. *Pediatrics* **19**, 303.

Park, W. P., and Watkins, A. L. (1949). Facial paralysis: analysis of 500 cases. *Arch. Phys. Med.* **30**, 749.

Peer, L. A. (1955). *Transplantation of tissues, Vol. I.* Williams and Wilkins, Baltimore.

Pettit, J. (1975). Leprosy. In *Tropical neurology* (ed. J. D. Spillane). Oxford University Press.

Poppi, A., and Morganite, P. (1961). In *Neurological symptoms in blood disease*, (ed. N. d'Eramo and M. Levi). Miller and Metcalf, London.

Prasad, U. (1976). Malignant otitis externa. *J. Laryng.* **90**, 10.

Pulec, J. (1966). Total decompression of the facial nerve. *Laryngoscope* **76**, 1015.

——. (1974). Bell's palsy. *Laryngoscope* **79**, 2119.

——. (1976). Geniculate neuralgia. *Laryngoscope* **86**, 955.

Puvanendran, K., Vitharana, M., and Wong, P. K. (1977). Delayed facial palsy after head injury. Prospective study. *J. Neurol. Neurosurg. Psychiat.* **40**, 342.

Ramamurthi, B. (1970). Tuberculoma of the brain. *J. Int. Coll. Surg.* **35**, 605.

Rauch, S. (1959). Das salivo-suidostpare Syndrome. *Z. Leprosy U.S.W.* **38**, 259.
Rees, R. Pearson, J., and Waters, M. (1970). Experimental and clinical studies on rifampicin in treatment of leprosy. *Brit. Med. J.* **1**, 89.
Rhoton, A. (1974). Microscopy of the internal auditory meatus. *Surg. Neurol.* **2**, 311.
Ridley, A. (1969). The neuropathy of acute intermittent porphyria. *Quart. J. Med.* **38**, 307.
Riskaer, N. (1946). The course of otitic facial palsy under adequate treatment of the disease of the ear. *Acta Otolaryng.* (*Stockh.*) **34**, 280.
Rosen, G., and Konak, S. (1973). Tympanic neurectomy in the crocodile tears syndrome. *Ann. Otolaryng. Chir. Cervicofacial* **90**, 723.
Sadé, J. (1975). Facial nerve reconstruction and its prognosis. *Ann. Otol.* **83**, 343.
Saidi, F. (1977). A new approach to the surgical treatment of hydatid cyst. *Ann. roy. Coll. Surg.* (*Engl.*) **59**, 715.
Shafar, J., Tallett, E. R., and Knowlson, P. (1971). Evaluation of clonidine in the prophylaxis of migraine. A double-blind trial. *Lancet* **ii**, 403.
Shambaugh, G. (1959). In: *Surgery of the ear.* Saunders, Philadelphia.
Sheehy, J. L. (1968). Facial nerve decompression. Two interesting cases. *Arch. Otolaryng.* **87**, 241.
——. (1970). The intact canal wall technique in management of aural cholesteatoma. *J. Laryng.* **84**, 1.
Sklansky, B. D., Jafek, B. W., and Wiernick, P. H. (1974). Oto-laryngological manifestations of leukaemia. *Laryngoscope* **84**, 210.
Smith J. W. (1966). Microsurgery: review of the literature and discussion of microtechniques. *Plast. reconst. Surg.* **37**, 227.
Smith, D. F., and Rawlins, M. D. (1973). *Variability in human drug response.* Butterworths, London.
Smith, J. W. (1971). A new technique of facial animation. In *Transactions of the Vth International Congress in Plastic and Reconstructive Surgery*, p. 83. Butterworths, Australia.
——. (1972). Advances in facial nerve repair. *Surg. Clins. N. Amer.* **52**, 1287.
Smythe, G. D. L., Kerr, A. G., and Gordon, D. S. (1976). Vestibular nerve section in Ménières disease. *J. Laryng.* **90**, 823.
Spiro, R. H., and Martin, H. (1967). Gustatory sweating following parotid surgery and neck dissection. *Ann. Surg.* **165**, 118.
Stookey, B. P. (1922). *Surgical and mechanical treatment of peripheral nerves.* W. B. Saunders, Philadelphia.
Tandon, P. N. (1975). In: *Tropical neurology* (ed. J. D. Spillane). Oxford University Press.
Taverner, S. (1955). Bell's palsy: a clinical and electromyographic study. *Brain* **78**, 209.
——. (1971). Comparison of corticotraphin and prednisolone in treatment of Bell's palsy. *Brit. Med. J.* **4**, 20.
——. (1973). Medical management of idiopathic (Bell's) palsy. *Proc. roy. Soc. Med.* **66**, 554.
The Lancet (1976). Leader. Microsurgery. *Lancet* **i**, 1223.
The Leprosy Mission. (1976). The net. 16 mm colour film. Available for showing by members of Leprosy missions, regional staff, from 50 Portland Place, London, W1H 3DE.
Thompson, H. (1961). Motor function in the Abbe flap. A histo-chemical study of motor re-innervation in transplanted muscle tissue of the lips in man. *Brit. J. Plast. Surg.* **14**, 66.

——. (1971). Autogenous free grafts of skeletal muscle. A preliminary experimental and clinical study. *Plast. Reconst. Surg.* **48**, 11.
——. (1971). Treatment of facial paralysis by free skeletal muscle grafts. *Transactions of the Vth International Congress of Plastic and Reconstructive Surgery*, p. 68. Butterworths, Australia.
——. (1974). A new technique to correct facial paralysis. *Clin. Plast. Surg.* **1**, 349.
Tos, M. (1969). Facial palsy in Hand–Schuller–Christian disease. *Arch. Otolaryng.* **90**, 563.
Totsuka, G., Hitose, H., and Kobayashi, T. (1972). Selective facial nerve branch blocking. *Arch. Otolaryng.* **95**, 360.
Vejjajiva, A. (1975). Vaccination against rabies. In: *Tropical neurology* (ed. J. D. Spillane). Oxford University Press.
Vernier, V. G. (1969). The toxicologic and pharmacologic properties of amantadine hydrochloride. *Toxicology and Appl. Pharmacology* **15**, 642.
Wagasuki, B. (1972). Facial nerve block in the treatment of facial spasm. *Arch. Otolaryng.* **95**, 356.
Walters, J. B., and Israel, M. S. (1974). *General pathology* (ed. J. B. Walters and M. S. Israel). Churchill Livingstone, London.
Ward, C. M. (1975). Injury to facial nerve during surgery of the parotid gland. *Brit. J. Surg.* **62**, 401.
Wells, J. H. (1977). Corr. of hemi-facial atrophy with a flap from the lower abdomen. *Plast. Reconst. Surg.* **59**, 223.
Wilcocks, C. (1972). Manson's tropical diseases (ed. C. Wilcocks and P. H. Manson). p. 68. Baillière Tindall, London.
Wolf, S. M., Wagner, J. H. Jnr., Davidson, S., Forsythe, A. (1978). Treatment of Bell's palsy with prednisone: a prospective randomized study. *Neurology* **28**, 158.
Wolferman, A. (1974). The present status of therapy of Bell's paralysis: a critical evaluation. *Ann. Otol.* **83**, *Suppl.* **12**, 1.
Wullstein, H. (1957). Decompression des Nervus Facialis, nach Wullstein. Arch. *Ohr.-Nas-H. Kehlk-Heilk.* **171**, 138.
Yanekawa, (1976). quoted in Microsurgery. *Lancet* **i**, 1223.
Yuill, G., Swinburn, W. R., and Liversedge, L. A. (1970). Treatment of polyneuropathy with azothioprine. *Lancet* **ii**, 854.

Index